Physical Therapy Clinical Handbook for PTAs

Olga Dreeben, PT, PhD, MPT
Director and Professor
Physical Therapist Assistant Program
Lake City Community College
Lake City, FL

D1561387

JONES AND BARTLETT PUBLISHERS
Sudbury, Massachusetts
BOSTON   TORONTO   LONDON   SINGAPORE

World Headquarters
Jones and Bartlett
Publishers
40 Tall Pine Drive
Sudbury, MA 01776
978-443-5000
info@jbpub.com
www.jbpub.com

Jones and Bartlett Publishers
Canada
6339 Ormindale Way
Mississauga, Ontario L5V 1J2
Canada

Jones and Bartlett Publishers
International
Barb House, Barb Mews
London W6 7PA
United Kingdom

Jones and Bartlett's books and products are available through most bookstores and online booksellers. To contact Jones and Bartlett Publishers directly, call 800-832-0034, fax 978-443-8000, or visit our website www.jbpub.com.

Substantial discounts on bulk quantities of Jones and Bartlett's publications are available to corporations, professional associations, and other qualified organizations. For details and specific discount information, contact the special sales department at Jones and Bartlett via the above contact information or send an email to specialsales@jbpub.com.

Copyright © 2008 by Jones and Bartlett Publishers, LLC.

All rights reserved. No part of the material protected by this copyright may be reproduced or utilized in any form, electronic or mechanical, including photocopying, recording, or by any information storage and retrieval system, without written permission from the copyright owner.

The authors, editor, and publisher have made every effort to provide accurate information. However, they are not responsible for errors, omissions, or for any outcomes related to the use of the contents of this book and take no responsibility for the use of the products and procedures described. Treatments and side effects described in this book may not be applicable to all people; likewise, some people may require a dose or experience a side effect that is not described herein. Drugs and medical devices are discussed that may have limited availability controlled by the Food and Drug Administration (FDA) for use only in a research study or clinical trial. Research, clinical practice, and government regulations often change the accepted standard in this field. When consideration is being given to use of any drug in the clinical setting, the health care provider or reader is responsible for determining FDA status of the drug, reading the package insert, and reviewing prescribing information for the most up-to-date recommendations on dose, precautions, and contraindications, and determining the appropriate usage for the product. This is especially important in the case of drugs that are new or seldom used.

Production Credits
Executive Editor: David Cella
Production Director: Amy Rose
Production Editor: Daniel Stone
Editorial Assistant: Lisa Gordon
Marketing Manager: Jen Bengtson

Manufacturing and Inventory Coordinator:
  Amy Bacus
Cover Design: Kristin E. Ohlin
Printing and Binding: Malloy, Inc.
Cover Printing: Malloy, Inc.

Library of Congress Cataloging-in-Publication Data
Dreeben, Olga.
  Physical therapy clinical handbook for PTAs / Olga Dreeben.
    p. ; cm.
  Includes bibliographical references and index.
  ISBN-13: 978-0-7637-4667-4
  ISBN-10: 0-7637-4667-3
  1. Physical therapy assistants—Handbooks, manuals, etc. 2. Physical therapy—
Handbooks, manuals, etc. I. Title.
  [DNLM: 1. Physical Therapy Modalities—Handbooks. 2. Allied Health Personnel—
Handbooks. 3. Emergency Treatment—Handbooks. 4. Interpersonal Relations—Handbooks.
5. Safety Management—Handbooks. WB 39 D771p 2008]
  RM705.D75 2008
  615.8'2—dc22   2007000639
6048

Printed in the United States of America
12 11 10 09 08   10 9 8 7 6 5 4 3 2

Contents

Preface

In physical therapy practices, physical therapists and physical therapist assistants encounter patients who need a variety of interventions based on the patient's specific impairments and functional limitations. In contemporary research-based practices, the range and amount of information in regard to interventions and data collection is substantial and demanding, even for the most prepared and experienced physical therapist and physical therapist assistant. Some interventions that are not used regularly may require the clinician to seek a quick reminder to help obtain a successful patient outcome. This concise and condensed clinical pocket guide was designed specifically to assist the busy physical therapist assistant who might require a rapid reference source in the clinic. This book is also valuable to the physical therapist assistant student to consider and further access important material when in clinical rotations or in the classroom. Although primarily directed to the physical therapist assistant and the physical therapist assistant student, physical therapist can also benefit from these pages, especially in facilitating the most patient-advantageous interventions and outcomes.

This book makes no claim to be a comprehensive reference work on physical therapy, but it is meant as a concise, condensed pocket-guide, offering immediate information concerning regular interventions and data collection elements in various physical therapy clinical settings and categories including musculoskeletal, neurologic, geriatric, pediatric, cardiopulmonary, and integumentary. With its portable user-friendly design, it includes the basic facts that a physical therapist assistant or a physical therapist assistant student needs. This handbook embodies as much research-based information as possible in regard to physical therapy interventions. It also contains terminology that reflects current physical therapy practice according to the APTA's "Guide to Physical Therapist Practice."

This book is organized into eight parts with sections for each part, and five appendices. The appendices contain a balance assessment form, and four cardiac and integumentary patient education explanations that may be duplicated for the patient's home use.

Part I, *Safety*, contains eight sections describing the collaborative relationship between the physical therapist and the physical therapist assistant, patient communication elements, patient education topics, patient confidentiality, cultural competence and domestic violence issues, infection control guidelines, and safety fundamentals during interventions.

Part II, *Clinical Documentation*, contains four sections relating to documentation guidelines and elements, a description of SOAP notes, and examples of approved abbreviations and symbols.

Part III, *Musculoskeletal Interventions*, is the largest segment containing seven sections that include musculoskeletal data collection, basic musculoskeletal clinical impairments and functional limitations of arthritic and other orthopedic conditions, musculoskeletal interventions and patterns, and a review of musculoskeletal anatomy.

Part IV, *Neurologic Interventions*, has five sections that impart information about neurological data collection, clinical impairments and functional limitations, neurologic conditions, neurologic interventions and patterns, and a review of the nervous system and its anatomy and physiology.

Part V, *Cardiopulmonary Interventions*, is a six-section segment that contains cardiopulmonary data collection elements, cardiopulmonary clinical impairments and functional limitations, cardiopulmonary conditions, cardiopulmonary interventions and patterns, and a review of cardiopulmonary anatomy and physiology.

Part VI, *Integumentary Interventions*, has six sections that include integumentary data collection, clinical impairments and functional limitations of integumentary conditions, types of integumentary interventions and patterns, wound documentation elements, and a review of integumentary system anatomy.

Part VII, *Geriatric Interventions*, includes four sections: geriatric data collection, age related impairments and functional limitations and suggestions for interventions, geriatric disorders and diseases and interventions, and a Medicare reimbursement overview.

Finally, Part VIII, *Pediatric Interventions*, has three sections: pediatric data collection, pediatric interventions, and pediatric disorders and diseases and interventions.

Part I

Safety in the Clinical Environment

Physical Therapist and
Physical Therapist Assistant
Relationship

The Collaborative Path Between the PT and the PTA[1]

- The physical therapist (PT) performs an initial examination of the patient. The physical therapist assistant (PTA) helps the PT with the initial examination, gathering specific data that the PT requested. The PTA accepts the delegated tasks within the limits of his or her capabilities and considering legal, jurisdictional, and ethical guidelines.

- The PT evaluates the results of data collection and makes a judgment about data value. The PTA does not interpret the results of initial examination.

- The PT establishes the goals or outcomes to be accomplished by the plan of care and the treatment plan.

- The PT performs the patient's interventions. The PTA performs the selected patient's interventions as directed by the PT.

- The PTA may perform data collection during the course of the patient's interventions to record the patient's progress or lack of progress since the initial examination and evaluation. The PTA may ask the PT for a re-examination.

- The PT performs the re-examination and establishes new outcomes and a new treatment plan.

- The PT performs the new patient's interventions. The PTA performs the new selected patient's interventions as directed by the PT.

- The PT performs the discharge examination and evaluation of the patient.

PTA Duties (as Per the American Physical Therapy Association—APTA)

Table 1-1   PTA Duties[2]

Perform selected physical therapy interventions under the direction and at least general supervision of the PT. The ability of the PTA to perform the selected interventions as directed shall be assessed on an ongoing basis by the supervising PT.

Make modifications to selected interventions either to progress the patient as directed by the PT or to ensure patient safety and comfort.

Document the patient's progress.

Perform routine operational functions, including direct personal supervision, where allowable by law, of physical therapy aide and the PTA student and other personnel.

PTA's Clinical Considerations During Interventions[1]

- The complexity, criticality, acuity, and stability of the patient
- The accessibility to the PT
- The type of setting where services are provided
- Federal and state statutes
- The available PT supervision in the event of an emergency
- The mission of physical therapy services for that specific clinical setting
- The needed frequency of reexamination

Patient Communication

General Recommendations for Verbal Communication

Table 1-2   General Recommendations[1]

Verbal commands should focus the patient's attention on specifically desired actions for intervention.

Instruction should remain as simple as possible and must never incorporate confusing medical terminology.

General sequence of events should be explained to the patient before initiating the intervention.

The PTA should ask the patient questions before and during the intervention in order to establish a rapport with the patient and to provide feedback as to the status of the current intervention.

The PTA should speak clearly in moderate tones and vary his or her tone of voice as required by the situation.

The PTA should be sensitive to the patient/client's level of understanding and cultural background.

Methods of Effective Patient Communication[1]

- Greet the patient and provide a nonthreatening environment for the patient so that he or she feels welcome and valued.
- Display sensitivity to cultural influences by a careful selection of words and actions.
- When introducing yourself to the patient, position yourself to greet the patient at eye level.
- Be aware of cultural differences when establishing eye contact with the patient, as this may not be appropriate in some cultures.
- Introduce yourself by your name and title, and refer to the patient by his or her last name and title. Avoid using first names, and do so only if deemed appropriate by the patient. Ask the patient what he or she would prefer to use to avoid offending and showing disrespect for the patient.
- Explain to the patient your role in the therapeutic relationship.
- Inform the patient of what you plan to do initially.
- Advise the patient in regard to options for therapeutic interven-

tions. If there are more than one option, share possibilities, and invite the patient's input.

- Obtain informed consent from the patient for the intervention that is to be rendered.
- Advise the patient about the intervention's effects, indications, contraindications, and alternatives.
- Actively involve the patient in the intervention by determining the patient's participation during and after the intervention.
- Respond to the patient's questions and concerns throughout interactions.
- Promote patient autonomy and responsibility throughout interactions.

SAFETY IN THE CLINICAL ENVIRONMENT

Informed Consent

Table 1-3   Intervention Elements of Informed Consent for the Patient[1]

Clear description of proposed intervention
Reasonable alternatives to proposed intervention
Risks, benefits, and concerns of proposed intervention
Assessment of patient understanding
Patient's acceptance of intervention

Methods of Effective Listening[1]

- The PTA focuses his or her attention on the patient.
- The PTA helps the patient to feel free to talk by smiling and looking at the patient.
- The PTA pays attention to patient's nonverbal communication, such as gestures, facial expressions, tone of voice, and body posture.
- The PTA asks the patient to clarify the meaning of words and the feelings involved or to enlarge the statement.
- The PTA reflects to patient's message to understand completely the meaning and the content of the message.
- The PTA takes notes as necessary to help remember or document what was said.

- The PTA uses body language such as nonverbal gestures (nodding the head, keeping eye contact, or keeping hands at side) to show involvement in the patient's message.
- The PTA does not abruptly interrupt the patient, giving adequate time to present the full message.
- The PTA empathizes with the patient.

Patient Education

The PTA's Responsibilities During Patient Education

- To communicate clearly and simply by using everyday words, repeating the information as necessary and explaining new words
- To gain the learner's attention, motivation, and active participation
- To provide an overview of the learning process such as the objectives, the purposes, and the nature of the task and the procedures to follow
- To stimulate the learner's recall of previous learning
- To relate present learning to past and future learning
- To monitor and control the learning
- To organize learning units over a period of time
- To break down learning into a series of steps or units
- To determine the best sequence(s) of learning units and experiences such as a sequence from familiar to unfamiliar, simple to complex, or concrete to abstract
- To provide ample opportunity for practice and repetition
- To progress at a comfortable pace for the learner
- To give timely feedback
- To provide accurate knowledge of results
- To reward successful behaviors
- To monitor and control the environment
- To reduce conditions that have a negative impact on learning, such as pain or discomfort, anxiety, fear, frustration, feelings of failure, humiliation, embarrassment, boredom, or time pressures

Patient Education for Patients (Clients) Who Have Difficulty Reading

Table 1-4   Recommendations[1] for Patients/Clients Having Difficulty Reading

Materials need to be written in plain language, consistently using the same words. New health care terms need to be defined, and repetition can be used to reinforce the information. Sentences have to be written short and simple, marking each item with a bullet point.

Five or six bullet points should be on each list.

Attention can be drawn to essential information by making circles or arrows or adding dividers or tabs to the material.

Patient (Client) Education for Older Adults

Table 1-5   Recommendations[1] for Older Adults

Assess how and when the patient (client) is ready to learn by finding out the patient's (client's) interest and level of motivation to learn and tying in new information to past experiences.

Enhance the learning process by teaching the patient (client) in an environment conducive to learning, such as a quiet place, sitting near the patient (client), speaking clearly, and teaching in brief sessions. Instructions can be taught one step at a time by demonstrating and describing the intervention and encouraging the patient (client) to practice each step.

Adjust the teaching method to the patient's (client's) learning style and special needs. For example, if the patient (client) is a visual learner, the PTA may need to give the patient (client) a picture of the exercise that he or she learned today. Considering the patient's vision, the PTA should give the patient a large-sized print (at least 16 points) of the exercise picture.

Find out the patient's (client's) preference to learn such as reading, listening, watching, or doing.

Encourage bringing a family member or a friend to the teaching session for support and to reinforce and clarify information.

Patient Education for Patients (Clients) Who Have Visual Impairments

Table 1-6   Recommendations[1] for Patients/Clients Having Visual Impairments

Introduce yourself and other people present in the room.

Ask whether the patient (client) wants assistance, and provide directions.

For a home exercise program (HEP), write the material in large print size (16 points).

Use simple fonts. Avoid italics. Write clearly and concisely, or print information in Braille.

Patient Education for Patients (Clients) Who Have Hearing Impairments

Table 1-7   Recommendations[1] for Patients/Clients Who Have Hearing Impairments

Move a chair closer to face the patient (client). Get the patient's (client's) attention by touching him or her; speak clearly and distinctly, not loudly.

Do not exaggerate pronunciation.

Reduce distracting and interfering sounds.

Have adequate light in the room because many patients (clients) having hearing impairments read lip movements when looking at the mouth and further speech read when looking at gestures, expressions, and pantomime actions.

Patient Education for Patients (Clients) Who Cannot Speak English

Table 1-8   Recommendations[1] for Patients/Clients Who Cannot Speak English

Use certified interpreters to communicate key information to the patient (client).

The patient (client) must be comfortable with the interpreter, especially when concerning embarrassing topics.

Greet the patient (client) in his/her native language. Pronounce the patient's (client's) name correctly.

Speak clearly, and concentrate on the most important message(s) for the patient (client).

Considering cultural diversity, understand the patient's (client's) values and beliefs, and pay attention to nonverbal communication such as voice volume, postures, gestures, and eye contact. Working with the family decision maker, who may be different from the patient (client), is essential for the success of intervention. The intervention has to be creative, and considering patient's cultural background, it may involve having the patient's spiritual advisor helping with the intervention (as long as the spiritual healing method is not antagonistic to the intervention).

Basic Requirements for the Home Exercise Program (HEP)

Table 1-9   HEP Basic Requirements[1]

The HEP should be organized, concise (short), and written in layman terms. The words must make sense to the patient (client) and be consistent with the therapist's verbal explanations and demonstrations.

When a caregiver is involved, he or she must be involved earlier in the HEP to allow an easier transition at the discontinuation of physical therapy.

The HEP represents an extension of the interventions. The HEP starts in the first day of interventions and continues through the day of discontinuation of physical therapy. HEP should be presented in context of the total process of patient education and rehabilitation.

In regard to exercises or activities, they should be simple and clear. HEP should contain approximately three to five exercises or activities. These should include the number of repetitions, the number of sets, how long to hold, the amount of exercise resistance, positions for performing the exercises or activities, the duration of exercises or activities, the frequency, and the method of progression. The exercises and activities must be sorted in a logical manner so that the patient (client) does not have to change positions too much.

The HEP may include diagrams, drawings, or pictures of exercises or activities. These should be uncomplicated.

The HEP should be written in the patient's (client's) primary language.

Technical terms must be avoided, and short sentences must be used as much as possible. Complex words (such as inflammation) must be replaced with simple ones (such as redness).

Each sentence in the HEP must present only one idea and contain no more than one three-syllable word.

Lines of copy should be no longer than five inches wide, and the type size should be 12 points or larger.

For patients (clients) with vision impairments, the handouts must have a high contrast between the foreground and the background and include large amounts of blank space on the page.

The HEP should be written at a fifth- or sixth-grade reading level.

SECTION 1-4

Patient Confidentiality

Situations When Patient's Written Authorization for Release of Medical Information Is Required

- For patient's attorney or insurance company
- For patient's employer (unless a workers compensation claim is involved)
- For any member of the patient's family (except where a member of the family received durable power of attorney for health care agencies)

Cultural Competence

General Methods to Increase Cultural Competence

Table 1-10   Methods[1] to Increase Cultural Competence

Identify personal cultural biases (ethnocentrism) and personal values and beliefs
Understand general cultural differences
Accept, respect, and value cultural differences
Apply cultural understanding

Guidelines to Cultural Competence

- Providing training to increase cultural awareness, knowledge, and skills
- Recruiting and retaining minority staff
- Providing interpreter services
- Providing linguistic competency that extends beyond the clinical encounter to the appointment desk, advice lines, medical billing, and other written material
- Coordinating evaluations and interventions with traditional healers
- Using community health workers
- Incorporating culture specific attitudes and values into health promotion tools
- Including family and community members in health care decision making
- Locating clinics in geographic areas that are easily accessible for certain populations
- Expanding hours of operation

Religious Beliefs and Health Concepts

Table 1-11   Selected Religious Beliefs and Health Concepts[3]

Patients/clients who are members of the Baha'i religious conviction essentially believe that "all healing comes from God." In regard to concepts of health, they have the following beliefs: abortion is forbidden. Birth control is acceptable. Alcohol or drugs are forbidden. Medications can be used as necessary. Healing beliefs are that there is harmony between religion and science. There are no restrictions for medical healing practices. Religious healing practices include prayer. Family and community members assist and support the patient/client. Organ donations are permitted. Surgical procedures are acceptable. Autopsy is not restricted if necessary (from the legal or medical perspective).

Patient/clients who are members of the Buddhist Churches of America religious conviction essentially believe that "to keep the body in good health is our duty—otherwise we shall not be able to keep our mind strong and clear." In regard to concepts of health, they have the following beliefs: abortion is determined by the patient's condition. Birth control is acceptable. Food combinations are restricted, and extremes of diets must be avoided. Medications can be used as necessary. Healing beliefs are that people should not believe in healing through faith. There are not restrictions for medical healing practices. Family and community members assist and support the patient/client. Organ donations are considered an act of mercy, and if there is a hope for recovery, all means may be taken. Surgical procedures are acceptable, avoiding the extremes. Autopsy is a matter of individual practice.

Patient/clients who are members of the Roman Catholic American religious conviction essentially believe that "the prayer of faith shall heal the sick, and the Lord shall raise him up." In regard to concepts of health, they have the following beliefs: abortion is prohibited. Birth control is unacceptable. Food must be used in moderation. Medications may be taken if the benefits outweigh the risks. Healing beliefs are various considering the regional religious belief system. There are no restrictions for medical healing practices. Religious healing practices include sacrament taken by the sick, praying by lighting candles, and having the priest laying on of hands. Family, friends, the priest, and many outreach programs through the church are ready to assist and support the patient/client. Organ donations are permitted if are justifiable. Most of the surgical procedures are acceptable, except for abortion and sterilization. Autopsy is permissible.

Patient/clients who are members of the Christian Science religious conviction believe the following in regard to concepts of health: abortion is prohibited being incompatible with the faith. Birth control has to do with the individual judgment.

There are not food restrictions except alcohol, tobacco, and some tea and coffee. Medications are not permitted at all. Healing belief is that there is acceptance of the physical and moral healing. No medical healing practices are permitted. Religious healing practices are permitted only by the full time healing ministers. Also, spiritual healing practices are advocated. Family, friends, and members of the Christian Science Community and Healers and Christian Science Nurses are providing health care to the sick. Organ donations depend on the individual decision. Surgical medical procedures are all prohibited. Autopsy is not an usual event, but may be decided by the individual and the family.

Patient/clients who are members of the Church of Jesus Christ of Latter Day Saints religious conviction believe the following in regard to concepts of health: abortion is forbidden. Birth control is unacceptable, as it is in contrast to the Mormon religious belief. Alcohol, tea (except for herbal teas), coffee, and tobacco are forbidden. Fasting (being 24 hours without food and drink) is required once a month. Medications are not restricted, but patients/clients may use herbal folk remedies. Healing beliefs are that the power of God can bring healing. Medical healing practices are permitted. Religious healing practices are anointing with oil, sealing, prayer, and laying on of hands. Family, friends, church members (such as the Elder and the Sister), and the Relief Society help the members in case of sickness. Organ donations are permitted. Surgical medical procedures are permitted being a matter of individual choice. Autopsy is permitted with consent from the next of kin.

Patient/clients who are members of the Hinduism religious conviction essentially believe that "Enricher, Healer of disease, be a good friend to us." In regard to concepts of health, they have the following beliefs: there is no policy in regard to abortion. All forms of birth control are acceptable. Eating meat is forbidden. Medications are acceptable. Healing beliefs are various—some believe in medical interventions and some in faith healing. Considering the regional religious belief system, there are no restrictions for medical healing practices. Religious healing practice includes traditional faith healing system. Family, friends, the priest, and the community provide support to the sick. Organ donations are permitted. Surgical procedures are acceptable. If a member needs an amputation, the loss of the limb is seen as a consequence of sins from a previous life. Autopsy is permissible.

Patient/clients who are members of the Islam religious conviction essentially believe that "the Lord of the world created me—and when I am sick, He healeth me." In regard to concepts of health, they have the following beliefs: abortion is not permitted. Birth control is acceptable. Food made with pork and those containing alcohol are forbidden. Medications are acceptable, except insulin, which may be refused if it is made from a pork base (made from the pancreas of the pig). Med-

continues

Table 1-11 (continued)

ical interventions are acceptable. Faith healing generally is not acceptable. Considering the regional religious belief system, religious healing practices differ. Some use herbal remedies, and some use faith healing (although faith healing is not acceptable). Family and friends provide support to the sick. Organ donations are permitted. Most of the surgical procedures are permitted. Autopsy is permissible for medical and legal purposes.

Patient/Clients who are members of the Jehovah's Witnesses religious conviction believe the following in regard to concepts of health: abortion is forbidden. Birth control and sterilization are prohibited. Tobacco is restricted, and alcohol can be consumed in moderation. Medications are accepted if are not derived from blood or blood products. Medical interventions are acceptable if they do not involve blood or blood products. Faith healing is forbidden. Religious healing practices involve reading the scriptures to comfort the individual and to lead to mental and spiritual healing. Members of the congregation and Elders pray for the sick. Organ donations are forbidden. Surgical medical procedures are not opposed, but the administration of blood during surgery is strictly prohibited. Autopsy is acceptable if it is required by the law.

Patient/clients who are members of the Judaism religious conviction essentially believe that "O Lord, my God, I cried to Thee for help and Thou has healed me." In regard to concepts of health, they hold the following beliefs: abortion is therapeutically permitted, and some groups accept abortion on demand. Birth control is acceptable, except for the Orthodox Judaism. Strict dietary laws prohibit mixing of milk and meat. Food made with pork, meat of predatory animals, fowl, and shellfish are forbidden. Kosher products are required in the diet. Medications are not restricted. Medical interventions are expected. Religious healing practices include prayers for the sick. Family, friends, rabbi, and many community services are available to provide support to the sick. Organ donations are not permitted, being a very complex issue. However, some practice organ donations. Most of the surgical procedures are permitted. Autopsy is permissible under certain circumstances.

Patient/clients who are members of the Mennonite religious conviction believe the following in regard to concepts of health: abortion is acceptable for therapeutic reasons. Birth control is acceptable. There are not specific dietary restrictions. Medications are not restricted. Healing beliefs are considered part of God's work. To pray for the sick is the common practice. Medical interventions are acceptable. Religious healing practices include prayers and anointing with oil. Family and the community are available to support the sick. Organ donations are acceptable. Surgical medical procedures are acceptable. Autopsy is acceptable.

Patient/clients who are members of the Seventh-Day Adventists religious conviction believe the following in regard to concepts of health: abortion is acceptable for therapeutic purposes. Birth control is an individual choice. Vegetarian diet is encouraged. Medications are not restricted. Healing beliefs are that there is Divine healing. Medical interventions are permitted. Religious healing practices are anointing with oil and prayer. Family, the Pastor, and the Elders pray and anoint the sick person. Worldwide health system includes hospitals and clinics. Organ donations are permitted. Surgical medical procedures are permitted. Autopsy is acceptable.

Patient/clients who are members of the Unitarian/Universalist Church religious conviction believe the following in regard to concepts of health: abortion is acceptable, is therapeutic, and can be offered on demand. All types of birth control are acceptable. Medications are not restricted. Healing beliefs are that faith healing is superstitious. Medical interventions are permitted. Religious healing practices believe that the use of science facilitates healing. Family, friends, and the church members support the sick. The Pastor and the Elders pray and anoint the sick person. Organ donations are permitted. Surgical medical procedures are permitted. Autopsy is acceptable and recommended.

* The PTA is urged not to generalize from this guide but to show respect, sensitivity, and understanding to the patient/client.

Intervention Strategies Considering Cultural Diversity

Table 1-12   Intervention Strategies[1] Considering Cultural Diversity

When providing intervention to Native American patients, the therapist needs to recognize the importance of nonverbal communication. For example, for Navajo Native Americans, sustained eye contact when speaking directly with someone is rude and possibly confrontational, whereas avoiding eye contact is deemed a sign of respect. The therapist needs to focus on positive facial expressions without frowning or negative expression such as the flat affect. First, the therapist needs to address the older member of the family, not the patient. Often, Native American patients observe the provider and say very little. They expect the provider to figure out their health problem through instinct rather than through the use of questioning. The conversation must be in a very low tone of voice. It is impolite to say, "I beg your pardon" or to imply that the communication was not heard. The therapist must speak with the patient or the older member of the family in a quiet setting. Note taking is taboo. The therapist needs to use memory skills and not to record

continues

Table 1-12   (continued)

patient's history on a writing pad. If the therapist needs to take patient history, he or she has to use a conversational approach while taking the history. Native American patients respond to interventions using silence; other times, they leave and do not return. Also, consideration must be given to a very accessible, open schedule for the patient because time orientation is not a priority for the Native American patient. In addition, Native American patients believe that health and wellness exist in a harmonious relationship with all other living things, including spirits. Problem solving and decision making are group experiences. Respected elders or the family have to make decisions about rehabilitation.

When providing interventions or administering tests and measures to brown or black-skinned patients, the therapist is required (for safety purposes) to consider the patient's physiological and integumentary needs. For example, to identify pallor the therapist should consider that there is an absence of underlying red tones, and the skin of the brown-skinned patient appears yellow-brown, whereas the black-skinned patient appears ashen gray. Mucous membranes also appear ashen, and the lips and nailbeds are similar. Erythema (redness) can be detected by palpation. The skin is usually warmer in the area, is tight, and edematous, and the deeper tissues are hard. Cyanosis can be seen by close inspection of lips, tongue, conjunctiva (of the eyelids), palms of the hands, and the soles of the feet. One method of testing is pressing the palms. Slow blood return indicates cyanosis. Another sign is ashen gray lips and tongue. Ecchymosis (superficial bleeding under the skin) from trauma can be detected by swelling of the skin surface. Keloids are scars that form at the site of the wound. Keloids appear on a wound highly elevated and irregular continuing to enlarge.

Also, when providing interventions to African American patients, the therapist should consider the patient's beliefs and practice of folk medicine. Physical therapy interventions can be combined with folk treatments as long as they are not antagonistic to each other. The patient's background, income, religious practices, and accessibility to health resources need also to be included. For example, when suggesting an assistive device or an orthosis, the therapist must be familiar with formal and informal sources of help in the African American community. Including patient's family in the rehabilitation process is essential for patient's motivation and positive outcomes. Because African Americans are verbally expressive, family members should be encouraged to discuss who will take responsibility as the primary caregiver. The therapist should keep an open line of communication and be sensitive to the need of African American patients to operate in a family unit.

When providing interventions to the Asian American patients, the therapist should keep in mind the importance of communication and possible difficulties in communication. Many Asian American cultures value silence and talking too much can give a negative impression. When patients cannot understand specific patient education topics, they may agree to follow through to "save face," and not to embarrass the authority figure (such as the health care provider). An interpreter can be used if the interpreter is able to understand the patient's dialect and regional language differences. Also, the interpreter's gender can be a problem if the interpreter is of the opposite gender and the patient is not comfortable sharing personal or intimate information with a stranger. As with any other patients, the therapist needs to establish a partnership with the patient. This will allow the patient to share information about use of alternative therapies and alert the therapist of any antagonist effects with medications or interventions. In addition, the therapist needs to help the patients understand that they have a choice in making health care decisions. The patient or the patient family may make decisions based on family needs and not the medical needs, considering also the financial and physical hardship faced by the family. In regard to interventions, the therapist should include patient's extended family and the environmental context in which the patient lives. The interventions may have to integrate the Asian American patients' values that are different than of the Western ideology. These may include interdependence, social belonging, and agreement with their illness-related conditions.

When providing interventions to the Hispanic American patients, the therapist should consider the importance of nonverbal communication, the patient's practice of folk medicine, the language barriers, the time-orientation issues, and the caregiver performing self-care or activities of daily living for the patient. Communication strategies such as a smile that expresses warmth and concern, arms relaxed at sides (not crossed), good eye contact (not to members of the opposite sex), shaking hands, and speaking first with the male patient or caregiver are important customs. The therapist must consider that common folk remedies for patients of Puerto Rican and Mexican backgrounds can be found in the "botanicas," which are stores that sell folk remedies such as herbs, potents, ointments, amulets, candles, medals, relics, and religious statues. A spiritualist may be present in the "botanica" and recommend certain herbs for the patient's illness. Other Hispanic American patients may visit a "santeria," which is a form of Latin American magic using spirits to treat illness, or a "curandero," a traditional holistic healer. Physical therapy interventions can be combined with folk treatments as long as they are not antagonistic. The language barrier can be remedied using certified interpreters who are generally accurate and nonjudgmental. The time

continues

Cultural Competence **25**

SAFETY IN THE CLINICAL ENVIRONMENT

Table 1-12   (continued)

orientation issue can be accommodated by an open or a "walk in" schedule. Regarding activities of daily living, the therapist may need to explain to the caregiver the importance of patient's independence with activities of daily living and work with the caregiver by showing how to help the patient (without doing all the work for the patient).

* The PTA is urged to consider that each patient/client is unique; the previous strategies may help to maximize a culturally competent approach to delivering physical therapy interventions.

SECTION 1-6

Infection Control

Centers for Disease Control (CDC) Recommended Standard Precautions[4]

Table 1-13   Centers for Disease Control Standard Precautions

Handwashing: Wash hands after touching blood, body fluids, secretions, excretions, and contaminated items, whether or not gloves are worn. Wash hands immediately after gloves are removed, between contact with patients, and when otherwise indicated to avoid transfer of microorganisms to other patients or environments (it may be necessary to wash hands between tasks and procedures on the same patient to avoid cross-contamination of different body sites). Use plain soap (nonantimicrobial) for routine handwashing. Use antimicrobial agent or waterless antiseptic agent for specific circumstances (such as control of outbreaks of Methicillin-resistant Staphylococcus Aureus—MRSA) as defined by the infection control program in your area.

Gloves: Wear clean, nonsterile gloves when touching blood, body fluids, secretions, excretions, and contaminated items. Put on clean gloves just before touching mucous membranes and nonintact skin. Change gloves between tasks and procedures on the same patient after contact with material that may contain a high concentration of microorganisms. Remove gloves promptly after use, before touching noncontaminated items and environmental surfaces and before going to another patient, and wash hands immediately to avoid transfer of microorganisms to another patient or environments.

Mask, Eye Protection, Face Shield: Wear a mask and eye protection or a face shield to protect mucous membranes of the eye, nose, and mouth during procedures and patient care activities that are likely to generate splashes or sprays of blood, body fluids, secretions, and excretions.

Gown: Wear a clean, nonsterile gown to protect skin and to prevent soiling of clothing during procedures and patient care activities that are likely to generate splashes or sprays of blood, body fluids, secretions, and excretions. Select a gown that is appropriate for the activity and amount of fluid to be encountered. Remove a soiled gown as promptly as possible, and wash hands to avoid transfer of microorganisms to other patients or environments.

Patient Care Equipment: Handle used patient-care equipment soiled with blood, body fluids, secretions, and excretions in a manner that prevents skin and mucous membrane exposures, contamination of clothing, and transfer of microorganisms to other patients or environments. Ensure that reusable equipment is not used for the care of another patient until it has been cleaned and reprocessed appropriately. Ensure that single-use items are discarded properly.

Environmental Control: Ensure that the hospital has adequate procedures for the routine care, cleaning, and disinfection of environmental surfaces, beds, bedrails, bedside equipment, and other frequently touched surfaces, and ensure that these procedures are being followed.

Linen: Handle, transport, and process used linen soiled with blood, body fluids, secretions, and excretions in a manner that prevents skin and mucous membrane exposures and contamination of clothing, and avoid transfer of microorganisms to other patients and environments.

Occupational Health and Bloodborne Pathogens: Take care to prevent injuries when using scalpels, needles, and other sharp instruments or devices, when handling sharp instruments after procedures, when cleaning used instruments, and when disposing of used needles. Never recap used needles or otherwise manipulate them using both hands or use any other technique that involves directing the point of a needle toward any part of the body; rather, use either a one-handed scoop technique or a mechanical device designed for holding the needle sheath. Do not remove used needles from disposable syringes by hand, and do not bend, break, or otherwise manipulate used needles by hand. Place used disposable syringes and needles, scalpel blades, and other sharp items in appropriate puncture resistant containers, which are located as close as practical to the area in which the items were used, and place reusable syringes and needles in a puncture resistant container for transport to the reprocessing area.

Resuscitation: Use mouthpieces, resuscitation bags, or other ventilation devices as an alternative to mouth-to-mouth resuscitation methods in areas where the need for resuscitation is predictable.

Patient Placement: Place a patient who contaminates the environment or who does not (or cannot be expected to) assist in maintaining appropriate hygiene or environmental control in a private room. If a private room is not available, consult with infection control professionals regarding patient placement or other alternatives.

CDC Guidelines for Airborne, Droplet, and Contact Transmission Based Precautions

Table 1-14   Airborne Transmission Guidelines—Infections: Tuberculosis, Measles, Chickenpox

1. Respiratory isolation room
2. Mask when entering the room
3. Limitation of patient movement out of the room
4. Patient's mask when transporting the patient out of the room

Table 1-15   Coughing, Sneezing, and Talking Transmission Guidelines—Infections: Mumps, Rubella, Pertussis, Influenza

1. Isolation room
2. Mask when entering the room
3. Limitation of patient movement out of the room
4. Patient's mask when transporting the patient out of the room

Table 1-16   Direct Contact Transmission Guidelines

1. Isolation room
2. Gloves and gown (when touching the patient or the patient's environmental surfaces)
3. Single-patient use equipment
4. Limitation of patient movement out of the room

Occupational Safety and Health Administration's Universal Precautions Recommendations

Table 1-17   Universal Precautions Recommendations[4]

Use protective equipment and clothing whenever in contact with bodily fluids.

Dispose of waste in proper containers having knowledge of handling of infectious waste.

Dispose of sharp instruments and needles into proper containers.

Keep the work area and the patient area clean.

Wash hands immediately after removing gloves and at all times, as required by the agency policy.

Immediately report any exposure to needle sticks or blood splashes or any personal illness to the direct supervisor and receive instructions about follow up action.

Asepsis Methods

1. Sterilization of instruments using
   - Heat (250°F to 270°F) and water pressure
   - Ionizing radiation to sterilize medications, plastics, or sutures
   - Boiling water (212°F) for non–spore-forming organisms
   - Dry heat and gas (ethylene oxide, or formaldehyde gas)

2. Disinfection—reducing microorganisms—using
   - Filtration (for water purification)
   - Ultraviolet light—for air and surface disinfection
   - Ultrasonic cleaning—for instruments
   - Washing with antimicrobial products—for surfaces and hands
   - Chemicals such as chlorination, iodines, phenols, quaternary ammonia, formaldehyde. Hydrotherapy disinfection includes draining and cleaning tanks, and scrubbing pumps and equipment with a germicidal agent such as bleach, povidone-iodine, or Chloramine-T.
3. Antisepsis—inhibiting or destroying microorganisms—using
   - Antiseptic solutions: alcohol and iodines
   - Quaternary ammonia
   - Germicidal soaps
   - Mercurials
   - Antibacterial additives to whirlpools, tubs, tanks, or pools

Types of Nosocomial Infections

1. Urinary tract infections
2. Surgical site infections
3. Respiratory tract infections
4. Blood stream infections
5. Intestinal tract infections
6. Central nervous system infections
7. Nosocomial fungal infections
8. Nosocomial pneumonia such as Bacterial pneumonia, Legionnaires' Pulmonary aspergillosis, mycobacterium tuberculosis, viral pneumonias, or influenza
9. Other nosocomial infections by pathogens are Staphylococci, Pseudomonas, *Escherichia coli*, antibiotic-resistant nosocomial infections such as methicillin-resistant *Staphylococcus aureus*, vancomycin-resistant *Staphylococcus aureus*, vancomycin-resistant enterococci

Infectious Diseases

A. AIDS caused by the human immunodeficiency virus[5] (HIV)—
   loss of immune system function resulting in

   • Opportunistic infections: pneumocystis carinii pneumonia,
     esophageal candidiasis, cytomegalovirus infection, cryptococ-
     cus, atypical mycobacteriosis, chronic herpes simplex, toxo-
     plasmosis, or mycobacterium tuberculosis

   • Neurologic dysfunctions: AIDS dementia complex, central
     nervous system toxoplasmosis, cryptococcal meningitis,
     encephalopathy, peripheral neuropathy

   • Unusual cancers: Kaposi's sarcoma, non-Hodgkin's lymphoma,
     primary brain lymphoma

Table 1-18   Possible Transmission of AIDS

Direct contact with infected body fluids: blood, semen, cerebrospinal fluid, breast milk, and vaginal/cervical secretions

Table 1-19   High-Risk Behaviors for AIDS

Unprotected sexual contact, needle sharing or injections with contaminated nee-dles, and maternal fetal transmission before and during birth or through breast milk

Table 1-20   Low-Risk Behaviors for AIDS

Needle sticks and casual contacts such as hugging and kissing

Table 1-21   Medical Management of AIDS—To Stop HIV Replication

Multidrug therapy, patient education to prevent the spread of the disease and live a healthy lifestyle, and supportive care

B. Hepatitis—inflammation of the liver caused by viral or bacterial infection or by chemical agents. Types of Hepatitis:
- Hepatitis A virus (HAV)—acute infectious hepatitis transmitted through fecal–oral transmission, contaminated food or water, and infected food handlers.
- Hepatitis B virus (HBV)—serum hepatitis transmitted through contact with infected body fluids or tissues via oral or sexual contact, blood and blood product exposure, maternal fetal transmission, and contaminated needles.
- Hepatitis C virus (HCV)—transmitted in the same manner as HBV. It can cause liver damage and liver cancer.

Table 1-22   Prevention of HAV

Good hygiene, hand washing after using the toilet, sanitation, and immunization

Table 1-23   Medical Management of HAV

Intravenous fluids, analgesics, and treatment of acute symptoms

Table 1-24   Prevention of HBV

HBV vaccine, education, lifestyle changes, and healthy habits
Remember that the HBV is more contagious than HAV and can survive on the surface for up to seven days.

Table 1-25   Medical Management of HBV—No Cure

Interferon for chronic HBV

Table 1-26   Prevention of HCV

Lifestyle changes and patient education to decrease the spread of the disease and to encourage healthy habits

Table 1-27   Medical Management of HCV

Interferon and treatment of acute illness

C. Tuberculosis (TB)—airborne respiratory infection that is highly contagious
   Tuberculosis is
   • Transmitted through mycobacterium tuberculosis from contact with an infected person
   • Spreads from coughing and sneezing through droplets or sputum

Table 1-28   Medical Management of TB

Isolation until cleared from the contagious stage and chemotherapy using anti-TB medications for acute illness (Rifampin and Isoniazid)

SECTION 1-7

Domestic Violence

How to Recognize Forms of Domestic Abuse

Table 1-29   Forms of Domestic Abuse[1]

Using sexual violence such as forcing the victim to have sexual intercourse or to engage in other sexual activities against the intimate partner's will

Using children as pawns such as accusing the intimate partner of bad parenting, threatening to take the children away, or using the children to relay messages to the partner

Using denial and blame such as denying that the abuse occurred or shifting responsibility for the abusive behavior onto the partner

Using coercion and threats such as threatening to hurt other family members, pets, children, or self

Using economic abuse such as controlling finances, refusing to share money, sabotaging the partner's work performance, making the partner account for money spent, or not allowing the partner to work outside of the home

Using intimidation such as using certain actions, looks, or gestures to instill fear, and breaking things, abusing pets, or destroying property

Using emotional abuse such as insults, criticism, or name calling

Using isolation, such as limiting the partner's contact with family and friends, requiring the partner's permission to leave the house, not allowing the partner to attend work or school, or controlling the partner's activities and social events

Using privilege such as making all major decisions, defining the roles in the relationship, being in charge of the home and social life, or treating the partner as a servant or possession

Difficulties Identifying/Helping Victims of Domestic Violence[1]

1. Health care provider's fears or experiences of exploring the issue of domestic violence
2. Health care provider's lack of knowledge of community resources
3. Health care provider's fear of offending the victim and jeopardizing the provider–patient relationship
4. Health care provider's lack of time or lack of training
5. Health care provider's unresponsiveness, feeling powerless, and not being able to fix the situation
6. Infrequent victim's visits as a patient

7. Victim's unresponsiveness to questions (asked by the health care provider)

Methods to Overcome Difficulties Identifying/Helping Victims of Domestic Violence

Table 1-30   Methods to Overcome Difficulties Identifying/Helping Victims of Domestic Violence

Observe the victim for physical and behavioral clues.

Question the victim and validate domestic abuse.

Respect the victim's privacy and use confidentiality measures.

In physical therapy, the PT examines and treats the victim. If a PTA suspects a patient to be a victim of domestic abuse, the PTA should immediately report the findings to the PT of record.

Keep accurate records and concise documentation about the victim's abuse.

Support and follow up the victim's care.

Signs Indicating a Victim of Domestic Abuse

1. The abuser accompanies the victim to all appointments and refuses to allow the victim to be interviewed alone. Also, the abuser can use verbal or nonverbal communication to direct the victim's responses during appointments.

2. The patient is noncompliant with physical therapy treatment regimens and/or frequently missing appointments.

3. The patient makes statements about not being allowed to take or obtain medications (prescription or nonprescription medication).

4. The abuser cancels the victim's appointments or sabotages the victim's efforts to attend appointments (by not providing child care or transportation).

5. The patient engages in therapist hopping.

6. The patient lacks independent transportation, access to finances, or ability to communicate by phone.

Domestic Abuse Signs That Need Screening

- The victim's chronic pain, and injuries during pregnancy
- The victim's repeated and chronic injuries and gynecological problems
- The victim's exacerbated or poorly controlled chronic illnesses such as asthma, seizure disorders, diabetes, hypertension, and heart disease
- The victim's physical symptoms related to stress, anxiety disorders, or depression; hypervigilant signs such as easily startled or very guarded; the victim experiencing nightmares or emotional numbing
- The victim's suicide attempts and eating disorders
- The victim's self-mutilation and car accidents where the victim is the driver or the passenger
- The victim's overuse of prescription pain medications and other drugs

Joint Commission on Accreditation of Healthcare Organizations' (JCAHO's) Guidelines and Goals Identifying Victims of Domestic Violence

Table 1-31   JCAHO's Guidelines/Goals[1]

All physical therapy facilities should develop objective criteria for identifying victims of domestic violence.

All individuals who may be involved in screening, evaluating and examining, re-evaluating, and caring for patients should be knowledgeable in the criteria for identifying and caring for victims of domestic violence.

Supervisors are responsible, either personally or through delegation, for orienting and for providing in-service training and continuing education to all such individuals.

The evaluation and examination of victims of alleged or suspected domestic violence should be conducted with the consent of the patient or the parent or legal guardian or as otherwise provided by the law.

The examination and evaluation of victims of alleged or suspected domestic violence should be conducted in accordance with the facility's policies for the collection, the retention, and the safeguarding of evidentiary material released by the patient.

The evaluation and examination of victims of alleged or suspected domestic violence includes as legally required, the notification and release of information to the proper authorities.

A list of appropriate referrals to community agencies should be available on-site for patients.

A domestic violence protocol for emergencies should be developed and implemented in all physical therapy practice settings (such as a clinic or private practice department).

Patient Safety During Interventions

Vital Signs Normatives[1]

Table 1-32 Blood Pressure (BP) Normatives—Adult

Category	Systolic BP	Diastolic BP
Normal BP	120 mm Hg or less	80 mm Hg or less
Prehypertension	120–140 mm Hg	80–90 mm Hg
Stage I hypertension (HTN)	140–159 mm Hg	90–99 mm Hg
Stage II hypertension	160–179 mm Hg	100–109 mm Hg
Stage III hypertension	More than 180 mm Hg	More than 110 mm Hg

Table 1-33 BP Normatives Infant/Child/Adolescent

Normal BP infant = 80/50 mm Hg
Normal BP child = 100/55 mm Hg
Normal BP adolescent = 115/70 mm Hg

Table 1-34 Heart Rate (HR) Normatives Adult/Infant/Child/Adolescent

Normal HR adult = 70 beats per minute (bpm) (range = 60–100)
Abnormal HR adult = bradycardia = less than 60 bpm; tachycardia = more than 100 bpm
Normal HR infant = 120 bpm (range = 70–170)
Normal HR child = 125 bpm (range = 75–140)
Normal HR Adolescent = 85 bpm (range = 50–100)

Table 1-35 Temperature and Respiratory Rate for Adult/Infant/Child/Adolescent

Temperature adult/infant/child/adolescent	Respiratory rate (RR) adult/infant/child/adolescent
Normal temperature adult = 98.6°F	Normal RR adult = 12–18 breaths/min
Normal temperature infant = 98.2°F	Normal RR infant = 30–50 breaths/min
Normal temperature child = 98.6°F	Normal RR child = 20–40 breaths/min
Normal temperature adolescent = 98.6°F	Normal RR adolescent = 15–22 breaths/min

Table 1-36   Elements That Increase/Decrease BP/HR/RR/Temperature

Increase BP/HR/RR/temperature: infection, anxiety, pain, exercise (only systolic BP and HR), high blood sugar, low blood sugar, and low potassium (only HR), low hematocrit, and hemoglobin (only HR and RR), acute myocardial infarction, coronary artery disease, asthma, and anemia

Decrease BP/HR/RR/temperature: decreased hemoglobin and hematocrit (only SBP and temperature), decreased potassium (only SBP), acute myocardial infarction (only HR and SBP), narcotics, increased potassium (only HR), decreased blood sugar (only temperature), and anemia (only SBP)

Patient's Emergency Situations

1. BP = 160/100 and/or 90/60 (may not need to call the emergency medical services; the PTA must take into consideration patient/client's age, medications, and interventions; may need to stop the interventions, inform the PT, and monitor the patient/client carefully)

2. Resting HR = 110 bpm and/or 60 bpm (may not need to call the emergency medical services; the PTA must take into consideration patient/client's age, medications, and interventions; may need to stop the interventions, inform the PT, and monitor the patient/client carefully)

3. Resting RR = 30 breaths/min (may not need to call the emergency medical services; the PTA must take into consideration patient/client's age, medications, and interventions; may need to stop the interventions, inform the PT, and monitor the patient/client carefully)

4. Absent or decreased breath sounds

5. Sudden cognitive changes

6. Chest discomfort, shortness of breath, sweating, and/or faintness

7. Sudden severe headache and facial pain

8. Abdominal discomfort, nausea, and/or bloody or dark, tarry stools

General Signs and Symptoms to Discontinue Physical Therapy Interventions

Table 1-37   Signs/Symptoms[5] to Discontinue Interventions

Temperature of more than 100°F
Systolic BP of more than 240 mm Hg
Diastolic BP of more than 110 mm Hg
Fall in systolic BP of more than 20 mm Hg; rise in HR of more than 20 bpm
Resting HR of more than 130 bpm and/or less than 40 bpm
Chest pain, palpitations, and/or irregular pulse
Oxygen saturation of less than 90%
Blood glucose of more than 250 mg/dL
Cyanotic and/or diaphoretic
Dizziness and/or syncope
Bilateral leg/foot edema

Signs and Symptoms of Hyperglycemia: High Blood Sugar of More than 200 mg/dL[5]

- Extreme thirst and frequent urination
- Blurred vision and dry skin
- Nausea, vomiting, or abdominal pain
- Fatigue and lethargy
- Dizziness and increased appetite
- Weight loss and infections
- Glucose and ketones in the urine

Table 1-38   Emergency Treatment: Hyperglycemia and/or Ketoacidosis

Call for medical assistance; monitor the patient until help arrives; inform the PT
Hyperglycemia can cause ketoacidosis and ultimately diabetic coma (and death)

Signs and Symptoms of Hypoglycemia: Low Blood Sugar of Less than 50 mg/dL[5]

- Increased heart rate and lightheadedness
- Sweating, unsteadiness, and weakness
- Headache, fatigue, and impaired vision
- Confusion, pallor, and behavior changes
- Clumsiness and tingling sensation in the mouth

Table 1-39   Emergency Treatment: Hypoglycemia

Patient needs sugar: half of cup of orange juice, or four or five candies, or three glucose tablets, or a glass of milk

Intervention Precautions for Patients with Diabetes

Table 1-40 Intervention Precautions for Diabetes

Plan the patient's exercises in conjunction to food intake and insulin administration. Ask the patient about his or her nutritional status prior to interventions.

Monitor the patient's glucose levels before exercises. Do not exercise patients with blood glucose of 250 mg/dL or higher.

Monitor the injection site before exercises. Do not exercise at or near the muscles where the injection of insulin was administered. Do not administer interventions such as physical agents at the injection site.

Exercise at or around the same time of day.

Do not administer interventions such as physical agents without testing the patient's superficial sensations.

Do not exercise patients with a high level of ketones in urine or high blood levels.

Inform the PT if the patient experienced hypoglycemia or hyperglycemia.

Educate the patient about avoiding exercising or activities late at night or just before sleep (can cause hypoglycemia at night).

Educate the patient about diabetic foot care.

Educate the patient about eating a slowly absorbed carbohydrate snack (pasta, crackers, or bread) after exercises. Educate the patient about eating a fast absorbing carbohydrate snack (fruit) after prolonged activities (for every 30 minutes of activity).

Signs and Symptoms of Electrolyte Disturbances: Hyperkalemia (High Potassium Level in Blood)

- Muscle weakness and/or flaccid paralysis
- Bradycardia and/or arrhythmia
- Diarrhea and/or abdominal cramps

Table 1-41   Possible Causes of Hyperkalemia

High-potassium diet, kidney failure, Addison's disease (hyposecretion of adrenocortical hormones secondary to infections such as TB or hemorrhage), trauma to muscle, decreased aldosterone insulin

Table 1-42   Clinical Safety Measures for Hyperkalemia

Monitor the patient's cardiopulmonary response to physical therapy interventions; inform the PT

Signs and Symptoms of Electrolyte Disturbances: Hypokalemia (Low Potassium Level in Blood)

- Muscle fatigue and/or cramps in the legs
- Slow reflex and/or orthostatic hypotension
- Dizziness and/or arrhythmia
- Irritability and/or confusion
- Depression and/or respiratory distress
- Nausea and/or lack of appetite
- Diarrhea and/or vomiting

Table 1-43   Possible Causes of Hypokalemia

Poor nutrition, decreased food intake, Cushing's disease (hypersecretion of adrenal cortex and excessive production of glucocorticoids secondary to tumor or excessive stimulation of adrenal gland), diuretic medications, and kidney disease

Table 1-44   Clinical Safety Measures for Hypokalemia

Monitor the patient's cardiopulmonary response to interventions; watch patient for orthostatic hypotension; inform the PT

Signs and Symptoms of Electrolyte Disturbances: Hypernatremia (High Sodium Level in Blood)

- Weight gain and/or pitting edema
- Pulmonary edema and/or hypertension
- Tachycardia and/or agitation
- Restlessness and/or convulsions

Table 1-45   Possible Causes of Hypernatremia

Cushing's disease, salt water ingestion, decreased fluid intake, dehydration, kidney disease

Table 1-46   Clinical Safety Measures for Hypernatremia

Observe the patient for the signs and symptoms of hypernatremia. Monitor the patient's cardiopulmonary response to interventions. Inform the PT.

Signs and Symptoms of Electrolyte Disturbances: Hyponatremia (Low Sodium Level in Blood)

- Muscle weakness and/or muscle twitching
- Hypotension and/or tachycardia
- Anxiety and/or headache
- Restlessness and/or convulsions
- Cyanotic and/or cold and clammy skin
- Shock

Table 1-47   Possible Causes of Hyponatremia

Addison's disease, excessive fluid loss (due to sweating, vomiting, diarrhea, and/or diuretic medications)

Table 1-48   Clinical Safety Measures for Hyponatremia

Observe the patient for the signs and symptoms of hyponatremia. Monitor the
patient's hypotension. Inform the PT.

Signs and Symptoms of Electrolyte Disturbances: Hypercalcemia (High Calcium Level in Blood)

- Generalized weakness and/or decreased muscle tone
- Weight loss and/or anorexia
- Bone pain and/or fractures
- Drowsiness and/or lethargy
- Headache and/or confusion
- Hypertension and/or cardiac arrest

Table 1-49   Possible Causes of Hypercalcemia
Hyperparathyroidism, bone cancer, or bone atrophy

Table 1-50   Clinical Safety Measures for Hypercalcemia

Monitor the patient's cardiopulmonary response to interventions; inform the PT.

Signs and Symptoms of Electrolyte Disturbances: Hypocalcemia (Low Calcium Level in Blood)

- Muscle cramps and spasms and/or tetany
- Tingling and numbness
- Irritability and/or anxiety
- Convulsions and/or hypotension
- Arrhythmia

Table 1-51   Possible Causes of Hypocalcemia
Renal disease, renal failure, hyperparathyroidism, decreased absorption of calcium
in the gastrointestinal system, decreased vitamin D, and infantile diarrhea

Table 1-52   Clinical Safety Measures for Hypocalcemia

Monitor the patient's cardiopulmonary system, especially for orthostatic hypotension; inform the PT.

Signs and Symptoms of Respiratory Acidosis: CO_2 Retention and Impaired Alveolar Ventilation

- Dyspnea and/or cyanosis
- Headache and/or disorientation
- Decreased deep tendon reflexes (DTRs) and/or possible coma
- Restlessness and/or anxiety

Table 1-53   Possible Causes of Respiratory Acidosis

Hypoventilation, chronic obstructive pulmonary disease (asthma, bronchitis, pneumonia, and emphysema), Guillaine Barre, myasthenia gravis, hypermetabolism (in burns or sepsis), diabetes, renal insufficiency, and renal failure

Table 1-54   Clinical Safety Measures for Respiratory Acidosis

Observe the patient for the signs and symptoms of respiratory acidosis. Monitor the patient's cardiopulmonary system. Inform the PT.
Respiratory acidosis may lead to disorientation, stupor, and coma or death.

Signs and Symptoms of Respiratory Alkalosis: Low CO_2 and Alveolar Hyperventilation

- Tachypnea and/or anxiety
- Dizziness and/or paresthesia
- Blurred vision and/or diaphoresis
- Arrhythmia and/or numbness and tingling
- Tetany and/or convulsions

Table 1-55   Possible Causes of Respiratory Alkalosis

Decreased oxygen (due to emphysema, or pneumonia), anxiety attacks and hyperventilation, CHF, pulmonary embolism, aspirin poisoning, stress, liver disease, central nervous system disease, scoliosis, sepsis, and excessive exercise

Table 1-56   Clinical Safety Measures for Respiratory Alkalosis

Observe the patient for the signs and symptoms of respiratory alkalosis. Monitor the patient's cardiopulmonary system. Inform the PT.

Signs and Symptoms of Overhydration: Excess of Body Fluid

- Swelling or edema in the interstitial tissues
- Shortness of breath with activities
- Increased BP and HR
- Lethargy and/or headache
- Muscle cramps and/or stiffness and twitches
- Weight gain and pitting edema of the extremities

Table 1-57   Possible Causes of Overhydration

Excessive fluid intake, CHF, renal failure, cirrhosis

Table 1-58   Clinical Safety Measures for Overhydration

Observe the patient for the signs and symptoms. Monitor the patient's cardiopulmonary system. Elevate extremities. Inform the PT.

Signs and Symptoms of Dehydration: Extreme Decrease of Body Fluid

- Skin turgor and poor skin integrity
- Headache and/or lethargy
- Increased body temperature and/or muscle cramps
- Vertigo and/or orthostatic hypotension
- Irritability and/or confusion and disorientation
- Rapid HR and RR and/or incoordination
- Diarrhea and/or vomiting

Table 1-59   Possible Causes of Dehydration

Heat, emesis, diuretics, sodium deficiency, and sweating

Table 1-60   Clinical Safety Measures for Dehydration

Monitor the patient's cardiopulmonary system especially for orthostatic hypotension. Monitor the patient for fainting or fatigue. Inform the PT.

Medications and Patient's Adverse Reactions in the Clinic

See Table 1-61.

Contraindications and Precautions of Physical Agents/Modalities

See Table 1-62.

Table 1-61 Medications and Patient's Adverse Reactions in the Clinic[6]

Medication Group	Most Used Brand Names	Adverse Reactions
Nonnarcotic Analgesic	Abenal, Anacin – 3, Datril, Dolanex, Exdol, Halenol, Liquiprim, Panadol, Tempra, Tylenol, Valadol	Gastrointestinal (GI) distress, dizziness, lethargy, chills, and diaphoresis. Chronic use: may cause renal damage or renal failure
Analgesic	Acetylsalicylic Acid (ASA): Aspirin, Astrin, Ecotrin Acetic Acid: Clinoril	ASA: GI distress, GI bleeding, anemia, tinnitus, hearing loss, dizziness, easy bruising, skin rash Clinoril: GI distress, skin rash
Nonsteroidal Antiinflammatory (NSAID) and NSAID Analgesic	Advil, Aleve, Anaprox Motrin, Nuprin, Trendar, Daypro, Dolobid, Feldene, Lodine, Nalfon, Actron, Orudis, Tolectin, Voltaren, Relafen, Celebrex, Vioxx	Headache, dizziness, somnolence (Feldene and Relafen), vertigo, lightheadedness, fatigue, drowsiness, confusion, HTN (Advil, Motrin, Nuprin, and Trendar), blurred vision, skin eruptions, pruritus, rash, fluid retention with edema, GI bleeding, nausea, tinnitus, hearing loss
Narcotic Analgesic	Hycodan, Vicodin, Tylenol # 3, Paveral, Empirin, OxyContin, Percolone, Roxicodone, Darvon	Nausea, vomiting, lethargy, lightheadedness, drowsiness, dyspnea, bradycardia, orthostatic hypotension and facial flushing (Tylenol # 3, Paveral, and Empirin), dizziness
Muscle Relaxant	Rela, Soma, Lioresal, Paraflex, Parafon Forte, Cyclofel, Flexeril, Valium, Apo-Diazepam, Vivol, Marbaxin, Robaxin	Orthostatic hypotension, facial flushing, tachycardia, bradycardia, nausea, vomiting, drowsiness, dizziness, lightheadedness, ataxia, tremor, headache, vertigo, irritability, diplopia, blurred vision, skin rash, fatigue

Antihypertensive and Cardiac (CHF): Ace Inhibitor Agent	Capoten, Vasotec, Prinivil, Zestril, Monopril, Accupril	Skin rash, cough, headache, dizziness, fatigue, orthostatic hypotension, GI distress, impaired taste
Antihypertensive and Cardiac (Angina): Calcium Channel Blocking Agent	Cardizem, Dilacor XR, Tiamate, Tiazac, Calan, Isoptin, Verelan, Norvasc, Adalat, Procardia	Headache, fatigue, dizziness, lightheadedness, vertigo, drowsiness, nervousness, insomnia, confusion, gait abnormality, tremor, edema, hypotension, palpitations, skin flushing, GI distress, skin rash, dyspnea, peripheral edema
Antihypertensive and Cardiac (Angina, Arrhythmia, Acute MI): Beta-Blocker Agent	Apo-Propranolol, Inderal, Novopranol, Apo-Atenolol, Tenormin, Apo-Metoprolol, Lopressor, Toprol	Confusion, agitation, fatigue, vertigo, drowsiness, weakness, insomnia, bradycardia, hypotension, cold extremities, GI distress, paresthesia of hands, dyspnea
Antidepressant	Amitril, Elavil, Meravil, Norpramine, Pertofrane, Sinequan, Triadapin, Zonalon, Wellbutrin, Zyban, Prozac, Sarafem, Zoloft	Drowsiness, dizziness, fatigue, headache, orthostatic hypotension, tachycardia, dry mouth, GI distress, urinary retention, tinnitus, blurred vision, skin rash, HTN and dyspnea (Zoloft)

SAFETY IN THE CLINICAL ENVIRONMENT

Patient Safety During Interventions **53**

Table 1-62 Contraindications and Precautions of Physical Agents/Modalities[7]

Physical Agent or Modality	Contraindications	Precautions
Therapeutic Heat	Acute inflammation/trauma; deep vein thrombosis (DVT) and malignant tumors; edema and open wounds; hemorrhage and bleeding; loss of sensory capability; inability to communicate; ischemia and immature scar; atrophic and infected skin.	Monitor sensory capability of pediatric and geriatric patients.
Whirlpool	Chronic wounds (eschar); nonlocalized infection wounds; clean granulating wounds; epithelializing wounds; migrating epidermal cells; new skin grafts; new tissue flaps; venous ulcers; nonnecrotic diabetic ulcers; bowel/bladder incontinence; Patients with: skin infections; unstable BP; severe epilepsy; upper respiratory infections; TB and cellulitis; edema of the extremities; lethargy; unresponsiveness; wound maceration; febrile conditions; compromised cardiovascular and pulmonary function; acute phlebitis; renal failure; dry gangrene; incontinence (in full body whirlpool).	Check: Whirlpool ground fault circuit interrupter. Check whirlpool water temperature: Limbs = 103°–110°F; Open wound = 92°F–96°F; MS = 88°F;PVD = 95°F–100°F; Insert tank liner for hepatitis and open wounds; burns and HIV; Hubbard Tank—closely monitor patient's physiological responses.

Paraffin Bath	Open wounds and allergic rash; skin infections and recent scars and sutures.	Wash patient's hands or feet prior to application of paraffin bath.
Aquatic Therapy	Bowel or bladder incontinence (except patients who are catheterized); urinary tract infection (UTI) and severe epilepsy; unprotected wounds; Unstable BP and severe cardiorespiratory dysfunctions.	Patients to shower before immersion. Check water temperature: General pool temperature = 92°F–98°F; MS = 84°F; Spasticity (20–45 min) = 86°F– 94°F; RA/OA (10–20 min) = 96.8°F–98.6°F.
Ultraviolet Radiation	Acute eczema and psoriasis; herpes simplex; lupus erythematosus; generalized dermatitis.	Antibiotics such as tetracycline or sulfonamides and diuretics can increase photosensitivity and burn the skin.
Ultrasound (US)	Acute infections; impaired circulation and sensation; cognitive impairments; malignancy; very old or very young patients; specific ultrasound contraindications: healing fractures; thrombophlebitis; epiphysis of growing bones (of young children); over eye, heart, carotid sinuses; cervical ganglia and spinal cord; reproductive organs; cardiac pacemaker and pregnant uterus.	Metal implants in the treatment area; osteoporosis; plastic implants; over scar tissue; postsurgically after repairs of tendons and ligaments. Thermal US periosteal pain must be stopped by decreasing intensity; increasing treatment surface area. Thermal US temperature increases at tissue interfaces: bone/ligaments; bone/joint capsule; bone/muscle. US "hot spot" must be stopped by applying more coupling agent; decreasing the intensity; moving the transducer. Use plastic container for US in the water.
Fluidotherapy	Acute traumatic and inflammatory conditions; impaired circulation; impaired sensation and cognitive function; DVT and malignant tumors; hemorrhage and edema; pediatric or older patients.	Cover with a plastic barrier: open wounds; lesions.

Patient Safety During Interventions **55**

Table 1-62 (continued)

Physical Agent or Modality	Contraindications	Precautions
Diathermy	Cardiac insufficiency; older adults and young children (under 4 years old); peripheral vascular disease (PVD) and infections; applications over metal, cardiac pacemaker, pregnant uterus, and epiphyses of growing bones.	Check patient often during treatment—treated area is not visible.
Therapeutic Cold	Impaired circulation and sensation; Raynaud's disease and PVD; sensitivity/allergic reaction to cold; prolonged application over superficial nerves (can result in neurapraxia).	Monitor patients first time for urticaria = erythema of the skin with wheal formation and severe itching (remove cold); facial flush = eyelids puffiness and respiratory problems (remove cold); anaphylaxis = decreased BP, increased HR, syncope (call emergency services). Monitor the patient's normal physiological response to ice: cold, burning, aching, and numbness (CBAN).
Contrast Baths	Same contraindications as therapeutic cold/heat. Specific contraindications: advanced arteriosclerosis; arterial insufficiency; loss of sensation to heat or cold.	Check water temperature: • Hot (warm) = 100°F–110°F • Cold = 55°F–65°F

Therapeutic Massage	Acute inflammation in the treatment area; acute febrile conditions; severe atherosclerosis; severe varicose veins; phlebitis and recent surgery; thrombophlebitis; cardiac arrhythmia; severe RA and hemorrhage; edema secondary to kidney dysfunction, heart failure, and venous insufficiency.	Therapeutic massage is a passive modality and should be used for a short period of time as an adjunct, not as a substitute, to active interventions such as therapeutic exercises and activities and patient education.
Intermittent Compression	Acute inflammation; acute DVT and arterial insufficiency; peripheral arterial disease (PAD) and arterial ulcers; cancer and acute pulmonary edema; cardiac insufficiency; kidney insufficiency and HTN; diminished skin sensation; cognitive dysfunction; very young and very old patient.	Check the patient's blood pressure carefully. Position the patient in a comfortable position with the upper or lower extremity abducted between 20 and 70 degrees, and elevated at approximately 40 degrees.
Electrical Stimulation	Healing fractures; demand-type pacemaker; over superficial metal implants; areas of active bleeding; distal to an area of thrombophlebitis; pregnancy and malignancy; active tuberculosis; cardiac arrhythmias and heart conduction dysfunction; application over carotid sinuses, pharyngeal or laryngeal muscles.	Obesity and areas of decreased or absent sensation; severe edema and diabetes; patients with thin fragile skin; peripheral neuropathies; broken or not biannually certified electrical stimulators; patients with external or internal metal devices, denervated muscle, spinal cord injury (can acquire dysreflexia), diminished cognition

continues

Table 1-62 (continued)

Physical Agent or Modality	Contraindications	Precautions
Iontophoresis	The same as for ES; previous allergic reactions to medication or to direct current; cuts, bruises or broken skin; metal near treatment area; recent scars.	Check for intact skin; no scratches or abrasions in treatment area. REMINDER: Use negative medication for (−) electrode and positive medication for (+) electrode; Use low levels of current intensity for (−) electrode; (−) electrode must be twice as large as (+) electrode.
Transcutaneous Electrical Nerve Stimulation (TENS)	The same as for ES; do not apply TENS over eyes, mucosal membranes, laryngeal or pharyngeal muscles, head and neck following a CVA, on very young or very old patients, or on patients with epilepsy.	Patient education for TENS units: not to be used in shower or when sleeping; electrode placement; skin inspection—skin irritation; checking adherence of electrodes to the skin; accommodation to ES (patient to contact PT/PTA—needs modulation).
Traction	Spinal traction contraindicated for: meningitis; spinal cancer; spinal cord pressure; spondylolisthesis; RA; osteoporosis and recent fracture; hiatal hernia; HTN; cardiovascular disease; osteopenia; acute soft tissue injury; Down's syndrome; joint hypermobility; very young and very old patients; acute whiplash injury.	Spinal traction: acute inflammation aggravated by traction; acute strains and sprains; claustrophobia and joint instability; pregnancy and temporomandibular joint (TMJ) syndrome (when using cervical halter). Cervical traction—observe patient for discomfort in the TMJ—adjust head halter and insure force is applied to occipital region; in general, traction force not to exceed weight of patient's head (can start 7% of patient's body weight).

Acute Care Safety

Table 1-63   Acute Care Safety

Check with nursing personnel to temporarily remove suction tubes or disconnect tube feedings.

Do not dislodge peripheral or central lines. Ask for nursing assistance.

Do not disrupt the setup of vital medical equipment. Endotracheal tubes, nasogastric tubes, and arterial and central venous catheters contribute to the patient's morbidity and mortality. Ask for nursing assistance.

Before transfer and ambulation, ensure that the patient is properly dressed. Loose clothing and/or inappropriate footwear (such as slippers, socks without shoes, or sandals) are not safe. Shoes need to be nonslip, to fit snugly, and to have a low, wide heel.

A safety belt should always be used in transfers and ambulation. The transfer surfaces need to be secured by locking the wheelchair (and stabilizing the wheelchair against a wall or using a wooden block under the wheelchair wheels to increase stability). Transfer surfaces should be at the same height or level as possible.

The therapist should not hold onto the patient's joints or fragile areas.

During ambulation and transfers, the urinary (Foley) catheter drainage bag must be secured below the patient's bladder and 2 inches above the floor. The bag must be repositioned after interventions.

Before ambulation and transfers, inspect the Foley catheter. The tubing must be straight and not twisted.

When working with patients who suffered fractures and are in traction (such as Bryant's traction or external traction), do not bump the bed or disturb the traction devices (weights). Team up with the nursing staff to reposition the patient and prevent decubitus ulcers.

References

1. Dreeben, O. *Introduction to Physical Therapy for Physical Therapist Assistants*. Sudbury, MA: Jones and Bartlett Publishers; 2007.
2. The American Physical Therapy Association. *APTA Governance*. The American Physical Therapy Association Web site. Available at www.apta.org. Accessed November 2006.
3. Spector, RE. *Cultural Diversity in Health & Illness* (6th ed.). Upper Saddle River, NJ: Pearson Prentice Hall; 2004.
4. Centers for Disease Control. *Standard Precautions*. Centers for Disease Control Web site. Available at http://www.cdc.gov. Accessed November 2006.
5. Rothstein, JM, Scalzitti, DA, Mayhew, TP. *The Rehabilitation Specialist's Handbook* (3rd ed.). Philadelphia: F.A. Davis Company; 2005.
6. Ciccone, CD. *Pharmacology in Rehabilitation* (3rd ed.). Philadelphia: F.A. Davis Company; 2002.
7. Hecox, B, Tsega, AM, Weisberg, J, Sanko J. *Integrating Physical Agents in Rehabilitation* (2nd ed.). Upper Saddle River, NJ: Pearson Education; 2006.

Part II

Clinical Documentation

CLINICAL
DOCUMENTATION

Documentation Guidelines

General Documentation Guidelines

Table 2-1   General Guidelines[1]

The patient's right to privacy should be respected regarding written information in the SOAP examination and evaluation, re-examination, and re-evaluation and in the SOAP note.

The release of the medical information, including written physical therapy documentation, must be authorized by the patient in writing.

All inquiries for medical information to the PTA should be directed to the supervising PT.

Written physical therapy records should be kept in a safe and secure place for seven years.

American Physical Therapy Association's (APTA's) Documentation Guidelines

Table 2-2   APTA's Guidelines[1]

The documentation must be consistent with the APTA's Standards of Practice.

All documentation must be legible and use medically approved abbreviations or symbols.

All documentation must be written in black or blue ink, and the mistakes must be crossed out with a single line through the error, initialed, and dated by the PTA.

Each intervention session must be documented. The patient's name and identification number must be on each page of the documentation record.

Informed consent for the interventions must be signed by a competent adult.

If the adult is not competent, the consent must be signed by the patient/client's legal guardian.

If the patient is a minor, the consent must be signed by the parent or an appointed guardian.

Each document must be dated and signed by the PT/PTA using the first and the last name and the professional designation; professional license number may be included but can be optional.

All communications with other health care providers or health care professionals must be recorded.

The PTA students' notes should be co-signed by the PTA (clinical instructor) or by the PT (clinical instructor).

Nonlicensed personnel notes should be co-signed by the PT.

APTA's Documentation Guidelines on Domestic Violence[2]

- The medical records must be written in the regular course of business during the examination or the interview.
- The medical records must be legible.
- The medical records must be properly stored and be accessed only by the appropriate staff.
- The medical records must include the following information:
  A. Patient's date and time of arrival at the clinic or the treatment site
  B. Patient's name, address, and the phone number of the person(s) accompanying the victim (if possible)
  C. Patient's own words about the cause of her or his injuries
  D. A detailed description (with explanations) of injuries, including the type, number, size, location, and resolution, a description of a chronology of the violence asking about the first episode, the most recent, and the most serious episode
  E. Any documentation of inconsistency between the injury and the explanation about the injury
  F. Documentation that the clinician asked about domestic violence and of the patient's response
  G. A color photograph(s), including the patient's informed consent for the photograph(s); photographs should be taken from different angles including the patient's face in at least one picture; two pictures are necessary for each major trauma area; the photographs must be marked, including the patient's name, location, and names of the person taking the pictures
  H. If police were called, documentation about the investigating officer's name, badge number, phone number, and any actions taken
  I. Documentation about the name of the PT or the PTA or the physician or the nurse who treated the patient (if applicable)

SECTION 2-2

Documentation Elements

Initial Examination and Evaluation Elements

- Referral, including the reason for referral and the specific intervention requested by the referral source
- Data accompanying referral: primary medical diagnosis (or onset date), secondary medical diagnoses, medical history, medications, other complications or precautions
- Physical therapy history: patient's date of birth, age, gender, start of care, and primary complaint
- Referral diagnosis: mechanism of injury, prior diagnostic imaging (or testing)
- Prior physical therapy history
- Tests and measures (data collection): patient's cognition, vision, hearing, vital signs, vascular signs, sensation and proprioception, coordination, balance, posture, pain, edema, active range of motion (AROM), passive range of motion (PROM), strength, bed mobility, transfers, ambulation (level and stairs), wheelchair use, orthotic/prosthetic devices, durable medical equipment used or needed, activity tolerance, special tests, architectural considerations, requirements to return to prior activity level (including work, school, or home), wound description (for wound care, including the incision status)
- Prior level of function: mobility at home and in the community, employment and/or school
- Physical therapy diagnosis
- Assessment: reason for skilled care
- Problems
- Plan of care: specific interventions strategies, frequency, duration, patient instruction/home program, caregiver training, short-term goals (STGs) and dates of achievement, long-term goals (LTGs) and dates of achievement, patient's rehabilitation potential

Patient's History Elements

Table 2-3   Patient History Elements

Personal information including patient's age, gender, and occupation

Medical diagnosis and any precautions related to physical therapy

Patient's chief complaint, including the patient's description of his or her condition and the reason seeking assistance, identification of patient's primary problem

Patient's present illness including the symptoms associated with the patient's primary problem such as location of the problem (may use a body chart), severity, nature (such as aching, burning, or tingling), persistence (constant versus intermittent), and aggravated by activity versus relieved by rest

Onset of the patient's primary problem including mechanism of injury (if traumatic), sequence and progression of symptoms, date of the initial onset and status to the current visit, prior interventions and results, and associated disability

Patient's past history, including prior episodes of the same problem, prior interventions and responses, other affected areas (or body parts), familial, developmental, and congenital disorders, general health status, medications, and x-rays or other pertinent tests

Patient's lifestyle, including patient's profession or occupation, assistance from family or friends, occupational and family demands (spouse, children, job expectations), activities of daily living (hobbies, sports), and patient's concept of the impact of functional (including cosmetic) and socioeconomic factors

Progress Report Elements

- Attendance
- Current baseline data: patient's cognition, vision, hearing, vital signs, vascular signs, sensation and proprioception, coordination, balance (sit and stand), posture, pain, edema, AROM, PROM, strength, bed mobility, transfers, ambulation (level and stairs), wheelchair use, orthotic/prosthetic devices, durable medical equipment used or needed, activity tolerance, special tests, architectural considerations, requirements to return to prior activity level (including work, school, or home), wound description (for wound care and including the incision status)
- Physical therapy diagnosis
- Assessment: reason for skilled care

- Problems
- Plan of care: specific interventions strategies, frequency of interventions, duration of interventions, patient instruction/home program, caregiver training, STGs and dates of achievement, LTGs and dates of achievement, patient's rehabilitation potential

Discontinuation of Physical Therapy Report Elements

- Attendance
- Current baseline data: patient's cognition, vision, hearing, vital signs, vascular signs, sensation and proprioception, coordination, balance (sit and stand), posture, pain, edema, AROM, PROM, strength, bed mobility, transfers, ambulation (level and stairs), wheelchair use, orthotic/prosthetic devices, durable medical equipment used or needed, activity tolerance, special tests, architectural considerations, requirements to return to prior activity level (including work, school, or home), wound description (for wound care, including the incision status)
- Physical therapy diagnosis
- Assessment: reason for skilled care
- Problems
- Plan of care: specific interventions strategies, frequency of interventions, duration of interventions, patient instruction/home program, caregiver training, STGs and dates of achievement, LTGs and dates of achievement, discontinuation of physical therapy prognosis

Possible Indications for Patient's Discontinuation of Physical Therapy

Table 2-4   Possible Indications

Patient's desire to stop treatment

Patient's inability to progress toward goals because of medical or psychosocial complications or because financial/insurance resources have been expended

PT's decision that the patient will no longer benefit from physical therapy

SECTION 2-3

Daily/Weekly SOAP Note Elements

Subjective Data

Table 2-5 Examples of Subjective Data

Patient's complains of pain

Patient's response to the previous treatment

Patient's description of functional improvements such as being able to do activities of daily living

Patient's lifestyle situation such as being able to go out to dinner or entertain friends (like he or she used to do before this condition)

Patient's goals such as to be able to drive his or her car in two to three weeks

Patient's compliance or difficulties with the home exercise program (HEP)

Strategies for Writing Subjective Data

- Do not use irrelevant information; use information that affects the interventions and goals, describes a change in patient's condition, and proves effectiveness/ineffectiveness of interventions.
- Include patient's pain information in the subjective data.

Objective Data

Table 2-6 Examples of Objective Data

The results of the physical therapy measurements and tests such as manual muscle testing, goniometry, gait assessment, and specific neurological assessments (such as balance, sensation, or proprioception)

The description of the interventions provided to the patient such as physical agents and modalities, therapeutic exercises, wound care, functional training (such as gait using assistive devices), patient education/instruction (such as post surgery precautions), discussion and coordination with other disciplines (such as occupational therapy that gave the patient a shoe horn to be able to put his or her shoes on)

The description of the patient's function such as performing transfers, gait (with or without assistive devices, on even or uneven surfaces and stairs), or bed mobility (such as turning from supine to side lying to sitting)

The PTA's objective observations of the patient during interventions (such as the increase in the number of exercise repetitions), tests and measurements (such as compensating for muscular weakness), and patient education/instruction (such as understanding the HEP on the first performance)

CLINICAL DOCUMENTATION

Objective Data Guidelines

Table 2-7   Guidelines

Describe the reason(s) for interventions and the interventions provided to the patient in enough detail that another PT or PTA could read the description and replicate the interventions (improves different therapists' follow-up, quality, and consistency of intervention).

Describe patient's response to each intervention; in this way, the most effective patient's intervention response can be found and used during physical therapy.

Do not write what the PTA[3] did, such as "applied moist hot pack to the patient's lower back;" write patient's response to moist hot pack, such as "patient had decreased muscular spasm of right erector spinae at L2–L4 level after application of moist hot pack to the muscles for 20 minutes, patient in prone position."

After repeating tests and measurements that were performed in the initial examination, describe the results by relating them with the initial results.

Use words that describe patient performing a function in order for the reader to visualize the function.

Organize the information in a logical manner.

Use words that portray skilled physical therapy services.

Include any copy of written information that was given to the patient (such as the home exercise program).

Examples of Impairments and Related Functional Limitations

Table 2-8   Examples of Impairments and Related Functional Limitations

Impairment	Functional Limitation
Weakness in the lower extremity	Knee buckles on heel strike Decreased speed during gait training Decreased safety during transfers and gait training Unable to ambulate on uneven terrain
Incoordination in both upper extremities	Unable to comb hair within tolerable timeframe Unable to don clothes without continuous guidance Unable to toothbrush teeth without continuous guidance
TMJ dysfunction	Limited bite and chewing Unable to consume full meals without food alteration
Left knee effusion	Unable to ascend/descend 10 steps Unable to ambulate 20 feet in 9 seconds Unable to tolerate 30 minutes of unassisted walking

Strategies for Writing Objective Data

- The results of tests and measures must be documented considering the PT's initial evaluation. Do not introduce new tests and measures. Consider the patient's starting and ending positions and points of measurement from the initial evaluation.
- Detail patient's function considering elements such as type of assistive device, type of equipment, distance, speed, time, repetitions, sets, type of gait pattern, amount of assistance, reason for assistance, and the environment.
- Do not write what the PTA did[3] but what the patient did.
- Organize the information.

- Detail the interventions considering elements such as type of intervention, type of equipment and/or machine, position of patient, description of treated area, patient's physiologic response, parameters, settings, intensity, sets, number of repetitions, number of sets, and purpose of intervention.

Assessment Data

Table 2-9   Examples of Assessment Data

Overall patient's response to interventions
Patient's progress toward STGs and LTGs (from the PT's initial evaluation)
Explanations why the interventions are necessary
Effects on interventions on the patient's impairments and functional limitations

Strategies for Writing Assessment Data

- Be consistent in regard to relating the information in the assessment with information from the subjective data and objective data in the daily/weekly SOAP note and the initial evaluation.
- Do not make generalized statements but be specific describing patient's progress/lack of progress toward STGs and LTGs.
- Do not introduce new information (such as tests or measures) that is not mentioned in the initial evaluation.

Plan Data

Table 2-10   Examples of Plan Data

Plan for next intervention session.
Plan for consultation with another discipline.
Plan for the frequency of the interventions.
Plan for reevaluation or discontinuation of physical therapy by PT.
Plan to discuss with PT changes in patient's condition, introduction of new exercises, or specific patient's goals or complaints to the PTA.

Strategies for Writing Plan Data

- Do not forget to include information about working as a team with the PT.
- Write relevant information and suggestions considering STGs and LTGs and that the content reflects what will happen next intervention session.
- Include the numbers of remaining intervention sessions.

Documentation Tips

Table 2-11   Documentation Tips[4]

Always write on every line in the chart.

Write using one pen. In cases where a pen runs out of ink in the middle of an entry, indicate in parenthesis that the first pen ran out of ink.

Correct mistakes by drawing a single line through the error, initial it, and date it (where required by law). You may also consider writing "incorrect entry" by the error.

Write legibly or print if necessary.

Do not backdate an omission in the intervention record. Document any omitted prior entry as a new entry.

Do not write expressing personal feelings about a patient/client such as "this patient seems to be malingering."

Do not write expressing disapproval or denigrating other health care providers or personnel.

Do not include extraneous verbiage not related to interventions.

Avoid using terms or abbreviations except for the ones approved to be used in the medical record.

Telephone Referral Documentation

Table 2-12   Telephone Referral Guidelines[4]

Date and time of the call

Name of the person calling and name of the health care provider who referred the patient

Name of the PTA who took the referral

Name of the patient and all other details in regard to the referral

Date when a written copy of the referral would be sent to physical therapy

Name of the PT who will be responsible for the referred patient

Health Insurance Portability and Accountability Act (HIPAA) and Documentation

Table 2-13   HIPAA Documentation Requirements[4]

Patient records are considered Protected Health Information (PHI).

PHI needs to be secured in locked file cabinets or records rooms.

PHI stored in the computer needs to be secured using additional passwords.

In physical therapy facility, during physical therapy practice, the PT/PTA must take safeguards to limit access to areas where patient's chart is located by ensuring that the area is supervised, by keeping the chart face down or facing a wall if stored vertically, or by escorting nonemployees in the area.

PT/PTA can share patient information with students (for training purposes). When students return to the academic institution, the patient information should be deidentified before it is shared. Alternatively, the student could obtain an authorization from the patient to use patient's protected health information at the academic institution.

During the customary and necessary health care communications or practices, the PHI can be used or disclosed if the PT/PTA applied reasonable safeguards and implemented the minimum necessary standards. It means that the PT/PTA must make every effort to limit the disclosure to the minimum necessary to accomplish the intended purpose.

Physical therapy facility needs to develop and implement policies and procedures that reasonably minimize the amount of PHI used, disclosed, and requested. The policies and procedures must establish standard protocols for routine or recurring requests and disclosures of PHI. For special requests, the policies and procedures must establish a protocol that the requests will be reviewed individually by one person called the (chief) privacy officer.

The patient (client) has the right to access his or her PHI that was generated during the six years before the date of the request. The patient (client) has also the right to access any piece of information that reflects a decision the provider made regarding the patient (client) and an accounting of PHI disclosures (including the date of each disclosure, the name of the person who received PHI, a brief description of the PHI disclosed, and a brief statement of the purpose of the disclosure). The patient (client) has the right to examine his or her chart and other records (of his or her), even records the provider thinks that the patient (client) will never see (such as a letter to a collection agency to collect the copayment). The patient (client) has the right on request to get a copy of his or her records in 30 days (if the records are onsite) and in 60 days (if the records are off–site). The provider can charge a reasonable copying cost (certain state laws require a certain amount per copy per page).

A PT/PTA can not use the PHI in marketing.

Patient (client) authorization for uses and disclosures of PHI is not needed for the following: patient (client) seeking his or her PHI; Department of Health and Human Services; uses and disclosures required by laws other than HIPAA (such as vital statistics, communicable diseases, OSHA, related workplace surveillance); victims of domestic violence, child abuse, or elder abuse; judicial and administrative proceedings (such as court of law orders or court of law subpoena); Medicare or Medicaid; law enforcement activities; Secret Service; emergency situations with serious threats to health or safety; Workers Compensation (to the extent required by state law).

Abbreviations and Symbols Used the Most in Physical Therapy

Abbreviations

Table 2-14 Abbreviations[3]

A	assistance	CBC	complete blood count
AAROM	active assistive range of motion	CCs	chief complaints
		CHF	congestive heart failure
ACL	anterior cruciate ligament	CHI	closed head injury
		CKC	closed kinetic chain
ADL	activities of daily living	cm	centimeter(s)
Ad lib	as desired	CNS	central nervous system
AE	above elbow	c/o	complains of, complaint(s) of
afib	atrial fibrillation		
AFO	ankle foot orthosis	coord	coordination
AK	above knee	COPD	chronic obstructive pulmonary disease
AM, a.m.	morning		
amb.	ambulation	CP	compression pump, chest pain and cerebral palsy
ANS	autonomic nervous system		
		CPM	continuous passive motion machine
AP	anterior–posterior		
Appts	appointments	CPR	cardiopulmonary resuscitation
AROM	active range of motion		
ASIS	anterior superior iliac spine	CSF	cerebrospinal fluid
		C-tx	cervical traction
assist	assistance	CVA	cerebral vascular accident
B	bilateral, both		
BE	below elbow	CW	continuous wave
bid	twice a day	D1, D2	diagonal 1, diagonal 2
Bil.	bilateral	d/c	discharged, discontinued
BK	below knee	DDD	degenerative disc disease
BLE	both lower extremities		
BM	bowel movement	DEP	data, evaluation, performance goals
BMI	body mass index		
BP	blood pressure	DF	dorsiflexion
BPM	beats per minute	DJD	degenerative joint disease
Bx	biopsy		
Ca	cancer	DM	diabetes mellitus
CARF	Commission on Accreditation of Rehabilitation Facilities	DOB	date of birth
		DOE	dyspnea on exertion

CLINICAL DOCUMENTATION

Table 2-14 (continued)

DTR	deep tendon reflex	H/O	history of
DVT	deep vein thrombosis	HOB	head of bed
Dx	diagnosis	HP	hot pack
ECG/EKG	electrocardiogram	HPI	history of prior illness
EMG	electromyography	Hr	hour
ENT	ear, nose, throat	HR	heart rate
ER	external rotation	HTN	hypertension
E-stim, ES	electrical stimulation	HS	hamstring(s)
Ev, ev	eversion	Hx	history
Eval	evaluation	I/(I)	independent(ly)
Ex.	exercise	ICP	intermittent compression pump
ext.	extension		
F	frequency	ICU	intensive care unit
FAQ	full arc quads	IDDM	insulin-dependent diabetes mellitus
f/b	followed by		
FES	functional electrical stimulation	I/E	inspiratory/expiratory
		Int.	internal
flex	flexion	IV	inversion
ft	foot, feet	JCAHO	Joint Commission on Accreditation of Health Care Organizations
FVC	forced vital capacity		
FWB	full weight bearing		
FWW, fw/w	front-wheeled walker	JRA	juvenile rheumatoid arthritis
Fx	fracture		
F/U	follow-up	KAFO	knee ankle foot orthosis
Gluts	gluteals	L	left
GMT	gross muscle test	L5	5th lumbar vertebra
Gt.	gait	LAQ	long arc quadriceps
GTO	Golgi tendon organ	lat.	lateral
h/a	headache	lb	pound
Hams	hamstrings	LBP	lower back pain
HAV	hepatitis A virus	LCL	lateral collateral ligament
Hb/Hbg	hemoglobin		
HBV	hepatitis B virus	LDL	low-density lipoprotein
HCV	hepatitis C virus	LE	lower extremity
HDL	high-density lipoprotein	Lic	license
HEP	home exercise program	LLE	left lower extremity
HNP	herniated nucleus pulposus	LMN	lower motor neuron
		LOC	loss of consciousness

LTG	long-term goal	Pr	problem
M	male	PRE	progressive resistive exercise
max.	maximum		
mech	mechanical	PRN, prn	as needed
MCL	medial collateral ligament	PROM	passive range of motion
		pt.	patient
MHP	moist hot pack	PWB	partial weight bearing
MHz	MegaHertz	$q2^0$	every 2 hours
MI	myocardial infarction	quads	quadriceps
min	minutes	R	right
min.	minimal, minimum	RA	rheumatoid arthritis
mmHg	millimeters of mercury	reps	repetitions
mm(s)	muscle(s)	ret.	return
MMT	manual muscle test	RLE	right lower extremity
mod.	moderate	r/o	rule out
MOI	mechanism of injury	ROM	range of motion
MRI	magnetic resonance imaging	rot.	rotation
		RUE	right upper extremity
MS	multiple sclerosis	SAQ	short arc quadriceps
MVA	motor vehicle accident	SBA	standby assist
N/A	not applicable	SCI	spinal cord injury
neg.	negative	SEC	single-end cane
noc.	night	sec	second(s)
NPO	nothing per oral	SLR	straight leg raise
NWB	nonweight bearing	SOAP	subjective, objective, assessment, plan
occ	occasional		
OOB	out of bed	SOB	short of breath
OP	outpatient	s/p	status post
ORIF	open reduction internal fixation	STG	short-term goal
		Str.	strength
OT	occupational therapist	SLR	straight leg raise
PCL	posterior cruciate lig.	strep	Streptococcus
per	by	SWD	shortwave diathermy
PT	plantarflexion	Sx	symptoms
PM, p.m.	afternoon	S & S	signs and symptoms
POC	plan of care	TB	tuberculosis
POMR	problem-oriented medical record	TBI	traumatic brain injury
		TEE	Transesophageal echocardiography
pps	pulses per second		

continues

Abbreviations and Symbols Used the Most in Physical Therapy **81**

Table 2-14   (continued)

temp.	temperature	UMN	upper motor neuron
TENS	transcutaneous electrical nerve stimulation	US	ultrasound
		UTI	urinary tract infection
TFM	transverse friction massage	UV	ultraviolet
		VC	vital capacity
TFs	transfers	VMO	vastus medialis oblique
THA	total hip arthroplasty	V/O	verbal order
ther. Ex.	therapeutic exercise	WBAT	weight bearing as tolerated
Tid	three times a day		
TKA	total knee arthroplasty	WC, w/c	wheelchair
TKE	terminal knee extension	w/cm^2	watts per centimeter squared
TLC	total lung capacity		
TMJ	temporomandibular joint	WFL	within functional limits
trng.	training	wlp	whirlpool
TTP	tender to palpation	w/o	without
TTWB	toe touch weight bearing	WNL	within normal limits
TWB	touch weight bearing	wt.	weight
tx	treatment	X	times
UE	upper extremity	yr	year
UED1	upper extremity diagonal 1	YO	year(s) old

The PTA should use abbreviations that are approved (in his or her clinical facility) for utilization in the medical record.

Symbols

Table 2-15   Symbols[3]

↔	To/from	2^0	secondary to
↑	Increase	ā	before
↓	Decrease	p̄	after
//	parallel	c̄	with
&	and	<	less than
1×/1X	one time, one person	>	greater than
1^0	primary to		

References

1. The American Physical Therapy Association. *APTA's Documentation Guidelines*. Available at www.apta.org. Accessed November 2006.
2. The American Physical Therapy Association Web site. *APTA's Documentation Guidelines on Domestic Violence*. Available at: www.apta.org. Accessed November 2006.
3. Lukan M. *Documentation for Physical Therapist Assistants*. Philadelphia: F.A. Davis Company; 2001.
4. Dreeben O. *Introduction to Physical Therapy for Physical Therapist Assistants*. Sudbury, MA: Jones and Bartlett Publishers; 2007.

CLINICAL DOCUMENTATION

PART III

Musculoskeletal Interventions

Section 3-3: Types of Musculoskeletal Interventions
Therapeutic Exercises
Relaxation Exercises
PNF Exercises—Diagonal Patterns
Closed Kinetic Chain Exercises to Increase Weightbearing Control
  and Stability
Patient Education Topics for Lumbar Spine
Abdominal Strengthening Exercises
Exercise Topics for the Obstetric Patient
Physical Agents and Modalities: Indications and Applications
Therapeutic Massage Application
Orthotics
Orthotic Interventions
Transtibial (Below Knee) Prostheses
Transfemoral (Above Knee) Prostheses
Prosthetics: Levels of Amputation
Prosthetics: Pressure Tolerant and Pressure Sensitive Areas
Prosthetic Interventions
Phases of Gait Cycles
Muscle Activation Patterns
Common Gait Deviations: Stance Phase
Common Gait Deviations: Swing Phase
Gait Training Points
Wheelchair Measurements
Wheelchair's Postural Support System
Wheelchair Training

Section 3-4: Musculoskeletal Intervention Patterns
APTA's Guide to Physical Therapist Practice—APTA's
  Musculoskeletal Intervention Patterns
Arthritic Disorders and Intervention Patterns
Tendonitis and Bursitis and Intervention Patterns
Strains, Sprains, Dislocations, and Fractures and Intervention
  Patterns

MUSCULOSKELETAL
INTERVENTIONS

Musculoskeletal Data Collection

Goniometry—Joint Measurements: Body Position, Goniometer Alignment, and Normal Range of Motion Degrees (Per AAOS)

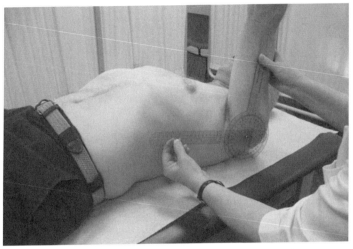

Figure 3-1   The alignment of the goniometer at the end of the ROM of GH flexion (Please see Table 3-1 on following page.)

Table 3-1 Goniometry—Joint Measurements: Body Position, Goniometer Alignment, and Normal ROM (Per AAOS)[1]

Joint	Supine	Prone	Sitting	Goniometer Alignment (Ending Position)	ROM Degrees (AAOS)
Shoulder	Flexion Abduction Internal Rotation (IR) External Rotation (ER)	Extension		Shoulder flexion (Figure 3-1) Shoulder extension (Figure 3-2) Shoulder abduction (Figure 3-3) Shoulder IR (Figure 3-4) Shoulder ER (Figure 3-5)	Flexion = 180° Extension = 60° Abduction = 180° IR = 70° ER = 90° Horizontal adduction = 135°
Elbow	Flexion			Elbow flexion	Flexion = 150°
Radioulnar (forearm)			Pronation Supination	Pronation (Figure 3-6) Supination (Figure 3-7)	Pronation = 80° Supination = 80°
Wrist			Flexion Extension Radial Deviation Ulnar Deviation	Wrist flexion (Figure 3-8) Wrist extension (Figure 3-9) Radial deviation (Figure 3-10) Ulnar deviation (figure 3-11)	Flexion = 80° Extension = 70° Radial deviation = 20° Ulnar deviation = 30°
Hip	Flexion Abduction	Extension	Internal Rotation (IR)	Hip flexion (Figure 3-12) Hip extension (Figure 3-13)	Flexion = 120° Extension = 30°

continues

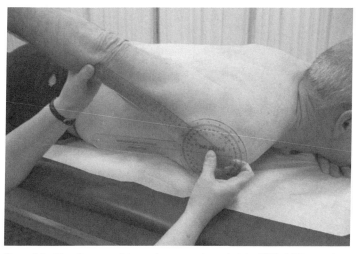

Figure 3-2   The alignment of the goniometer at the end of the ROM of GH extension

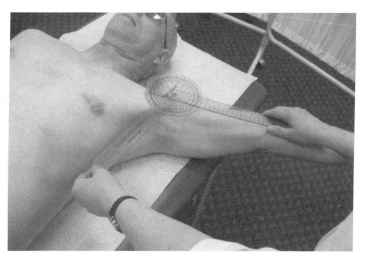

Figure 3-3   The alignment of the goniometer at the end of the ROM of GH abduction

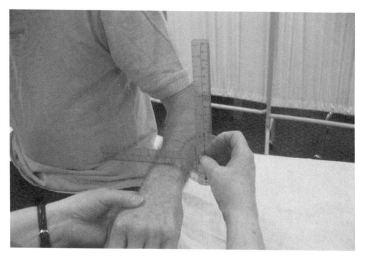

Figure 3-6　The alignment of the goniometer at the end of pronation ROM

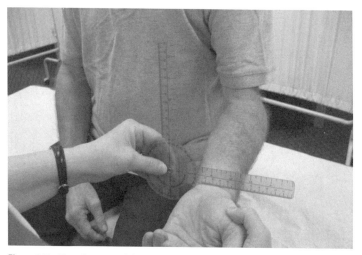

Figure 3-7　The alignment of the goniometer at the end of supination ROM

Musculoskeletal Data Collection　**92**

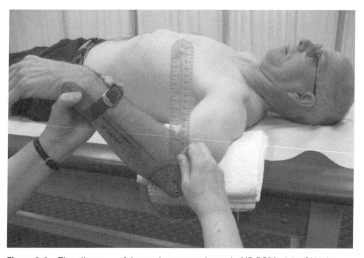

Figure 3-4   The alignment of the goniometer at the end of IR ROM of the GH joint

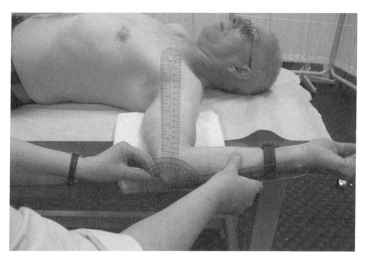

Figure 3-5   The alignment of the goniometer at the end of ER ROM of the GH joint

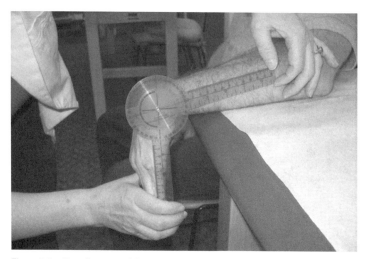

Figure 3-8 The alignment of the goniometer at the end of wrist flexion ROM

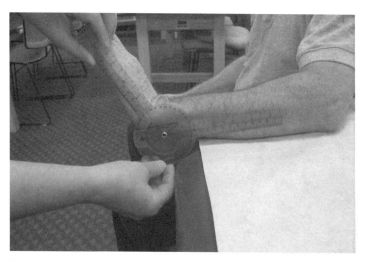

Figure 3-9 The alignment of the goniometer at the end of wrist extension ROM

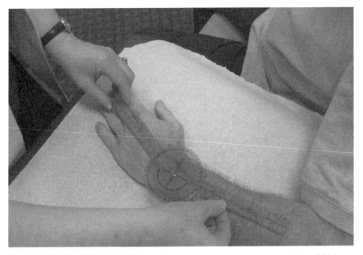

Figure 3-10 The alignment of the goniometer at the end of radial deviation ROM

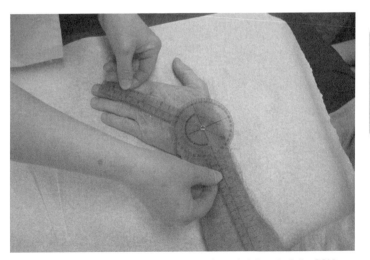

Figure 3-11 The alignment of the goniometer at the end of ulnar deviation ROM

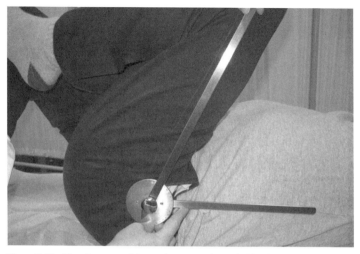

Figure 3-12 The alignment of the goniometer at the end of hip flexion ROM

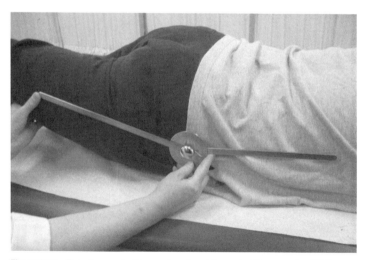

Figure 3-13 The alignment of the goniometer at the end of hip extension ROM

Table 3-1 (continued)

Joint	Supine	Prone	Sitting	Goniometer Alignment (Ending Position)	ROM Degrees (AAOS)
Hip	Adduction		External Rotation (ER)	Hip abduction/adduction (Figure 3-14) Hip IR (Figure 3-15) Hip ER (Figure 3-16)	Abduction = 45° Adduction = 30° IR/ER = 45°
Knee	Flexion			Knee flexion (Figure 3-17)	Flexion = 135°
Talocrural (ankle)			Dorsiflexion Plantarflexion	Dorsiflexion (Figure 3-18) Plantarflexion (Figure 3-19)	DF = 20° PF = 50°
Subtalar (rear foot)			Inversion Eversion	Inversion (Figure 3-20) Eversion (Figure 3-21)	Inversion = 35° Eversion = 15°

MUSCULOSKELETAL INTERVENTIONS

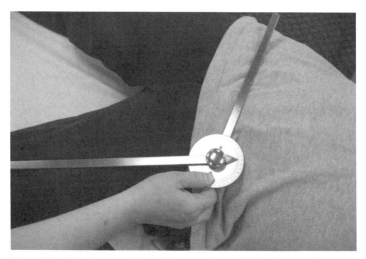

Figure 3-14 The alignment of the goniometer at the end of hip abduction ROM

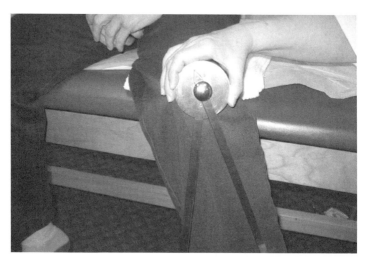

Figure 3-15 The alignment of the goniometer at the end of hip IR ROM

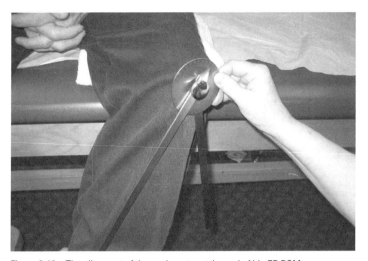

Figure 3-16 The alignment of the goniometer at the end of hip ER ROM

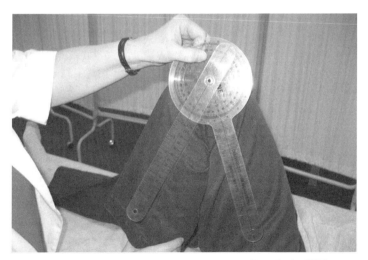

Figure 3-17 The alignment of the goniometer at the end of knee flexion ROM

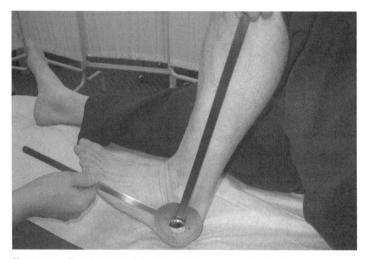

Figure 3-18   The alignment of the goniometer at the end of DF ROM

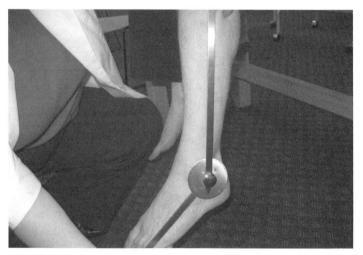

Figure 3-19   The alignment of the goniometer at the end of end of PF ROM

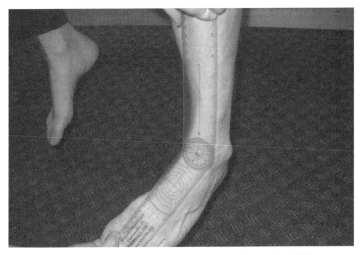

Figure 3-20 The alignment of the goniometer at the end of inversion ROM

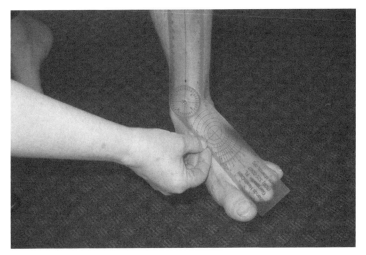

Figure 3-21 The alignment of the goniometer at the end of eversion ROM

Cervical and Thoracolumbar Range of Motion Normatives (Per AAOS)

Table 3-2   Cervical and Thoracolumbar ROM Normatives (Per AAOS)[1]

Cervical ROM	Flexion = 45° Extension = 45° Left lateral flexion = 45° Right lateral flexion = 45° Left rotation = 60° Right rotation = 60°
Thoracolumbar ROM	Flexion = 80° (tape measure = 4 inches) Extension = 20° to 30° Left lateral flexion = 35° Right lateral flexion = 35° Left rotation = 45° Right rotation = 45°

Manual Muscle Testing—Grading System of Hislop and Montgomery

Table 3-3   Grading System of Hislop and Montgomery[2]

Grade 5 (normal)—completes full ROM against gravity. Maintains end-range position against maximal resistance.

Grade 4 (good)—completes full ROM against gravity. Maintains end-range position against strong resistance. "Yields" (or "gives") at the end-range against maximal resistance.

Grade 3 + (fair +)—completes full ROM against gravity. Maintains end-range position against mild resistance and has functional implications.

Grade 3 (fair)—completes full ROM against gravity. Unable to maintain end-range position against any resistance.

Grade 2 (poor)—completes full ROM in a gravity eliminated position (in a horizontal plane of motion).

Grade 2 (–) minus (poor minus)—completes partial ROM in a gravity eliminated position (in a horizontal plane of motion).

Grade 1 (trace)—examiner visually detects or palpates contractile activity in the muscle(s). There is no movement of the part as a result of contractile activity.

Grade 0 (zero)—muscle is quiet, and no activity is detected.

Upper Extremity Manual Muscle Testing

Table 3-4   MMT Upper Extremity

Movement, Muscles, and Instructions to the Patient[2]	Patient/PTA Positions and Grades
Scapular Abduction and Upward Rotation Main Ms: Serratus anterior Others: Pectoralis minor Grades 4 and 5: "Raise your arm forward above your head; don't let me push your arm down." Grade 3: "Raise your arm forward above your head." Grade 2: "Hold your arm in this position (such as above 90°). Let it relax. Hold your arm up again. Let it relax." Grade 1: "Try to hold your arm in this position."	All grades: Patient sitting. Grades 4 and 5: PTA standing at test side, with one hand applies resistance to patient's arm proximal to elbow. Patient's arm needs to be elevated more than 60° to use the serratus. PTA other hand palpates edges of scapula (Figure 3-22).

continues

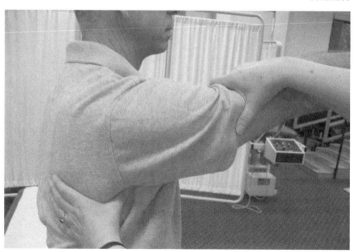

Figure 3-22   Scapular Abduction and Upward Rotation MMT

Table 3-4   (continued)

Movement, Muscles, and Instructions to the Patient[2]	Patient/PTA Positions and Grades
Scapular Elevation Main Ms: Upper trapezius Others: Levator scapulae and rhomboids Grades 4 and 5: "Raise your shoulders toward your ears. Hold it. Don't let me push them down." Grades 1, 2, and 3: "Raise your shoulders toward your ears."	Grades 1 and 2: Patient prone. Grades 3, 4, and 5: Patient sitting elevates shoulders. Grades 4 and 5: PTA standing behind patient with both hands over top of patient's shoulders gives resistance in downward direction (Figure 3-23).

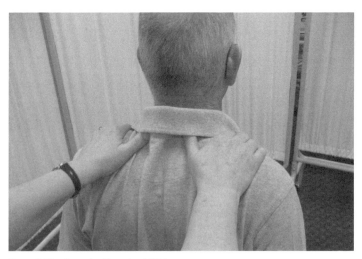

Figure 3-23   Scapular Elevation MMT

Scapular Adduction (Scapular Retraction)

Main Ms: Middle trapezius and rhomboid major

Others: Levator scapulae, rhomboid minor and upper and lower trapezius

Grades 4 and 5: "Lift your elbow toward the ceiling. Hold it. Don't let me push it down." Grade 3: "Lift your elbow toward the ceiling." Grades 1 and 2: "Try to lift your elbow toward the ceiling."

All grades: Patient prone.

Grades 4 and 5: PTA standing at test side, with one hand stabilizes contralateral scapula. PTA other hand applies resistance downward toward floor over distal humerus (deltoid must be grade of 3 or better) (Figure 3-24).

continues

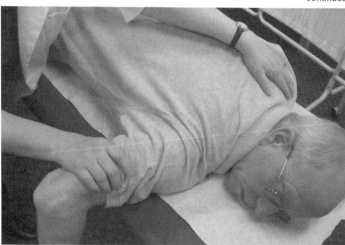

Figure 3-24   Scapular Adduction MMT

MUSCULOSKELETAL INTERVENTIONS

Table 3-4 (continued)

Movement, Muscles, and Instructions to the Patient[2]	Patient/PTA Positions and Grades
Scapular Depression and Adduction Main Ms: Middle and lower trapezius Others: Pectoralis and latissimus dorsi Grades 4 and 5: "Raise your arm from the table as high as possible. Hold it. Don't let me push it down." Grade 3: "Raise your arm from the table as high as possible." Grades 1 and 2: "Try to lift your arm from the table past your ear."	All grades: Patient prone. Grades 4 and 5: PTA standing at test side applies resistance downward toward floor over distal humerus (Figure 3-25).

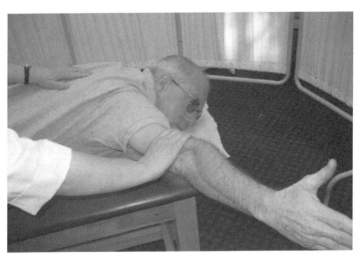

Figure 3-25 Scapular Depression and Adduction

Scapular Adduction and Downward Rotation

Main Ms: Rhomboids (major and minor)

Others: Levator scapulae

Grades 4 and 5: "Lift your hand. Hold it. Don't let me push it down." Grade 3: "Lift your hand." Grades 1 and 2: "Try to move your hand away from your back."

Grades 1 and 2: Patient sitting with shoulder in internal rotation and arm extended and adducted behind back. Grades 3, 4, and 5: Patient prone with shoulder in internal rotation and arm adducted across the back. Grades 4 and 5: PTA standing at test side, applies resistance downward and outward over humerus just above elbow (Figure 3-26).

continues

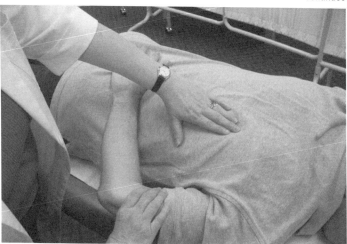

Figure 3-26 Scapular Adduction and Downward Rotation MMT

MUSCULOSKELETAL INTERVENTIONS

Table 3-4 (continued)

Movement, Muscles, and Instructions to the Patient[2]	Patient/PTA Positions and Grades
Shoulder Flexion Main Ms: Anterior deltoid and coraco-brachialis Others: Pectoralis major, middle deltoid, and serratus anterior Grades 4 and 5: "Raise your arm forward to shoulder height. Hold it. Don't let me push it down." Grade 3: "Raise your arm forward to shoulder height." Grades 1 and 2: "Try to raise your arm."	All grades: Patient sitting. Grades 4 and 5: PTA standing at test side, applies resistance downward over distal humerus just above elbow. PTA other hand stabilizes the shoulder (Figure 3-27).

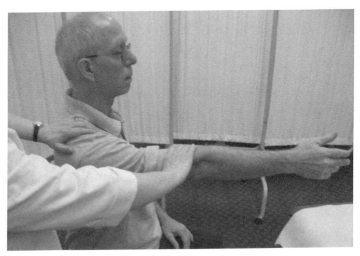

Figure 3-27   Shoulder Flexion MMT

Shoulder Extension
Main Ms: Latissimus dorsi, posterior deltoid, and teres major.
Other: Triceps brachii (long head)
Grades 4 and 5: "Lift your arm as high as you can. Hold it. Don't let me push it down." Grades 2 and 3: "Lift your arm as high as you can." Grade 1: "Lift your arm."

All grades: Patient prone. Grades 4 and 5: PTA standing at test side, applies resistance downward over posterior arm just above elbow (Figure 3-28).

continues

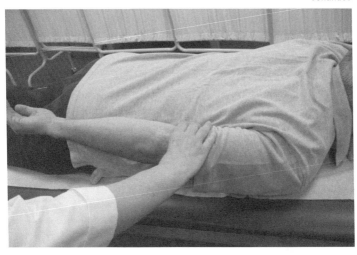

Figure 3-28   Shoulder Extension MMT

MUSCULOSKELETAL INTERVENTIONS

Table 3-4 (continued)

Movement, Muscles, and Instructions to the Patient[2]	Patient/PTA Positions and Grades
Shoulder Scaption Main Ms: Anterior and middle deltoid and supraspinatus Grades 4 and 5: "Raise your arm to shoulder height half way between straight and to the side. Hold it. Don't let me push it down." Grade 3: "Raise your arm to shoulder height half way between straight and to the side." Grades 1 and 2: "Try to raise your arm to shoulder height half way between straight and to the side."	All grades: Patient sitting. Grades 4 and 5: PTA standing in front and slightly to the side of patient, applies resistance downward over arm above elbow. Patient elevates arm halfway between flexion and abduction (Figure 3-29).

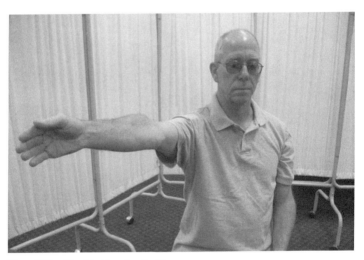

Figure 3-29 Shoulder Scaption Position

Shoulder Abduction
Main Ms: Middle deltoid and
supraspinatus
Grades 4 and 5: "Lift your arm out to the
side to shoulder level. Hold it. Don't
let me push it down." Grade 3: "Lift
your arm out to the side to shoulder
level." Grades 1 and 2: "Try to lift your
arm out to the side."

All grades: Patient sitting. Grades 4 and
5: PTA standing behind patient,
applies resistance downward over
arm just above elbow (Figure 3-30).

continues

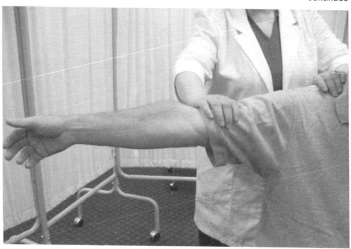

Figure 3-30   Shoulder Abduction MMT

MUSCULOSKELETAL
INTERVENTIONS

Table 3-4 (continued)

Movement, Muscles, and Instructions to the Patient[2]	Patient/PTA Positions and Grades
Shoulder External Rotation Main Ms: Infraspinatus and Teres Minor. Other: Posterior Deltoid Grades 4 and 5: "Raise your arm to the level of the table. Hold it. Don't let me push it down." Grade 3: "Raise your arm to the level of the table." Grades 1 and 2: "Turn your palm outward."	All grades: Patient prone. Grades 4 and 5: PTA standing at test side at level of patient waist, applies resistance with two fingers downward at the wrist. PTA other hand supports patient's elbow giving counterpressure at end of range (Figure 3-31).

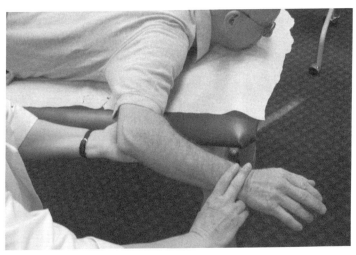

Figure 3-31   Shoulder ER MMT

Shoulder Internal Rotation
Main Ms: Subscapularis, pectoralis major (clavicular and sternal parts), latissimus dorsi, and teres major.
Other: Anterior deltoid.
Grades 4 and 5: "Move your forearm up and back. Hold it. Don't let me push it down." Grade 3: "Move your forearm up and back." Grades 1 and 2: "Turn your arm so that the palm faces away from the table."

All grades: Patient prone. Grades 4 and 5: PTA standing at test side, applies downward and forward resistance on anterior side of forearm just above the wrist. PTA other hand applies counterpressure backward and slightly upward (Figure 3-32).

continues

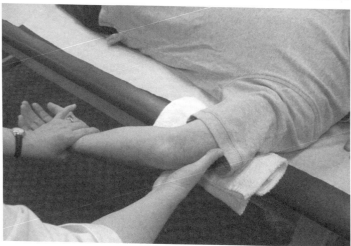

Figure 3-32   Shoulder IR MMT

Table 3-4 **(continued)**

Movement, Muscles, and Instructions to the Patient[2]	Patient/PTA Positions and Grades
Elbow Flexion Main Ms: Biceps brachii (short and long head), brachialis, and brachioradialis. Others: Pronator teres, extensor carpi radialis longus, flexor carpi radialis, and flexor carpi ulnaris Grades 4 and 5: "Bend your elbow. Hold it. Don't let me pull it down." Grade 3: "Bend your elbow." Grades 1 and 2: "Try to bend your elbow."	Grades 1 and 2: Patient supine (if cannot sit) with forearm supinated for biceps, pronated for brachialis, and in mid position for brachioradialis, and elbow flexed to 45°. Grades 3, 4, and 5: Patient sitting with arm abducted and forearm supinated for biceps, pronated for brachialis and in mid position for brachioradialis. Grades 4 and 5: PTA standing in front of patient, applies resistance over flexor surface of forearm proximal to wrist. PTA other hand applies counterforce cupping the palm over anterior superior surface of shoulder (Figure 3-33).

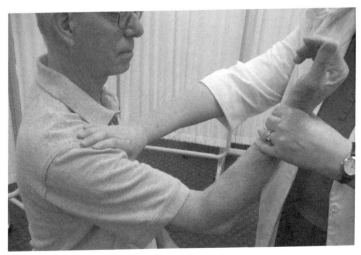

Figure 3-33 Elbow Flexion MMT

Elbow Extension
Main Ms: Triceps brachii (long, lateral, and medial heads).
Other: Anconeus.
Grades 4 and 5: "Straighten your elbow. Hold it. Don't let me bend it." Grade 3: "Straighten your elbow." Grades 1 and 2: "Try to straighten your elbow."

Grades 1 and 2: Patient sitting with arm abducted to 90°, shoulder in neutral rotation, and elbow flexed to about 45°. Grades 3, 4, and 5: Patient prone with arm in 90° abduction and forearm flexed hanging over table.
Grades 4 and 5: PTA supports patient's arm above the elbow. PTA applies resistance downward over dorsal surface of forearm (Figure 3-34).

continues

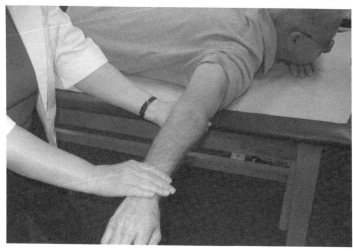

Figure 3-34 Elbow Extension MMT

MUSCULOSKELETAL INTERVENTIONS

Table 3-4   (continued)

Movement, Muscles, and Instructions to the Patient[2]	Patient/PTA Positions and Grades
Forearm Supination Main Ms: Supinator Others: Biceps brachii (short and long head). Grades 4 and 5: "Turn your palm up. Hold it. Don't let me turn it down. Keep your wrist and fingers relaxed." Grade 3: "Turn your palm up." Grades 1 and 2: "Turn your palm toward your face."	All grades: Patient sitting. Grades 1 and 2: Patient's shoulder flexed between 45° and 90° and elbow flexed to 90°. Grades 3, 4, and 5: Patient's elbow flexed 90° and forearm in pronation. Patient supinates until the palm faces the ceiling. Grades 4 and 5: PTA standing at patient's side, supports elbow, grasps the forearm, and applies resistance to anterior surface of forearm at wrist (Figure 3-35).

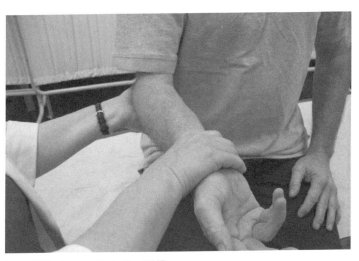

Figure 3-35   Forearm Supination MMT

Forearm Pronation

Main Ms: Pronator teres (humeral and ulnar heads) and pronator quadratus

Other: Flexor carpi radialis

Grades 4 and 5: "Turn your palm down. Hold it. Don't let me turn it up. Keep your wrist and fingers relaxed." Grade 3: "Turn your palm down." Grades 1 and 2: "Try to turn your palm down."

All grades: Patient sitting.

Grades 3, 4, and 5: Patient's arm at side with elbow flexed to 90°and forearm in supination. Patient pronates until the palm faces the floor. Grades 1 and 2: Patient's shoulder flexed between 45° and 90° and elbow flexed to 90°. Forearm in neutral. Grades 4 and 5: PTA standing at patient's side supports the elbow. PTA's other hand grasps the forearm, and applies resistance over posterior surface of forearm at wrist (the same as in Figure 3-35 but forearm is pronated).

Wrist Flexion

Main Ms: Flexor carpi radialis and flexor carpi ulnaris

Others: Palmaris longus, flexor digitorum superficialis, flexor digitorum profundus, abductor pollicis longus, and flexor pollicis longus

Grades 4 and 5: "Bend your wrist. Hold it. Don't let me pull it down. Keep your fingers relaxed." Grade 3: "Bend your wrist (for all muscles). Bend your wrist leading with the little finger (for FCU). Bend your wrist leading with the thumb side (for FCR)." Grade 2: "Bend your wrist. Keep your fingers relaxed." Grade 1: "Try to bend your wrist. Relax. Bend it again."

All grades: Patient sitting. Grades 1, 3, 4, and 5: Patient's forearm supinated, posterior side of forearm supported on table (or by examiner's hand), and wrist in neutral. Grade 2: Patient's elbow supported on table, forearm in mid position with hand resting on ulnar side. Grade 1: PTA supports patient's wrist in flexion with one hand while the other hand palpates the appropriate tendon. Grade 2: PTA supports patient's forearm proximal to the wrist. Grade 3: PTA supports patient's forearm under the wrist. Grades 4 and 5: PTA stands in front of patient, supports patient's forearm under the wrist. PTA's other hand applies resistance to the palm (Figure 3-36).

continues

MUSCULOSKELETAL INTERVENTIONS

Table 3-4   (continued)

Movement, Muscles, and Instructions to the Patient[2]	Patient/PTA Positions and Grades

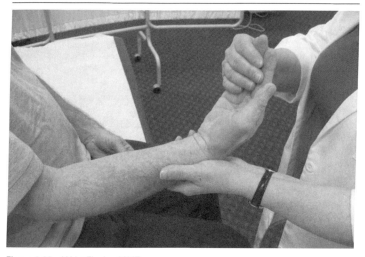

Figure 3-36 Wrist Flexion MMT

Wrist Extension

Main Ms: Extensor carpi radialis longus, extensor carpi radialis brevis, and extensor carpi ulnaris

Others: Extensor digitorum, extensor digiti minimi, and extensor indicis

Grades 4 and 5: "Bring your wrist up. Hold it. Don't let me push it down." Grade 3: "Bring your wrist up." Grade 2: "Bend your wrist back. Grade 1: "Try to bring your wrist back."

All grades: Patient sitting. Grades 3, 4, and 5: Patient's flexed elbow and fully pronated forearm supported on table (or by examiner's hand). Grade 2: Patient's forearm in neutral supported on table. Grade 1: Patient's fully pronated hand and forearm supported on table. Grade 1: PTA supports patient's wrist in extension with one hand while the other hand palpates the appropriate muscle. Grade

2: PTA supports patient's wrist in neutral (elevates it from the table).
Grades 3, 4, and 5: PTA stands in front of patient, supports patient's forearm under the anterior wrist. PTA's other hand applies resistance to the posterior surface of metacarpals (Figure 3-37).

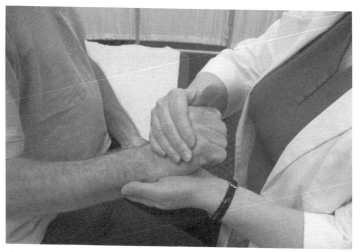

Figure 3-37   Wrist Extension MMT

Finger and Thumb Manual Muscle Testing

Table 3-5   Finger and Thumb MMT[2]

- Finger MP Flexion tests 1, 2, 3, 4 lumbricales, dorsal Interossei, and palmar interossei. Grades 3, 4, and 5: Patient sitting with forearm in supination, wrist in neutral, metacarpophalangeal (MP) joints fully extended, and interphalangeal (IP) joints fully flexed. Grades 4 and 5: Patient completes simultaneous MP flexion and finger extension and holds against maximal or moderate resistance. Resistance is given to fingers individually.

continues

Musculoskeletal Data Collection   **119**

Table 3-5 (continued)

- Finger PIP and DIP Flexion tests flexor digitorum superficialis and flexor digitorum profundus. Grades 3, 4, and 5: Patient sitting with forearm in supination, wrist in neutral, and finger to be tested in slight flexion at the MP joint. Grades 4 and 5: Patient completes ROM and holds against maximal or moderate finger resistance.
- Finger MP Extension tests extensor digitorum, extensor Indicis, and extensor digiti minimi. Grades 3, 4, and 5: Patient sitting with forearm in pronation, wrist in neutral, and MP and IP joints relaxed in flexed position. Grades 4 and 5: Patient completes active extension ROM with maximal and moderate finger resistance.
- Finger Abduction tests dorsal interossei and abductor digiti minimi. Grades 3, 4, and 5: Patient sitting with forearm in pronation, fingers in extension, and adduction. MP joints are in neutral. Grades 4 and 5: Patient completes finger abduction with as much resistance as the uninvolved finger. PTA's resistance is dependent on the uninvolved patient's finger abduction MMT.
- Thumb MP and IP Flexion tests fexor pollicis brevis and flexor pollicis longus. Grades 3, 4, and 5: Patient sitting with forearm in supination, wrist in neutral. Carpometacarpal (CPM) and IP joints of thumb are at 0°. Thumb is in adduction, lying relaxed by the second metacarpal. Grades 4 and 5: Patient completes ROM against maximal and moderate resistance.
- Thumb MP and IP Extension tests extensor pollicis brevis and extensor pollicis longus. Grades 3, 4, and 5: Patient sitting with forearm in mid position and wrist in neutral. CPM and IP joints of thumb are relaxed in slight flexion. MP joint of thumb is in abduction and flexion. Grades 4 and 5: Patient completes ROM with resistance. PTA resistance is dependent on the uninvolved patient's thumb MP and IP extension MMT.
- Thumb abduction tests mainly abductor pollicis longus and abductor pollicis brevis. Grades 3, 4, and 5: Patient sitting with forearm supinated, wrist in neutral, and thumb relaxed in adduction. Grades 4 and 5: Patient completes ROM against resistance. PTA resistance is dependent on the uninvolved patient's thumb abduction MMT.
- Thumb adduction tests mainly adductor pollicis. Grades 3, 4, and 5: Patient sitting with forearm in pronation, wrist in neutral, and thumb relaxed and in abduction. Grades 4 and 5: Patient completes ROM against maximal and moderate resistance.
- Opposition (Thumb to Little Finger) tests mainly opponens pollicis and opponens digiti minimi. Grades 3, 4, and 5: Patient is sitting with forearm in supination, wrist in neutral, and thumb in adduction with MP and IP flexed. Grades 4 and 5: Patient completes opposition with resistance at head of first metacarpal (in direction of external rotation, extension, and adduction) for opponens pollicis and at palmar surface of fifth metacarpal (in direction of internal rotation, flattening the palm) for opponens digiti minimi.

Lower Extremity Manual Muscle Testing

Table 3-6   MMT Lower Extremity

Movement, Muscles, and Instructions to the Patient[2]	Patient/PTA Positions and Grades
Hip flexion Main Ms: Psoas major and iliacus Others: Rectus femoris, sartorius, tensor fasciae latae, pectineus, adductors (brevis, longus, magnus), anterior gluteus medius Grades 4 and 5: "Lift your leg off the table and don't let me push it down." Grade 3: "Lift your leg straight up off the table." Grade 2: "Bring your knee up toward your chest. "Grade 1: "Try to bring your knee up to your nose."	Grade 1: Patient lying supine. Grade 2: Patient side lying with tested limb uppermost. Grades 3, 4 and 5: Patient sitting with thighs supported on the table. Grades 4 and 5: PTA standing next to limb to be tested, applies resistance over distal thigh proximal to the knee (Figure 3-38).

continues

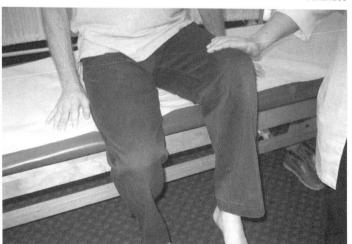

Figure 3-38   Hip Flexion MMT

MUSCULOSKELETAL INTERVENTIONS

Table 3-6   (continued)

Movement, Muscles, and Instructions to the Patient[2]	Patient/PTA Positions and Grades
Hip extension Main Ms: Gluteus maximus, semitendinous, semimembranous, and long head of biceps femoris Others: Adductor magnus and gluteus medius Grades 3, 4, and 5: "Lift your leg off the table as high as you can. Do not bend your knee." Grade 2: "Bring your leg back toward me. Keep your knee straight." Grade 1: "Try to lift your leg from the table."	Grades 1, 3, 4, and 5: Patient prone. Grade 2: Patient side lying with tested limb uppermost and knee straight. Grades 4 and 5: PTA standing at side of limb to be tested, applies with one hand resistance on posterior leg above the ankle. The other hand stabilizes the pelvis (Figure 3-39).

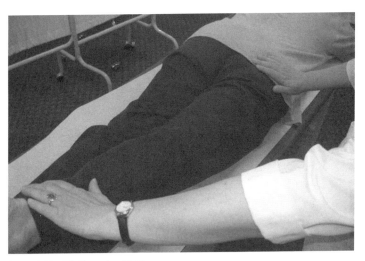

Figure 3-39   Hip Extension MMT

Hip abduction

Main Ms: Gluteus medius and gluteus minimus

Others: Gluteus maximus, tensor fasciae latae, obturator internus, gemellus inferior and superior, and sartorius

Grades 4 and 5: "Lift your leg up in the air. Hold it. Don't let me push it down." Grade 2: "Bring your leg out to the side." Grade 1: "Try to bring your leg out to the side."

Grades 1 and 2: Patient supine. Grades 3, 4, and 5: Patient side lying with tested limb uppermost and knee straight. Grades 4 and 5: PTA standing behind patient, palpates gluteus medius. PTA other hand applies resistance downward at the lateral surface of knee (Figure 3-40).

continues

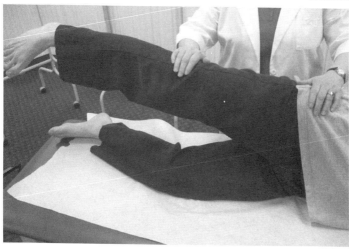

Figure 3-40 Hip Abduction MMT

Table 3-6 (continued)

Movement, Muscles, and Instructions to the Patient[2]	Patient/PTA Positions and Grades
Hip adduction Main Ms: Adductor magnus, adductor brevis, adductor longus, pectineus, and gracilis Others: Gluteus maximus and obturator externus Grades 4 and 5: "Lift your bottom leg up to your top one. Hold it. Don't let me push it down. Grade 3: "Lift your bottom leg up to your top one. Don't let it drop." Grade 2: "Bring your leg in toward the other one." Grade 1: "Try to bring your leg in."	Grades 1 and 2: Patient supine. Grades 3, 4, and 5: Patient side lying with the tested limb lowermost resting on the table. The uppermost limb is in 25° abduction and is supported by PTA. Grades 4 and 5: PTA standing behind patient, cradles the uppermost limb with forearm supporting it on medial knee. PTA other hand applies to lowermost limb resistance on medial distal femur proximal to knee (Figure 3-41).

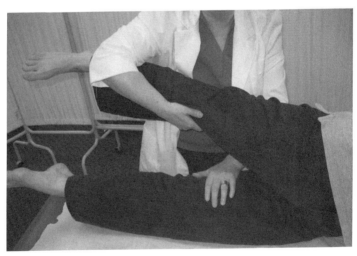

Figure 3-41 Hip Adduction MMT

Hip external rotation

Main Ms: Obturator externus, obturator internus, piriformis, gemelli superior and inferior, quadratus femoris, and gluteus maximus

Others: Sartorius, long head biceps femoris, gluteus medius, psoas major, adductor magnus and longus, and popliteus

Grades 4 and 5: "Don't let me turn your leg out." Grade 3: "Keep your leg in this position." Grades 2: "Roll your leg out." Grade 1: "Try to roll your leg out."

Grades 1 and 2: Patient supine with tested limb in internal rotation. Grades 3, 4, and 5: Patient sitting. Grades 4 and 5: PTA sitting besides limb to be tested, applies counter-pressure to lateral distal thigh above the knee giving resistance in a medially directed force at the knee. PTA other hand applies resistance in a laterally directed force at the ankle grasping the ankle above the medial malleolus (Figure 3-42).

continues

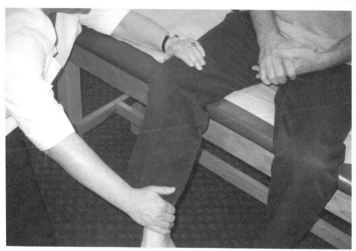

Figure 3-42   Hip ER MMT

MUSCULOSKELETAL INTERVENTIONS

Table 3-6 (continued)

Movement, Muscles, and Instructions to the Patient[2]	Patient/PTA Positions and Grades
Hip internal rotation Main Ms: Gluteus minimus, tensor fasciae latae, and gluteus medius Others: Semitendinous, semimembranous, adductor magnus, and adductor longus Grades 4 and 5: "Don't let me turn your leg in." Grade 3: "Keep your leg in this position." Grade 2: "Roll your leg in toward the other." Grade 1: "Try to roll your leg in."	Grades 1 and 2: Patient supine with tested limb in partial external rotation. Grades 3, 4, and 5: Patient sitting. Grades 4 and 5: PTA kneeling in front of tested limb, applies counterpressure to medial distal thigh above the knee giving resistance in a laterally directed force at the knee. PTA other hand applies resistance in a medially directed force at the ankle above the lateral malleolus (Figure 3-43).

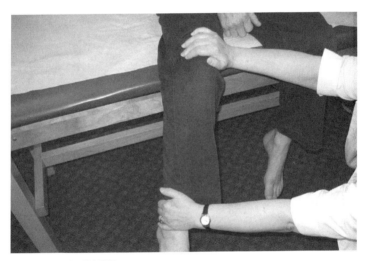

Figure 3-43 Hip IR MMT

Knee flexion

Main Ms: Long and short heads of biceps femoris, semitendinous, and-semimembranous

Other: Gracilis, tensor fasciae latae, sartorius, popliteus, gastrocnemius, and plantaris

Grades 4 and 5: "Bend your knee. Hold it. Don't let me straighten it." Grade 2 and 3: "Bend your knee." Grade 1: "Try to bend your knee."

Grade 1, 3, 4, and 5: Patient prone. Grade 2: Patient side lying with tested limb uppermost. Grades 4 and 5: PTA standing next to limb to be tested (showed here at opposite side not to obscure activity), applies resistance around posterior surface of leg above the ankle. PTA's other hand is placed over the hamstrings on posterior thigh (Figure 3-44).

continues

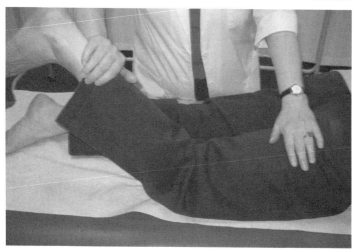

Figure 3-44   Knee Flexion MMT

Table 3-6 (continued)

Movement, Muscles, and Instructions to the Patient[2]	Patient/PTA Positions and Grades
Knee extension Main Ms: Rectus femoris, vastus intermedius, vastus lateralis, vastus medialis longus, and vastus medialis oblique Other: Tensor fasciae latae Grades 4 and 5: "Straighten your knee. Hold it. Don't let me bend it." Grade 2 and 3: "Straighten your knee." Grade 1: "Push the back of your knee down into the table."	Grade 1: Patient supine. Grade 2: Patient side lying with tested limb uppermost. Grades 3, 4, and 5: Patient sitting. Grades 4 and 5: PTA standing at side of tested limb with one hand giving resistance downward over anterior distal leg above ankle. PTA's other hand is under distal thigh not allowing patient to hyperextend the knee (Figure 3-45).

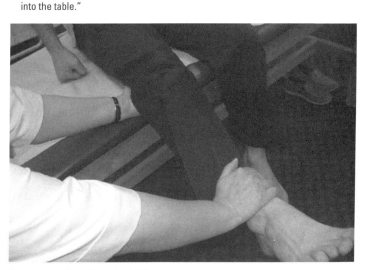

Figure 3-45 Knee Extension MMT

Ankle plantarflexion
Main Ms: Medial and lateral heads of gastrocnemius and the soleus
Others: Posterior tibialis, plantaris, peroneus longus, peroneus brevis, flexor digitorum longus, and flexor hallucis longus
Grades 4 and 5: "Stand on your right leg. Go up on your tiptoes. Now go down. Repeat this 20 times." Grade 3: "Stand on your right leg. Go up on your tiptoes. Now go down. Repeat this 9 times." Grade 2: "Stand on your right leg. Try to go up on your tiptoes." Grade 1: "Point your toes down."

Grade 1: Patient prone with feet at end of table. Grade 2: Patient standing on limb to be tested with knee extended, with two fingers on the table for balance assist. Grades 2, 3, 4, and 5: PTA standing with lateral view of patient's limb. Grades 3, 4, and 5: Patient standing on limb to be tested with knee extended with two fingers on a table for balance assist (Figure 3-46).

continues

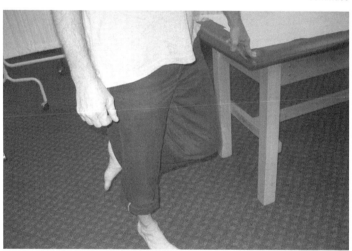

Figure 3-46   Gastrocnemius and Soleus Test

Table 3-6   (continued)

Movement, Muscles, and Instructions to the Patient[2]	Patient/PTA Positions and Grades
Foot dorsiflexion and inversion Main Ms: Tibialis anterior Others: Peroneus tertius, extensor digitorum longus, and extensor hallucis longus Grades 4 and 5: "Bring your foot up and in. Hold it. Don't let me push it down." Grades 1, 2, and 3: "Bring your foot up and in."	All grades: Patient sitting with heel resting on PTA's thigh. Grades 4 and 5: PTA sitting on stool in front of patient with patient's heel resting on his or her thigh. One hand is supporting around posterior leg above malleoli. PTA's other hand gives resistance over dorsal and medial aspect of the foot (Figure 3-47).

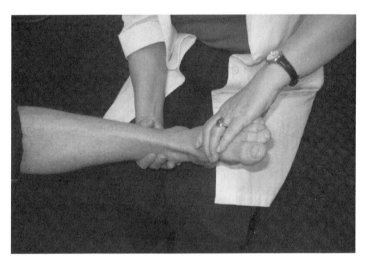

Figure 3-47   Foot DF and Inversion MMT

Foot inversion
Main Ms: Tibialis posterior
Other: Tibialis anterior, flexor digitorum longus, flexor hallucis longus, soleus, and extensor hallucis longus
Grades 4 and 5: " Turn your foot down and in. Hold it." Grades 2 and 3: "Turn your foot down and in." Grade 1: "Try to turn your foot down and in."

All grades: Patient sitting. Grades 2, 3, 4, and 5: Patient with ankle in slight plantarflexion. Grade 1: PTA palpates tibialis posterior tendon. Grades 4 and 5: PTA sitting on low stool in front of patient. One hand is stabilizing the ankle above malleoli. PTA's other hand gives resistance toward eversion and slight dorsiflexion at the dorsal and medial side of the foot at the metatarsal heads (Figure 3-48).

continues

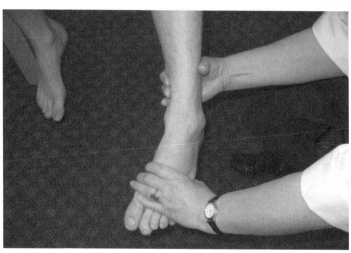

Figure 3-48   Foot Inversion MMT

Table 3-6 (continued)

Movement, Muscles, and Instructions to the Patient[2]	Patient/PTA Positions and Grades
Foot eversion with plantarflexion Main Ms: Peroneus longus and brevis Others: Extensor digitorum longus, peroneus tertius, and gastrocnemius Grades 4 and 5: "Turn your foot down and out. Hold it. Don't let me move it in." Grades 2 and 3: "Turn your foot down and out."	All grades: Patient sitting. Grades 2, 3, 4, and 5: Patient with ankle in neutral. Grade 1: PTA palpates main muscle's tendon. Grades 4 and 5: PTA sitting on low stool in front of patient. One hand is stabilizing the ankle above malleoli. PTA's other hand gives resistance toward inversion and slight dorsiflexion at the dorsal and lateral side of the forefoot (Figure 3-49).

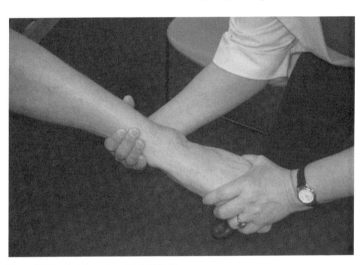

Figure 3-49 Foot Eversion with PF MMT

Big Toe and Other Toes Manual Muscle Testing

Table 3-7   Big Toe and Other Toes MMT[2]

- Hallux and Toe MP Flexion tests lumbricales and flexor hallucis brevis (two heads). All grades: Patient sitting with legs hanging over edge of table and ankle in neutral. Grades 4 and 5: Patient completes metatarsophalangeal (MP) flexion (for big toe or each lateral toe) and holds against strong or moderate resistance. Resistance is given with index finger placed beneath proximal phalanx of great toe or under the MP joints of four lateral toes.
- Hallux and Toe DIP and PIP Flexion tests flexor digitorum longus, flexor digitorum brevis, and flexor hallucis longus. All grades: Patient sitting with foot on PTA's lap. Grades 4 and 5: Patient completes ROM of toes and the big toe with minimal resistance. Resistance is given under the middle phalanges (for PIP) and under the distal phalanges (for the DIP).
- Hallux and Toe MP and IP Extension tests extensor digitorum longus, extensor digitorum brevis, and extensor hallucis longus. All grades: Patient sitting with foot on PTA's lap. Grades 4 and 5: Patient extends the big toe or the toes against minimal resistance. Resistance is given by PTA's thumb over the MP joint or over the IP joint.

Myotomes Testing

Table 3-8   Myotomes Testing

- Shoulder shrug: tests upper trapezius muscle. For CN XI (spinal accessory nerve) and spinal roots C2, C3 (posterior surface of neck), and C4 (AC joint).
- Shoulder abduction: tests deltoid muscle. For axillary nerve and spinal roots C5 (lateral aspect of arm) and C6 (lateral aspect of forearm; hand and thumb;index finger).
- Elbow flexion of supinated arm: tests biceps brachii muscle. For musculocutaneous nerve and spinal roots C5 and C6.
- Elbow flexion of neutral arm: tests brachioradialis muscle. For radial nerve and spinal roots C5 and C6.
- Elbow extension tests: triceps brachii muscle. For radial nerve and spinal roots C6, C7 (middle finger), and C8 (little and ring finger; medial aspect of hand and wrist).
- Radial wrist extension: tests ECU muscle. For radial nerve and spinal roots C6, C7, and C8.
- Wrist flexion: tests FCU muscle. For ulnar nerve and spinal roots C8 and T1 (medial forearm).

continues

Table 3-8   (continued)

- Thumb extension: tests EPL muscle. For radial nerve and spinal roots C6, C7, and C8.
- Fifth digit abduction: tests abductor digiti minimi muscle. For ulnar nerve and spinal roots C8 and T1.
- Hip flexion: tests iliopsoas muscles. For lumbar plexus and spinal roots L1 (proximal medial thigh), L2 (proximal anterior thigh), and L3 (distal anterior and medial thigh and knee).
- Knee extension: tests quadriceps femoris muscles. For femoral nerve and spinal roots L2, L3, and L4 (anterior and medial lower extremity).
- Ankle dorsiflexion: tests anterior tibialis muscle. For deep peroneal nerve and spinal roots L4 and L5 (anterior and lateral lower extremity; medial dorsal foot; plantar aspect of big toe).
- Big toe extension: tests EHL muscle. For deep peroneal nerve and spinal roots L5 and S1 (lateral dorsal foot; most of plantar foot).
- Knee flexion: tests hamstring muscles. For sciatic nerve and spinal roots L5, S1, and S2 (posterior thigh; proximal lower extremity).
- Ankle plantarflexion: tests gastrocnemius muscle. For tibial nerve and spinal roots S1 and S2.

Deep Tendon Reflexes and Grades

Table 3-9   Deep Tendon Reflexes and Grades

DTR Most Tested	DTR Grading
Biceps and brachioradialis: test C5–C6.	Absent DTR: grade is 0
Triceps: tests C7–C8.	DTR for hyporeflexia: grade is 1+
Quadriceps: tests L2–L4.	Normal DTR: grade is 2+
Hamstrings: tests L5–S3.	DTR for hyperreflexia: grade is 3+
Achilles tendon: tests S1–S2.	DTR for high hyperreflexia (clonus): grade is 4+ and 5+

Orthopedic Special Tests: Shoulder, Elbow, Wrist, and Hand

Table 3-10   Orthopedic Special Tests: Shoulder, Elbow, Wrist, and Hand

Area, Test, and Purpose	Interpretation	Procedure
Shoulder: Yergason's for bicipital tendonitis[3]	Tests: integrity of transverse humeral ligament (THL) that holds biceps tendon in bicipital groove of humerus. Positive for tendonitis: tenderness (or pain) in bicipital groove. Positive for THL tear: tendon felt to "pop out" of the groove.	Patient seating with elbow flexed to 90° and stabilized against thorax, forearm pronated. The therapist's one hand palpates biceps tendon in bicipital groove, while the other hand resists supination when patient laterally rotates the arm against resistance.
Shoulder: Adson's Maneuver for Thoracic Outlet Syndrome (TOS)[4]	Tests: presence of TOS. Positive for TOS: disappearance of radial pulse while patient holds a deep breath.	Patient seated with head rotated toward the tested shoulder, extends the head while taking a deep breath and holding it. The therapist's one hand palpates patient's radial pulse, while the other hand rotates and extends the patient's shoulder.
Shoulder: Neer impingement test for injury of supraspinatus muscle or biceps tendon tear	Tests: overuse injury of supraspinatus muscle. Positive: Patient's face shows pain.	Patient seated while his or her arm is forcibly flexed and internally rotated by the therapist. The passive stress causes compression of greater tuberosity of humerus against the acromion.

continues

Table 3-10 (continued)

Area, Test, and Purpose	Interpretation	Procedure
Shoulder: drop arm (Codman's) test for rotator cuff tear	Tests: tear of rotator cuff muscles. Positive: Patient drops his or her arm to the side.	Patient standing while the therapist abducts patient's shoulder to 90° and asks the patient to slowly lower his or her arm to the side.
Shoulder: apprehension test for anterior shoulder[3] dislocation	Tests: traumatic instability of anterior shoulder. Positive: Patient complains of pain or apprehensively resists the therapist's hand when moving patient's arm in external rotation.	Patient supine while the therapist abducts the patient's arm to 90° and laterally rotates the patient's shoulder slowly.
Elbow: lateral epicondylitis test (Cozen's test)[3]	Tests: inflammation of lateral epicondyle (tennis elbow). Positive: sudden severe pain in the area.	Patient seated with elbow extended, forearm pronated making a fist. The therapist's one hand stabilizes the patient's elbow palpating lateral epicondyle. The other hand resists patient's wrist extension and forearm supination.
Elbow: medial epicondylitis test	Tests: inflammation of medial epicondyle (golfer's elbow). Positive: sudden severe pain in the area.	Patient seated with elbow extended, forearm supinated. The therapist's one hand stabilizes the patient's elbow palpating medial epicondyle. The other hand passively extends and supinates patient's wrist and forearm.

Wrist: Phalen's test for carpal tunnel syndrome	Tests: pressure on median nerve secondary to carpal tunnel syndrome. Positive: tingling sensation in the thumb, index finger, and middle and lateral half of ring finger.	Patient standing. The therapist flexes the patient's wrist pushing the wrists together and holding them for 1 minute.
Wrist: Tinel's sign for carpal tunnel syndrome	Tests: pressure on median nerve and the rate of regeneration of sensory fibers of the nerve. Positive: tingling and paresthesia into thumb, index finger, middle and lateral half of ring finger, and distal to the point of pressure. The most distal point felt is the limit of nerve regeneration.	Patient seated with forearm supinated and hand relaxed. The therapist taps over the carpal tunnel.
Thumb: Finkelstein's test for DeQuervain's tenosynovitis	Tests: tendon inflammation of abductor pollicis longus and extensor pollicis brevis. Positive: pain in the area of these two tendons.	Patient seated with elbow extended making a fist with the thumb inside the fingers. The therapist's one hand stabilizes the patient's forearm. The other hand moves the patient's wrist toward the ulnar side.

MUSCULOSKELETAL INTERVENTIONS

Orthopedic Special Tests: Hip, Knee, and Ankle

Table 3-11   Orthopedic Special Tests: Hip, Knee, Ankle

Area, Test, and Purpose	Interpretation	Procedure
Hip: Ober test for TFL (iliotibial band) contracture[4]	Tests: contracture or tightness (shortness) of iliotibial band. Positive: tested leg remains abducted while patient's muscles are relaxed.	Patient side lying with lower leg flexed at the hip and knee. Patient's tested limb is uppermost with knee extended. The therapist passively abducts, extends the upper leg, and slowly lowers the limb.
Hip: Thomas test for hip flexion contracture	Tests: contracture or tightness (shortness) of hip flexors. Positive: patient's thigh lifts up from the table bending at the knee.	Patient supine. The therapist flexes the unaffected hip asking the patient to hold his or her knee to his or her chest (flattening the lumbar spine and stabilizing the pelvis). Patient holds the flexed hip against his or her chest.
Hip: Patrick's test (Fabere test or figure of four test)	Tests: arthritis of the hip or sacroiliac joint dysfunction. Positive: pain in the hip and the tested leg's knee remaining above the opposite knee.	Patient supine. The therapist flexes, abducts, and externally rotates the patient's hip until the lateral malleolus rests on the opposite knee above the patella. In this position, the therapist gently pushes the knee downward.

Knee: Valgus test (abduction test) for medial instability	Tests: instability of the medial collateral ligament (MCL). Positive: pain or excessive gapping of the joint (tibia moves away from the femur because gaps on medial side)	Patient supine with tested knee first in full extension, then in slight flexion (20° to 30°). The therapist stabilizes the ankle by sitting on it. The therapist's one hand palpates the knee joint line at the medial side, while the other hand at the lateral joint line pushes the knee medially by applying a valgus stress.
Knee: Varus test (adduction test) for lateral instability	Tests: instability of the lateral collateral ligament (LCL). Positive: pain or excessive gapping of the joint (tibia moves away from the femur because gaps on lateral side).	Patient supine with tested knee first in full extension, then in slight flexion (20° to 30°). The therapist stabilizes the ankle by sitting on it. The therapist's one hand palpates the knee joint line at the lateral side, while the other hand at the medial joint line pushes the knee laterally by applying a varus stress.
Knee: Lachman test for ACL instability	Tests: instability of the anterior cruciate ligament (ACL). Positive: "mushy" or soft end feel when tibia is moved forward on the femur. Caution of false negative if femur is not properly stabilized or meniscal tear is present.	Patient supine with tested knee in 30° of flexion. The therapist's one hand stabilizes the femur medially while the other hand laterally moves forward (translates) the tibia on femur.

continues

Table 3-11 (continued)

Area, Test, and Purpose	Interpretation	Procedure
Knee: McMurray test for loose meniscal fragments[4]	Tests: integrity of lateral and medial meniscus. Positive: snap or click (or feeling a crepitation) accompanied by pain as the knee is extended.	Patient supine with tested knee completely flexed. The therapist's one hand holds the patient's calcaneus (for internal or external rotation) while the other hand holds the knee joint for knee extension.
Ankle: Thompson's test for rupture of Achilles tendon	Tests: rupture of Achilles tendon. Positive: absence of plantar flexion when the calf muscles are squeezed.	Patient prone, relaxed, with feet over the edge of the table. The therapist squeezes the calf muscles.
Ankle: Homan's sign for deep vein thrombosis (DVT)	Tests: deep vein thrombosis (DVT). Positive: calf pain.	Patient supine with knee extended. The therapist's one hand holds and lifts the lower leg off the table, while the other hand passively dorsiflexes the foot.

Common Injuries of Brachial Plexus

Table 3-12   Common Injuries of the Brachial Plexus

Nerve and Its Origin	Motor Innervation	Musculoskeletal Injuries
Median Nerve Cords: Medial and lateral. Divisions: Anterior. Trunks: Upper, middle, and lower. Origin: Nerve Roots C6, C7, C8, and T1.	Motor Innervation Muscles: Pronator Teres; pronator quadratus; palmaris longus; FCR; FDS; FPL; lateral half of FDP; lumbricales 1 and 2; thenar muscles (abductor pollicis brevis; lateral half of FPB; and opponens pollicis).	Median Nerve Compression Injuries: (1) Thoracic Outlet Syndrome: presence of a cervical rib or narrowing of thoracic outlet; (2) Pronator Teres Syndrome: caused by trauma, humeral fracture, hypertrophy of muscle, or repetitive injury (such as using a screwdriver); (3) Anterior Interosseus Syndrome: caused by fibrous sheaths, thrombosis of vessels, or forearm fractures; (4) Carpal Tunnel Syndrome: caused by hormonal factors in pregnancy, hypothyroidism, congenital bone deformities, RA, or overuse syndrome. Median Nerve Trauma Injuries: Humeral Fractures, Wrist Lacerations, or Carpal Bones Trauma. Median Nerve Lesion Deformities: Ape Hand (paralysis and atrophy of thenar muscles; opposition is lost, thumb is permanently extended); Benediction Sign (inability to flex thumb, second, and third digit; they remain in extension because FDP and FPL are weak; ring and little finger are flexed while others are extended; cannot make a fist)[5].

continues

MUSCULOSKELETAL INTERVENTIONS

Table 3-12 (continued)

Nerve and Its Origin	Motor Innervation	Musculoskeletal Injuries
Ulnar Nerve Cord: Medial. Division: Anterior. Trunk: Lower. Origin: Nerve Roots C8 and T1.	Muscles: FCU; medial half of FDP; palmaris brevis; hand Interossei; third and fourth lumbricales; adductor pollicis; medial half of FPB; hypothenar muscles (opponens digiti minimi, abductor digiti minimi, and flexor digiti minimi).	Ulnar Nerve Compression Injuries: (1) Thoracic Outlet Syndrome: presence of a cervical rib or narrowing of thoracic outlet; (2) Crutches Injury: pressure on axillary region; (3) Cubital Tunnel Syndrome: entrapment at the elbow secondary to trauma, repetitive motion, or inflammatory conditions; (4) Guyon's Canal (or Ulnar Tunnel): secondary to RA or trauma (karate). Ulnar Nerve Lesion Deformity: Claw Hand (hyperextension of proximal phalanges of digits and extreme flexion of middle and distal phalanges; loss of opposition and inability to abduct little finger).[5]
Radial Nerve Cord: Posterior. Division: Posterior. Trunks: Upper, Middle, Lower. Origin: Nerve Roots C5, C6, C7, C8, and T1	Muscles: Brachioradialis, ECRL, triceps, anconeus, ECRB, supinator, ED, EDM, ECU, abductor pollicis longus, EPL, EPB, extensorindicis	Radial Nerve Compression Injuries: (1) Spiral Groove Syndrome: (called also Saturday Night Palsy) caused by falling asleep (inebriated) with spiral groove of the arm against a hard object or caused by direct trauma; (2) Crutches Injury: pressure on axillary region. Radial Nerve Trauma Injuries: Radial Neck Fractures; Humeral Fractures; Shoulder Dislocations.

Common Muscle Substitutions

Table 3-13   Examples of Common Muscle Substitutions

Scapular stabilizers initiate shoulder motion for weak shoulder abductors

Lateral trunk muscles or TFL take over for weak hip abductors

Long head of the biceps, coracobrachialis, and anterior deltoid take over for weak pectoralis major

Use of passive finger flexion by contracting wrist extensors for weak finger flexors

Lower back extensors, adductor magnus, and quadratus lumborum for weak hip extensors

Lower abdominals, lower obliques, hip adductors, and latissimus dorsi for weak hip flexors

Basic Clinical Impairments and Functional Limitations of Common Musculoskeletal Conditions

Clinical Impairments and Functional Limitations of Arthritic Disorders

Table 3-14 Clinical Impairments and Functional Limitations of Arthritic Disorders*

Osteoarthritis Impairments and Functional Limitations	Rheumatoid Arthritis Impairments and Functional Limitations
Sensory deficits: decreased proprioception and/or kinesthesia (such as during ambulation and/or ADLs); pain with weight bearing depending on the stages of the disease (or if it is a discal nerve root compromise); aching during sleep; hip pain can be prevalent depending on the stages of the disease; pain upon rising that eases through the morning with movement.	Sensory deficits: sharp pain with certain movements; paresthesia; decreased proprioception and/or kinesthesia.
Motor deficits: decreased muscular strength; decreased muscular endurance; decreased ROM; decreased flexibility (morning stiffness); sometimes a leg-length discrepancy; decreased balance; deformities such as valgus or varus in the knee joint; joint crepitus; joint swelling (moderate); increased muscular spasms; joint deformity (usually in abduction, flexion, and external rotation); postural deficits (such as increased kyphosis or lordosis); abnormal reflexes.	Motor deficits: decreased flexibility; decreased muscular strength; decreased muscular endurance; decreased flexibility (morning stiffness); decreased ROM; fatigue (lack of energy); joint swelling; increased joint laxity; crepitus; increased, joint hypermobility or hypomobility; increased skin and soft tissue temperature; edema; decreased balance and coordination; joint deformity especially in the second and third MP and PIP; may have Boutonniere deformity (PIP joint flexion and DIP joint extension); Swan neck deformity (PIP joint extension and MP and DIP joints flexion); valgus deformity at knees and ankles; clawed toes deformity.

continues

MUSCULOSKELETAL INTERVENTIONS

Table 3-14 Clinical Impairments and Functional Limitations of Arthritic Disorders

Osteoarthritis Impairments and Functional Limitations	Rheumatoid Arthritis Impairments and Functional Limitations
Functional deficits: antalgic gait pattern; may need assistive device in transfers and ambulation; decreased independence with ADLs (such as dressing) and home management activities; decreased independence with IADLs; inability to ambulate stairs (steps); inability to work/play/school or perform leisure activities.	Functional deficits: decreased independence with ADLs and home management activities; decreased independence with IADLs; inability to ambulate stairs (steps); inability to work/play/school or perform leisure activities; may need assistive devices in transfers and ambulation.
	Pulmonary deficits: may have pleural effusion or pleuritis; shallow breathing; chest pain during inspiration.

*This is a basic guide; PTA should consider PT's initial examination and evaluation.

Clinical Impairments and Functional Limitations of Other Musculoskeletal Conditions

Table 3-15   Impairments and Functional Limitations of Tendonitis, Bursitis, Sprains, Strains, Dislocations, and Fractures

Sensory deficits: pain at rest and with weight bearing; decreased sensation; decreased proprioception and/or kinesthesia. When cervical spine is involved (such as acceleration injury or cervical sprain of CS), patient can have neck pain; headaches, vertigo, dysesthesias (numbness, burning, prickling, or tingling) of face and upper extremities and changes in vision and hearing. In rib fractures, patient may have pain with deep inspiration. In brachial plexus lesions, patient may have sharp and burning pain in the upper extremity and numbness and pins and needles in the upper extremity. In cervical disk pathology, patient can have sensory changes in the respective dermatomes. In cervical faucet syndrome, patient can have paresthesia and pain with hyperextension and rotation of CS.

Motor deficits: increased muscular spasms; decreased muscular strength; decreased muscular endurance; decreased ROM; decreased flexibility; localized swelling; joint crepitus with active motion; decreased balance (if it is in the lower extremity); postural deficits; muscular substitutions (stronger muscles compensate for the loss of motion); postural changes (such as forward head kyphosis with cervical sprain). Colle's or Smith's fractures can have edema and ecchymosis, structural deformity (Colles' distal fragment is dorsal and Smith's is palmar), and limited ROM.

Functional deficits: decreased independence with ADLs (such as dressing) and home management activities, decreased independence with IADLs, inability to ambulate stairs or steps (if it is in the lower extremity), and inability to work/play/school or perform leisure activities.

Types of Musculoskeletal Interventions

Therapeutic Exercises

Table 3-16   Therapeutic Exercises: Indications and Contraindications

Exercises	Indications	Contraindications, Limitations, Precautions[6]
PROM Exercises (including the CPM device)	To demonstrate a movement, to prepare a patient for stretching, to maintain joint connective tissue mobility, to maintain elasticity of muscle, to increase synovial fluid for joint nutrition, to assist circulation, to prevent joint contracture, to decrease pain, to help in the healing process	Contraindication: Disruption of healing process. Limitations: Will not increase muscle strength or endurance, will not prevent or counteract muscle atrophy, will not assist in the blood circulation to the same extent as the active movement.
AROM exercises	For weak muscles, to promote bone and soft tissue integrity, to promote coordination and motor skills, to prevent DVT, to increase blood circulation, for aerobic conditioning, for preparation for functional activities	Contraindications: Disruption of healing process, harm to recent surgical procedure(s). Limitations: Will not increase strength in muscles that are already strong.
AAROM exercises using manual or mechanical assistance (wand, cane, finger ladder, or overhead pulleys)	To increase circulation and prevent DVT; to promote integrity of bone, muscles, ligaments and tendons; to promote coordination and motor abilities; to	Contraindications: Disruption of healing process, harm to recent surgical procedure(s) Limitations: will not increase strength in muscles already strong;

continues

MUSCULOSKELETAL INTERVENTIONS

Table 3-16   (continued)

Exercises	Indications	Contraindications, Limitations, Precautions[6]
	assist with learning a new movement pattern.	less effective than AROM exercises.
Muscle setting isometric exercises (quads sets; gluts sets; HS sets)	For very weak muscles, for acute stage of soft tissue healing, to increase circulation, to promote relaxation, to decrease pain	Precautions: cardiovascular disease, CVA, Valsalva maneuver (to prevent Valsalva, patient needs to count out loud or sing).
Resisted isometrics exercises (higher intensity than muscle setting): manual or mechanical (door frame or wall)	To increase strength throughout permitted ROM, and when manual or mechanical resistance is painful or harmful	Precautions: Cardiovascular disease, CVA, Valsalva maneuver (to prevent Valsalva, patient needs to count out loud or sing).
Stabilization Exercises (isometrics and rhythmic stabilization; cocontraction)	To develop muscle strength and stability, and to assist with postural control (muscles of trunk)	Precautions: Cardiovascular disease, CVA, Valsalva maneuver (to prevent Valsalva, patient needs to count out loud or sing).
Manual and Mechanical Resistance Exercises including also: PNF D1 Flexion; PNF D1 Extension; PNF D2 Flexion; PNF D2 Extension. For concentric contractions: the resistance must be applied in the	Manual resistance: For very weak muscles, for transition from manual to mechanical, where adjustment of resistance is indicated, when patient's muscles must work maximally at all points in ROM, when	Contraindications: Acute inflammation, acute diseases/disorders, pain, polio or post-polio syndrome, and Guillain-Barre syndrome. Mechanical resistance is not appropriate for very

opposite direction to the desired motion. For eccentric contractions: the resistance must be applied in the same direction to the desired motion.

protection of healing tissues is indicated, and when prevention of substitute motion is indicated.

Mechanical resistance: To increase strength and endurance, for independent training, and in intermediate and advanced stages of rehab.

weak muscles and in the early stages of healing.

Precautions: cardiovascular conditions, to monitor vital signs, Valsalva, DOMS

DeLorme PREs: (1) Determine patient's 10 RM, (2) patient performs one set of 10 reps at 50% of the 10 RM, (3) patient performs a second set of 10 reps at 75% of the 10 RM, (4) patient performs a final set of 10 reps at the full 10 RM

To increase strength and endurance

Contraindications: Acute inflammation, acute diseases/disorders, pain, polio or postpolio syndrome, Guillain-Barre syndrome.

Precautions: cardiovascular conditions, to monitor vital signs, Valsalva, DOMS

Oxford PREs: (1) Determine patient's 10 RM, (2) patient performs one set of 10 reps at the full 100% RM, (3) patient performs a second set of 10 reps at 75% of the 10 RM, (4) patient performs a final set of 10 reps at 50% of the 10 RM

To increase strength and endurance

Contraindications: Acute inflammation, acute diseases/disorders, pain, polio or postpolio syndrome, Guillain-Barre syndrome.

Precautions: cardiovascular conditions, to monitor vital signs, Valsalva, DOMS

DAPRE PREs: (1) Determine patient's 6 RM, (2) in set 1, patient performs 10 reps of 50% of

To increase strength and endurance

Contraindications: Acute inflammation, acute

continues

Table 3-16   (continued)

Exercises	Indications	Contraindications, Limitations, Precautions[6]
the 6 RM, (3) in set 2, patient performs 6 reps of 75% of the 6 RM, (4) in set 3, patient performs as many as maximum possible reps of 100% of the 6 RM, (5) in set 4, patient performs as many as possible reps of 100% of the "working weight" performed during set 3. The number of reps done in set 4 is used to determine the "working weight" for the next day.		diseases/disorders, pain, polio or postpolio syndrome, Guillain-Barre syndrome. Precautions: cardiovascular conditions, to monitor vital signs, Valsalva, DOMS
Circuit Weight Training: Using mechanical resistance for various muscle groups. Circuit Training Exercises: Using mechanical resistance for various muscle groups, flexibility exercises, and total body conditioning.	To increase muscular strength, to increase muscular endurance, to increase cardiovascular endurance	Contraindications: Acute inflammation, acute diseases/disorders, pain, polio or postpolio syndrome, Guillain-Barre syndrome. Precautions: cardiovascular conditions, to monitor vital signs, Valsalva, DOMS
Isokinetic Exercises (use accommodating resistance)	To increase muscular strength and endurance, for later stages of rehabilitation, when patient has full or	Contraindications: Acute inflammation, acute diseases/disorders, pain, polio or postpolio syndrome, Guillain-

	partial ROM in a pain-free mode	Barre syndrome. Precautions: Recent musculotendinous surgeries, cardiovascular diseases or disorders. Limitations: Resistance depends entirely on patient's efforts, does not accommodate all muscle groups, patient cannot perform exercises independently in his or her environment, are nonfunctional exercises, use specialized and expensive equipment. Precaution: Can increase BP.
OKC and CKC Exercises	OKC: For strengthening of individual muscle groups, and for NWB postures. CKC: For functionality, for WB postures, and to stimulate joint and mechanoreceptors.	Precautions: when using resistive OKC while terminal knee extension (TKE); when using CKC between 60° and 90° in nonoperative and operative ACL injuries; when using CKC in postop meniscal tears.
Stretching Exercises: manual passive stretching, self-stretching, prolonged mechanical or positional passive stretching, ballistic stretching (for athletes), cyclic mechanical stretching	To elongate structures, to improve ROM, for hypomobile joints	Contraindications: When a bony block limits joint motion; acute infectious and inflammatory processes; acute sharp pain; recent fracture; hematoma and joint hypermobility;

continues

MUSCULOSKELETAL INTERVENTIONS

Table 3-16   (continued)

Exercises	Indications	Contraindications, Limitations, Precautions[6]
		when contractures provide stability and functionality. Ballistic stretching is contraindicated: for sedentary individuals, for older patients, patients with musculoskeletal pathology or chronic contracture. Precautions: Do not stretch passively beyond normal ROM, newly united fractures, osteoporosis, prolonged immobilization, bone malignancy, total joint replacements.
Aerobic conditioning exercises (cardiopulmonary endurance exercises or total body endurance exercises) Can use: (1) Karvonen formula: total heart rate reserve (THRR) = maximal HR − resting HR (40% to 85%) + resting HR; (2) Age-adjusted maximal heart rate formula: THRR = (220 − age) × (65% to	To increase coronary arteries blood flow, to increase the heart wall thickness and muscle mass of the left ventricle, to increase blood cortisol level, to improve thermal regulation capability, to reduce risk of coronary artery disease, to increase aerobic enzymatic activity, to increase the maximum ventilatory ability	Contraindications: Unstable angina; resting systolic BP more than 200 mm Hg; resting diastolic BP more than 110 mm Hg; orthostatic hypotension; acute systemic illness or fever; tachycardia; thrombophlebitis; recent embolism; severe orthopedic problems; metabolic problems (such as thyroiditis). Precautions: swimming

85%); (3) MET method; (4) Borg's rate of perceived exertion (PRE) scale method		and cross-country skiing, dancing, basketball, racquetball, and competitive activities should not be used with patients who may have cardiorespiratory symptoms or are very deconditioned.
Aquatic Exercises	Poor standing balance, for stretching, for relaxation, for strengthening, for aerobic conditioning, for PWB gait training	Contraindications: Bowel and bladder incontinence, UTI, unstable BP, skin infections and water and airborne infections, unprotected open wounds, severe epilepsy, severe kidney disease, severe cardiac and respiratory dysfunction. Precautions: Patients who experience fear of water (need prior orientation).
Relaxation Exercises: (1) progressive relaxation (teaches voluntary contraction and relaxation of the muscles from distal to proximal), (2) one breathing technique (awareness on diaphragmatic breathing while silently repeating the word "one" with each exhalation)	Chronic pain (tension headache, vascular headache, or chronic neck and back pain) with biofeedback; cardiopulmonary stress or chronic pulmonary problems such as asthma or emphysema	Precautions: Patient with cardiopulmonary disorders performing progressive relaxation (when isometrically contracting the muscles).

Relaxation Exercises

Table 3-17   Relaxation Exercises

Relaxation exercises are performed with active participation from the patient to generate a relaxation response. The systemic effects of relaxation include decreased sympathetic nervous system (SNS) activity, respiratory rate, oxygen consumption, blood pressure, skeletal muscle blood flow, and muscle tension.

Relaxation techniques can be performed singly or incorporated into other exercise sessions such as part of the warm-up or cool-down of the aerobic conditioning exercises. The relaxation training is effective if it is acceptable to the patient, is easy to apply in different settings, helps to restore the patient's sense of control, and offers immediate reduction of pain.

Types of relaxation exercises include autogenic training, progressive relaxation, and Feldenkrais awareness through movement. Autogenic training involves conscious relaxation through autosuggestion and a progression of exercises as well as meditation. Progressive relaxation is one of the most common techniques that teaches voluntary contraction and relaxation of the muscles from distal to proximal. Feldenkrais awareness through movement combines self-massage, movements of the limbs and trunk, deep breathing, sensory awareness, and conscious relaxation procedures to adjust postural and muscular imbalances and decrease pain and tension.[7]

Other types of relaxation exercises include "one breathing technique," eye-movement breathing technique, cognitive relaxation techniques such as listening to audio tapes or watching videotapes with instructions or music for relaxation, guided imagery, hypnosis, and nontraditional psychophysical techniques such as Trager Psychophysical integration, TaiChi Chuan, and Hatha Yoga. "One breathing technique" is a form of meditation that involves passive focusing of awareness on the diaphragmatic breathing cycle while silently repeating the word "one" with each exhalation.[7] The patient or the client is instructed to maintain a passive attitude and allow but not force relaxation to occur at its own pace. Eye-movement breathing technique involves looking up toward the eyebrows (without head movement) during the inspiratory phase of diaphragmatic breathing, then holding the breath for 2 seconds, followed by looking down toward the chin (without head movement) while breathing out very slowly and completely. To promote relaxation, the expiratory phase of diaphragmatic breathing can be extended.

When applying progressive relaxation exercises the following procedures will take place: Relaxation training can be performed in a quiet environment with low lighting and soothing music. The therapist's voice has to be soft and soothing. The patient should be in a comfortable position and free of restrictive clothing. The procedure must be explained to the patient. The patient needs to breathe in (deep) and in a relaxed manner. The patient is asked to contract voluntarily for a few seconds the distal muscle of the hands or feet. The patient is asked to voluntarily relax for a few seconds the distal muscle of the hands or feet. The patient is asked to try to feel a sense of heaviness in the hands or feet. The patient is asked to try to feel a sense of warmth in the muscles just relaxed. The exercises can progress to a more proximal area of the body by asking the patient to voluntarily contract and relax for a few seconds the more proximal musculature. Finally, the patient is asked to voluntarily contract isometrically and relax the entire upper extremity or lower extremity. At the end of the procedures, the patient is asked to try to feel a sense of relaxation and warmth throughout the entire extremity and eventually throughout the entire body.

Relaxation exercises can be coupled with heating modalities such as hot packs, paraffin, ultrasound, or massage techniques such as light or deep stroking (effleurage).

PNF Exercises—Diagonal Patterns

Table 3-18   Description and Performance of PNF AROM Terminal Positions (Shoulder, Forearm, Wrist, Fingers, Hip, Knee, Ankle)[6]*

UE D1 Extension: Extension, Abduction, Internal Rotation (Scapular Depression, Abduction, and Downward Rotation); Pronation; Ulnar Extension of Wrist; and Abduction and Extension of Fingers including Thumb Abduction (Figure 3-50).

UE D1 Flexion: Flexion, Adduction, External Rotation (Scapular Elevation, Abduction, and Upward Rotation); Supination; Wrist Radial Flexion; and Fingers Flexion and Adduction including Thumb Adduction (Figure 3-51).

UE D2 Extension: Extension, Adduction, Internal Rotation (Scapular Depression, Abduction, and Downward Rotation); Pronation; Ulnar Extension of Wrist, and Flexion and Adduction of Fingers including Thumb Opposition (Figure 3-52).

UE D2 Flexion: Flexion, Abduction, External Rotation (Scapular Elevation, Adduction, and Upward Rotation); Supination; Radial Extension of Wrist; and Fingers Abduction and Extension including Thumb Extension (Figure 3-53).

LE D1 Extension: Extension, Abduction, Internal Rotation (Posterior Rotation of Pelvis); Knee Extension; and Ankle Plantaflexion and Eversion (Figure 3-54).

continues

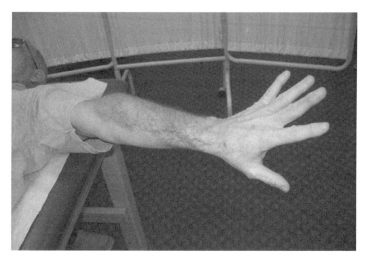

Figure 3-50 D1 UE Extension

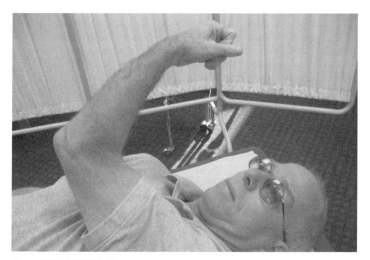

Figure 3-51 D1 UE Flexion

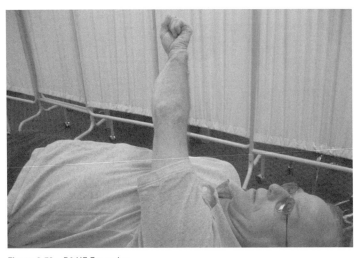

Figure 3-52 D2 UE Extension

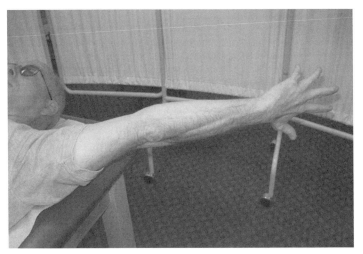

Figure 3-53 D2 UE Flexion

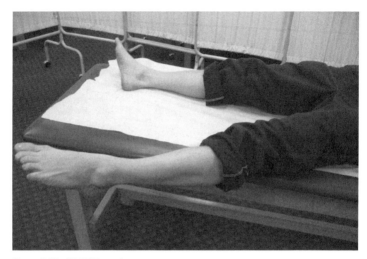

Figure 3-54 D1 LE Extension

Table 3-18 (continued)

LE D1 Flexion: Flexion, Adduction, External Rotation (Anterior Rotation of Pelvis);
   Knee Flexion; and Ankle Dorsiflexion and Inversion (Figure 3-55).
LE D2 Extension: Extension, Adduction, External Rotation (Depression of Pelvis);
   Knee Extension; and Ankle Plantarflexion and Inversion (Figure 3-56).
LE D2 Flexion: Flexion, Abduction, Internal Rotation (Elevation of Pelvis); Knee Flex-
   ion; and Ankle Plantarflexion (or Ankle Dorsiflexion) and Eversion (Figure 3-57).

---

*For musculoskeletal interventions, PNF can be performed as manual resistive
exercises.

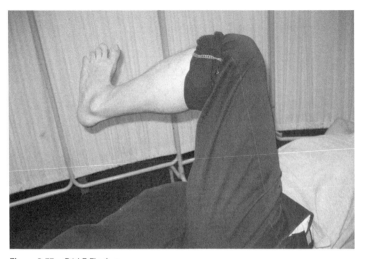

Figure 3-55 D1 LE Flexion

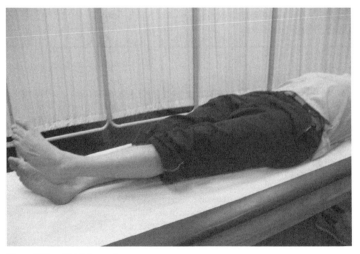

Figure 3-56 D2 LE Extension

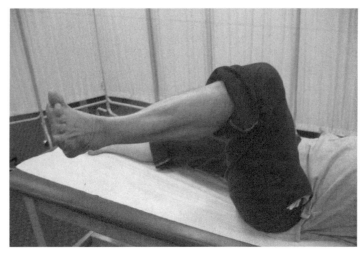

Figure 3-57 D2 LE Flexion

Closed Kinetic Chain Exercises to Increase Weight–Bearing Control and Stability

Table 3-19   CKC Exercises

CKC Isometric Exercises

Muscle setting exercises (to facilitate co-contraction of the quads and hamstrings): Position of patient: sitting on a chair with the knee extended or slightly flexed and the heel on the floor. Have the patient press the heel against the floor and the thigh against the seat of the chair and concentrate on contracting the quadriceps and hamstrings simultaneously to facilitate co-contraction around the knee joint. Hold the muscle contraction, relax, and repeat rhythmic stabilization.

Muscle setting exercises: Position of the patient: standing with bilateral weight bearing. Apply manual resistance to the pelvis in several directions as the patient holds the position. This will facilitate isometric contraction of muscles in the ankles, knees, hips, and trunk. Progress to rhythmic stabilization activity by having the patient bear weight only on the involved lower extremity while resistance is applied.

CKC Dynamic Exercises

Mini squats (short-arc training): begin by having the patient stand and bend both knees up to 30° to 45° and then ask the patient to extend the knees. Progress by using elastic resistance placed under both feet or by holding weights in the hands. Having the knees move anterior to the toes as the hips descend increases the shear forces on the tibia and strains the ACL. Squatting, as if sitting on a chair, in which the tibia remains relatively vertical requires greater trunk flexion to maintain balance and stronger quadriceps contraction to support the load of the pelvis posterior to the knee axis at an angle where patellar compressive loads are great (helping to reduce the stress on the ACL).

Forward, backward, and lateral step-ups and step-downs: begin with a low step, 2 to 3 inches in height, and increase the height as the patient is able. Make sure that the patient keeps the trunk upright. Emphasize control of body weight during concentric (step-up) and eccentric (step-down) quadriceps activity. Instruct the patient that the heel is to be the last to leave the floor and first to return (or to "keep the toes up").

Standing wall slides: The patient flexes the hips and knees and slides the back down and then up the wall, lifting and lowering the body weight. As control improves, the patient moves into greater knee flexion, up to a maximum of 60°. Knee flexion beyond 60° is not recommended in order to avoid excessive shear forces on ligamentous structures of the knee and compressive forces on the patellofemoral joint. Wall slides that are performed with a gym ball behind the back decrease stability and require more control.

Partial and full lunges: a step-forward stance position with weight acceptance on the forward foot. Have the patient rock body weight forward, allowing the knee to flex slightly, and then rock backward and control knee extension.

Patient Education Topics for Lumbar Spine

Table 3-20   Patient Education for Lumbar Spine

When supine, hook lying flexes the spine while legs extended extends the spine. A pillow under the head flexes the neck; a small roll under the neck stabilizes a mild lordosis with the head in neutral.

When prone, patient should use of a pillow under the abdomen (because it flexes the spine; without a pillow it extends the spine).

Sitting usually causes spinal flexion, especially if the hips and knees are flexed. To emphasize flexion, patient should prop the feet up on a small footstool (to increase

continues

Table 3-20   (continued)

hip flexion). To emphasize extension, patient should use a lumbar pillow (or support) in the low-back region.

Standing usually causes spinal extension. To emphasize flexion, patient should stand with a small stool under one of the feet.

If tolerated, the patient is taught to perform simple movements while protecting the spine in the functional position.

Gentle pelvic tilting or chin tucks should be taught in every position tolerated by the patient, including supine, prone, side lying, sitting, and standing.

Postlaminectomy or diskectomy (in hospital) the patient is taught to use the "log roll" technique to turn from supine to side lying to prone and return. The patient practices maintaining spinal alignment by keeping the shoulders aligned with the pelvis while rolling the trunk over as a unit (a log) and not twisting the spine. Then the patient is taught to sit from the supine-lying position by logrolling on to the side, pushing the body up with the hands while bringing the legs forward over the side of the bed. While moving through the sitting-up pattern, emphasis is placed on keeping the back in lordosis if there is an extension bias (or in flexion if there is a flexion bias). The patient is taught to go from standing to sitting and the reverse with spinal control. The trunk moves as a whole. Patient is taught the following: not to bend over; not to lift heavy or moderately heavy objects; not to twist his or her back; not to sit for prolong periods of time; not to climb long flights of stairs; to maintain proper body mechanics (to lessen strain and pressure on the spine), including proper body alignment and good posture; to sleep on a firm mattress; to start an exercise program (after 6 weeks post–op) of gradual abdominal muscles strengthening.

Abdominal Strengthening Exercises

Table 3-21   Abdominal Muscles Strengthening Exercises

Curl-ups: (1) Position of patient: hook lying, with the lumbar spine flat (posterior pelvic tilt). (2) First, have the patient lift the head off the mat (causing a stabilizing contraction of the abdominal muscles). (3) Patient progresses by lifting the shoulders until the scapulae and thorax clear the mat, keeping the arms horizontal. The patient does not come to a full sit-up because after the thorax clears the mat, the rest of the motion is performed by the hip flexor muscles. (4) Further progress the difficulty of the curl-up by changing the arm position from horizontal to folded across the chest and then to behind the head.[6]

Diagonal curl-ups: (1) To emphasize the external oblique muscles, the patient performs a diagonal curl-up by reaching one hand toward the outside of the opposite knee while curling up, then alternating. (2) The patient reverses the muscle action by bringing one knee up toward the opposite shoulder and then repeating with the other knee.

Double knee to chest: (1) To emphasize the lower rectus abdominis and oblique muscles, have the patient set a posterior pelvic tilt, then bring both knees to the chest and return. (2) Progress the difficulty by decreasing the angle of the hip and knee flexion.

Pelvic lifts: (1) The patient begins with the hips at 90° and knees extended. (2) The patient performs a posterior pelvic tilt and lifts the buttocks upward off the mat (small motion; the feet move also upward toward the ceiling). (3) The patient should not push against the mat with the hands.

Bilateral straight-leg raising (SLR): (1) This is a progression in difficulty of the double knee-to-chest exercise (it should be undertaken only if the muscles are strong enough to maintain a posterior pelvic tilt). (2) The patient begins with legs extended (the patient first performs a posterior pelvic tilt, then flexes both hips, keeping the knees extended; if the hips are abducted before initiating this exercise, greater stress is placed on the oblique abdominal muscles).

Exercise Topics for the Obstetric Patient

Table 3-22   Exercise Topics for the Obstetric Patient

Pregnancy-induced pathology: Diastasis Recti: separation of the rectus abdominis muscles in the midline at the Linea Alba. Any separation larger than 2 cm or two fingerwidths is considered significant. Diastasis Recti is not exclusive to childbearing women but is seen frequently in this population. The incidence increases as the pregnancy progresses, reaching a peak in the third trimester. Diastasis Recti does not always spontaneously resolve after childbirth and may continue past the 6-week postpartum period. Diastasis Recti can occur above, below, or at the level of the umbilicus but appears to be less common below the umbilicus.[6]

Diastasis Recti Test: The Diastasis is measured by the number of fingers that can be placed between the Rectus abdominis muscle bellies. A diastasis can also present as a longitudinal bulge along the Linea Alba.

Diastasis Recti Intervention: Perform corrective exercise for diastasis recti exclusive of other abdominal exercise until the separation is decreased to 2 cm or less.

Corrective Exercises for Diastasis Recti[6]

continues

Table 3-22 (continued)

Head lift corrective exercise: (1) Position of the patient is supine hook-lying with her hands crossed over midline at the diastasis to support the area. (2) As the patient exhales, the patient lifts only the head off the floor or until the point just before a bulge appears. (3) The patient's hands should gently pull the Rectus muscles toward midline. (4) Then the patient should lower the head slowly and relax.

Head lift with pelvic tilt corrective exercise: (1) Patient is positioned supine hook-lying. (2) If Diastasis Recti is present, the arms are crossed over the diastasis and pulled toward midline. (3) The patient slowly lifts the head off the floor while performing a posterior pelvic tilt. Then slowly lowers the head and relaxes. (4) All abdominal contractions should be performed with an exhalation so the intra-abdominal pressure is minimized.

Guidelines for Obstetric Exercise Instruction: It is suggested that supine positioning not exceed 5 minutes at any one time after the fourth month of pregnancy to avoid vena cava compression by the uterus. When supine, a small wedge or rolled towel should be placed under the right hip (to lessen the effects of uterine compression on abdominal vessels and to improve cardiac output by turning the patient slightly toward the left). Left side lying is the best position for pregnancy.

Recommendations for Obstetric Aerobic Exercise[6]: (1) It is preferable that the patient exercises regularly at least 3 times per week rather than intermittently. (2) Non-weight-bearing aerobic exercises such as stationary cycling or swimming should be used to minimize the risk of injury but, if able, the patient may continue activities such as running and aerobic dancing. (3) Resumption of pre-pregnancy exercise routines during the postpartum period should be gradually resumed. (4) Physiologic and morphologic changes of pregnancy continue for 4 to 6 weeks postpartum.

Absolute Contraindications to Obstetric Aerobic Exercises: Incompetent cervix, early dilation of the cervix before the pregnancy is full term, vaginal bleeding of any amount, placenta previa, rupture of membranes (loss of amniotic fluid prior to the onset of labor), premature labor, maternal heart disease, maternal diabetes or hypertension, intrauterine growth retardation.

Precautions to Obstetric Aerobic Exercises: multiple gestation, anemia, systemic infection, extreme fatigue, musculoskeletal complaints and/or pain, overheating, phlebitis, diastasis recti, uterine contractions.

Suggested Sequence for Obstetric Aerobic Exercise Class: warm up; gentle selective stretching exercises; aerobic activity for cardiovascular conditioning (15 minutes or less); upper and lower extremity strengthening; cool down activities.

Physical Agents and Modalities: Indications and Applications

Table 3-23   Physical Agents and Modalities: Indications and Applications

Physical Agent/ Modality	Indications	Applications
Note: For contraindications and precautions, see Part I, Section 8 (Table 1-62).		
Therapeutic heat (hot moist pack)	Joint stiffness; musculoskeletal pain and muscle spasm; preparation for electrical stimulation and massage; subacute, chronic, and traumatic conditions	Hot moist pack (HMP) is placed in terry cloth cover and wrapped in six to eight layers of dry towels; HMP is placed on patient's treated area. Another towel is placed over the hot pack to minimize heat loss. HMP must be secured well to the patient using towels, pillows, or straps if necessary. If patient is lying on the HMP, additional towels (more than eight layers) are necessary. The PTA monitors the patient's treated area after 5 to 10 minutes of HMP application. The patient receives a call bell to alert the PTA of any sensory changes.[8]
Whirlpool	Wound care; wound debridement; postsurgical orthopedic conditions such as for hip, knee, and ankle; subacute and chronic musculoskeletal conditions; rheumatoid arthritis	PTA assists patient immersing body or body part into the whirlpool tank. The PTA uses towels to pad any pressure points and minimize compression on tank edges. The PTA adjusts the agitator for position, force, direction, depth, and aeration. The PTA monitors the patient's response and tolerance

continues

Types of Musculoskeletal Interventions   **167**

MUSCULOSKELETAL INTERVENTIONS

Table 3-23   (continued)

Physical Agent/ Modality	Indications	Applications
		to treatment. Patients who have most of the body immersed in the whirlpool (such as in a Hubbard Tank) need close monitoring. The patient may also need a cold compress (and a cool drink). Insert tank liner for hepatitis and open wounds, burns, and HIV. Hubbard tank—closely monitor patient's physiological responses. Temperatures: limbs = 103°F to 110°F; open wound = 92°F to 96°F; MS = 88°F; PVD = 95°F to 100°F.[8]
Paraffin bath	Subacute and chronic inflammatory conditions such as RA, OA, joint stiffness, hand contracture, or scleroderma	Glove method: PTA washes patient's hands (or feet) prior to treatment. PTA inspects patient's hands (or feet) for infection, wounds, or cuts. The patient's sensation and heat tolerance is assessed. The patient is instructed not to touch sides or bottom of paraffin container and to avoid movements that could crack the paraffin. The patient is instructed first to dip the treated part into paraffin, creating a higher first layer of paraffin. Then other layers lower than the first one will follow. The patient is instructed to dip the treated part in paraffin until 6 to 12 layers are formed. The PTA wraps the treated part in plastic and towels.

Aquatic therapy	Relaxation and improvement of circulation; muscle strengthening; gait training with decreased stress on weight-bearing joints; mobility training for RA, OA, joint replacements, MS, and paraplegia	The patient needs to shower before immersion in the water. The type of water activity and duration of treatment are dependent on the patient's tolerance. General pool temperature = 92°F to 98°F; MS = 84°F; spasticity (20 to 45 minutes) = 86°F to 94°F; RA/OA (10 to 20 minutes) = 96.8°F to 98.6°F .
Ultraviolet (UV) radiation	Acne; subacute and chronic psoriasis; decubitus ulcers; infected wounds	Dependent on the MED test and types of UV lamps. MED = smallest UV exposure time to produce faint erythema 8 hours post exposure. MED subsides within 24 hours. First-degree erythema is 2.5 the MED (appears 6 hours after exposure). It presents with definite redness with desquamation, and lasts for 1-3 days. Second-degree erythema is 5.0 times the MED (appears 2 hours after exposure). It presents with intense erythema with edema and peeling, looking as severe sunburn. Third-degree erythema is 10.0 times the MED. It appears after the exposure test as erythema with severe blistering, peeling, and exudation. Treatment time = proportion of the MED.
Ultrasound (US): thermal US (TUS); pulsed US (PUS); phonophoresis	Thermal US: joint contractures; muscle spasm; musculoskeletal pain; subacute and chronic traumatic and inflammatory conditions; prior to stretch-	Can be applied: direct contact and indirect contact using water (or a balloon). Deeper tissues (2.5 to 5 cm) need 1-MHz frequency. Less deep tissues (1 to 2.5 cm) need 3-MHz frequency. PTA places transducer parallel to patient's skin

MUSCULOSKELETAL INTERVENTIONS

continues

Types of Musculoskeletal Interventions **169**

Table 3-23   (continued)

Physical Agent/ Modality	Indications	Applications
	ing shortened soft tissue; reduction of pain. Pulsed US: tissue healing of dermal ulcers, surgical skin incisions, tendon injuries, bone fractures; acute conditions (where thermal US is contraindicated)	moving it in slow circular movements. The transducer is always in firm contact (but not heavy) with patient's skin. Transducer must not be held in the air (without skin contact) when the US is on. For the TUS periosteal pain: decrease intensity; increase treatment surface area. For the TUS "hot spot:" apply more coupling agent; decrease intensity; keep the transducer moving. Use plastic container for US in the water (transducer must be 0.5 inch to 1 inch from patient's skin). TUS intensity = 0.2 watts/cm^2 to 3.0 watts/cm^2. PUS intensity = 0.2 watts/cm^2 to 1.0 watts/cm^2. Treatment time TUS/PUS = 5 to 10 minutes per treated area. PUS duty cycles: 10%, 20%, and 50%. Phonophoresis: applied direct contact continuous mode TUS or direct contact pulsed mode PUS. Apply US gel and the medication. Do not whip medication into US gel (air can be trapped in the mixture decreasing transmission of US). Phonophoresis intensities: direct contact continuous mode = 1.0 to 2.0 watts/cm^2; direct contact pulsed mode = 0.5 to 0.75 watts/cm^2 (20% duty cycle).[9]

| Fluidotherapy | Subacute and chronic musculoskeletal conditions such as rheumatoid arthritis, osteoarthritis, muscular pain, reflex sympathetic dystrophy; any other disorder where it promotes desensitization of hypersensitive tissues | Cover with a plastic barrier: open wounds; lesions. Safe to use with patients having splints, bandages, tape, metal implants, artificial tendons, or plastic joint replacements. Procedure: PTA places UE in a sleeve (of the machine) or LE over the treatment slot. The PTA sets the desired temperature and turns the unit on. The PTA adjusts agitation of cellulose (or silicone) particles to desired effect and patient's tolerance. The PTA instructs the patient in stretching or strengthening exercises during treatment. For desensitization, the PTA monitors the patient's response to treatment. Treatment time = 15 to 20 minutes. |
| Diathermy: short-wave (SW); microwave (MW) | Same as thermal US for thermal effects of SW/MW diathermy. Nonthermal or pulsed SW diathermy: wound care to decrease pain and edema, to increase oxygen to the tissue, and to increase muscle, bone, and nerve tissue repair by stimulation of protein synthesis at tissue cell level | Check patient often during treatment—the treated area is not visible. SW diathermy delivers thermal or pulsed electromagnetic field. SW frequency used most = 27.12 MHz. (1) SW diathermy treated area part of electrical circuit method: patient's area placed between two conducting electrodes for 15 to 30 minutes. (2) SW inductive field method: patient's treated area into a magnetic field of electrodes and current induced within patient's body tissues (are not part of circuit). Tissue resistance to current produces increased temperature in deep body tissues. (3) MW diathermy |

continues

Table 3-23 (continued)

Physical Agent/ Modality	Indications	Applications
		applied using electromagnetic radiation directed through a coaxial cable to an antenna mounted in the treatment applicator. Caution using MW diathermy: when energy is reflected at fat/muscle and muscle/bone interfaces; it can increase superficial tissues' temperatures (skin or fat). Treatment time MW Diathermy = 15 to 30 minutes
Therapeutic cold: cold pack (CP); ice pack (IP); ice massage with ice cube (IC)	CP/IP: acute and chronic traumatic and inflammatory conditions; edema; muscle spasm; musculoskeletal pain; thermal burns. Ice massage with IC: small areas of muscle guarding; muscle spasm; acute injuries to decrease pain, edema, and hemorrhage	First treatment: monitor adverse effects (such as urticaria; facial flush; anaphylaxis; call EMS for anaphylaxis). Patient's normal response to ice: cold, burning, aching, and numbness (CBAN). (1) CP wrapped in a warm moist towel placed on patient's treated area; place two to three dry towels over CP. Secure CP to patient with elastic bandages or towels. The PTA monitors the patient's treated area visually after 5 minutes. The patient receives a call bell. The patient should not lie on CP. Treatment time = 10 to 20 minutes. (2) IP the same as CP except IP should be placed in dry towels. (3) IC for ice massage must be round without sharp edges. IC applied in overlapping circles or overlap-

		ping longitudinal strokes, each stroke covering one half of the previous stroke. Treated area = 4 inches by 6 inches. The PTA should not do ice massage over bony area or superficial nerves (such as the peroneal nerve in the lower leg). The PTA uses a towel to wipe the excess water as it melts on the skin. Treatment time = 5 to 10 min.
Contrast Bath	Peripheral vascular disease; impaired peripheral blood circulation in the limbs; sprains and strains; edema; acute trauma.	Check water temperature: Hot (warm) = 100°F to 110°F; Cold = 55°F to 65°F. Select water based on patient's condition: PVD = 105° hot and 65° cold; open wounds add disinfectant. Prepare two pails of water. The PTA first immerses the patient's treated limb in hot water for 6 to 10 minutes. The PTA transfers the patient's treated limb in cold water for 1 minute. The PTA transfers the patient's treated limb in hot water again for 4 minutes. The PTA continues sequence of immersion for 20 to 30 minutes. The PTA ends treatment in hot water (condition determines ending in hot or cold water). For edema or acute sprains/strains is more beneficial to end in cold water.
Therapeutic Massage[9]	Subacute and chronic pain; muscle spasm; superficial scar formation and adhesions from trauma or burns;	Effleurage: PTA's hand molded over patient's body part, and movement is distal to proximal. Pétrissage is grasping, lifting, squeezing, or pressing of tissues

continues

MUSCULOSKELETAL INTERVENTIONS

Types of Musculoskeletal Interventions   **173**

Table 3-23   (continued)

Physical Agent/ Modality	Indications	Applications
	edema; postural drainage. Deep transverse friction can help to effect collagen fiber orientation in wound healing	(compression for sports massage). Friction is performed by rubbing repeatedly one surface over another. Deep friction is used to stretch scar tissues and loosen adhesions (cross-fiber friction are deep strokes across direction of muscle fibers; deep transverse friction is a specific cross fiber friction applied to site of a granulated wound for scar formation). Tapotement is a series of brisk percussive movements following each other in a rapid, alternating manner (hacking, cupping, slapping, tapping, and pincement). Cupping is applied to chest to mobilize bronchial secretions in pulmonary physical therapy. Vibration is an oscillating, trembling motion performed rapidly and repeatedly for postural drainage to loosen adherent secretions.
Intermittent Compression	Chronic edema; lymphedema (after mastectomies); venous stasis ulcer; traumatic edema; venous insufficiency; amputation	PTA takes patient's BP. The patient is positioned comfortably with UE or LE abducted between 20° and 70°, and elevated at approximately 40°. Before application of compression sleeve, a stockinette is put on removing all the wrinkles of the fabric. The compression sleeve is applied and the rubber tubing is attached to the sleeve and the pump. Set three

parameters: inflation pressure (to be set below the patient's diastolic BP), inflation and deflation time (to be set at ratio 3:1, inflating 80 to 100 seconds. and deflating 25 to 35 seconds), and total treatment time (2 to 3 hours). For amputation, inflate sleeve 40 to 60 seconds and deflate for 10 to 15 seconds. Lymphedema requires a treatment time of 2- to 3-hr daily sessions; venous stasis ulcer requires 2.5 hours, three times per week.

Electrical stimulation (ES): HVPC; NMES; FES; IFC[9]

Decrease muscle spasm using (1) tetanic contractions to fatigue the muscle, (2) muscle pump effect to obtain rhythmic contraction and relaxation of the muscle, and (3) muscle pump effect using ultrasound with electrical stimulation to increase muscle tissue temperature and obtain a pumping effect; increase or maintain joint ROM by decreasing joint pain and edema; increase muscle strength through muscle reeducation exercises; repair of the soft tissue in wound healing; decrease edema; decrease spasticity;

(1) High-voltage pulsed current (HVPC): (A) acute-stage edema control (frequency of 120 pps, continuous mode, with pulse between 20 to 100 msec for 30 min, four times per day); it has long-lasting effect; (B) postacute edema control (frequency of less than 20 pps, with a duty cycle of 2 to 10 seconds on and 2 to 10 seconds off, for 15 to 60 minutes, 2 to 3 times per week); it has muscle pumping effect; (C) wound healing (negative polarity for bactericidal effect; positive polarity for wound closure); a gauze pad with sterile saline solution applied first over wound; small active electrode is attached to gauze (dressing); large dispersive electrode is placed ipsilateral, proximal to wound. (2) Neuromuscular electrical stimulation (NMES): (A) muscular strengthening and reeducation (Russian stimulation)

continues

MUSCULOSKELETAL INTERVENTIONS

Table 3-23   (continued)

Physical Agent/ Modality	Indications	Applications
	denervated muscle. Interferential current (IFC): pain relief; muscle relaxation; edema control; increased circulation; tissue and bone healing	achieved using isometric muscular contractions (frequency between 50 to 80 pps; duty cycle = 1:5; treatment time = 10 to 30 minutes); (B) muscular endurance (frequency is 30 to 50 pps.; duty cycle is 6 to 15 seconds on and 6 to 15 seconds off; treatment time = 5 to 20 minutes and up to several hours per day); (C) spasticity (ES applied to antagonist of spastic muscle; frequency = 30 to 50 pps; duty cycle of 2 to 10 seconds on and 2 to 10 seconds off; treatment time = 10 to 30 minutes, two times per day); (D) for peripheral circulation (frequency of 50 to 200 pps; treatment time = 20 to 60 minutes); (E) stimulation of denervated muscle (controversial). (3) Functional electrical stimulation (FES): most common use is to control for foot drop (ankle dorsiflexors and evertor muscles during the swing phase of gait; frequency of 30 to 50 pps, with a duty cycle of 6 to 15 seconds on and 6 to 15 seconds off; AC carrier must have frequency of 2,500 Hz). (4) Interferential current (IFC): (A) pain relief (four electrodes placed diagonally to one another over large areas of treatment; frequency = 80 to 100 pps); (B) circulation and edema control (two electrode placement

over or around small areas of treatment; frequency = 20 to 40 pps); (C) for circulation through muscle contraction (frequency of 35 to 50 pps and pulse duration of 125 to 200 msec). Application of ES: PTA checks that all controls are at zero before turning on device. The PTA can shave patient's hair on top of treated skin or can rub alcohol on the skin to reduce amount of skin oil. The PTA selects two or four electrodes for size. The PTA prepares and places electrodes on patient's area that needs to be treated. The space between two electrodes must be at least the diameter of one electrode. The PTA secures electrodes to patient's treated area. The PTA sets appropriate frequency, waveform, and modulation rate. The PTA adjusts intensity to achieve optimal treatment effects. After 3 to 4 minutes of treatment PTA needs to slightly increase intensity due to patient's accommodation. At end of treatment, PTA slowly decreases intensity to zero before lifting electrodes from treated area. The PTA turns all controls to zero.

MUSCULOSKELETAL INTERVENTIONS

| Iontophoresis | Neuritis; bursitis; musculoskeletal inflammatory condition; calcific tendonitis; muscular relaxation; softening of scar tissue and adhesions; reducing | Check for intact skin; no scratches or abrasions. Use negative medication for (–) electrode and positive medication for (+) electrode; use low levels of current intensity for (–) electrode; (–) electrode must be twice as large as |

continues

Table 3-23 (continued)

Physical Agent/ Modality	Indications	Applications
	calcium deposits; decreasing edema; skin conditions such as ischemic ulcers, hyperhydrosis, and fungal infections	(+) electrode. Alkaline chemical reactions caused by negative polarity are stronger than acidic reactions. Carrier frequency = 2,500 Hz or 4,000 Hz. The electrical wave form is DC (monophasic, continuous current). Recommended dosage is: for positive electrode is 1.0 mA/cm^2 and for negative electrode is 0.5 mA/cm^2. The current must be started, terminated, or interrupted slowly, never abruptly. The current intensity must be lower than 4.0 mA. The treatment time varies from 10 to 40 minutes depending on medication dose. For example, if current intensity of 4.0 mA was comfortable to patient and a dosage of 80.0 mA/min of dexamethasone is applied, this dexamethasone dosage can be delivered in 20 min ($4 \times 20 = 80$). The PTA observes treated area every 3 to 5 minutes being alert for any adverse reactions. Negative meds: dexamethasone, acetate, salicylate (DAS). Positive med. used most: lidocaine.
Transcutaneous electrical nerve stimulation (TENS):	Pain management and pain modulation through activation of Gate Control Theory	Patient education for use of TENS units: not to be used in shower or when sleeping; electrode placement; skin inspection—skin irri-

conventional TENS; acupuncture-like or strong low rate TENS; point stimulation TENS	and endogenous opiate theory	tation; checking adherence of electrodes to the skin; accommodation to ES (patient to contact PT/PTA—modulation TENS). (1) Conventional TENS: frequency (between 50 to 200 pps); pulse duration (between 50 to 100 msec); uses gate theory mechanism; has fast pain relief; is short-lasting (approximately 1 hour). (2) Acupuncture-like or strong low rate TENS (frequency between 1 to 20 pps); Burst mode TENS (frequency between 50 to 100 pps sent in bursts or packets of 1 to 5 pps); point stimulation TENS or neuroprobe for trigger points or acupuncture points (frequency between 1 to 5 pps): all use the endogenous opiate theory, and all are long-lasting pain relief TENS.
Traction: cervical; lumbar	Spinal nerve root impingement caused by herniated nucleus pulposus (HNP) or spinal stenosis; muscle spasm; spinal hypomobility; muscle inflammation; subacute and chronic joint pain; spinal pain	Cervical traction—observe patient for discomfort in the TMJ—adjust head halter and insure force is applied to occipital region. For treated segment lower than C2, cervical spine must be positioned in 20° to 30° of spinal flexion. For nerve root impingement, cervical spine must be positioned in 15° of spinal flexion. Force of the traction not to exceed the weight of the patient's head. Start at 8 to 10 pounds (or 7% of patient's head weight). Increase force gradually up to 25 to 30 pounds. Research showed best force = 10 pounds. Maximum elongation occurs at

MUSCULOSKELETAL INTERVENTIONS

continues

Table 3-23   (continued)

Physical Agent/ Modality	Indications	Applications
		24° of spinal flexion. Treatment time = 5 to 10 minutes for HNP and 10 to 30 minutes for others. Initially static and then intermittent at 15 seconds on and 15 seconds off. Disc problems use 60 seconds on and 20 seconds off; muscular spasm use 5 seconds on and 5 seconds off. Lumbar traction—prone positions for posterior HNP. To increase L5-S1 space—use a small bench under patient's lower legs (45° to 60° of hip flexion). Start with low force traction—use split table and 25% of the patient's body weight. Increase force gradually to half of the patient's body weight (to effect intervertebral separation). Split table decreases leg/pelvis friction. Treatment time for HNP = 5 minutes at first and then increase to10 minutes; use 10 to 30 minutes for others. Initially begin with static and then intermittent (joint distraction) 15 seconds on and 15 seconds off. Muscle spasm use 5 seconds on and 5 seconds off; disc problems use 60 seconds on and 20 seconds off.
Electromyographic biofeedback	Muscle recruitment and strengthening in patients with periph-	Patients receiving EMG biofeedback must have good vision, good hearing, excellent communication abil-

| (EMG biofeedback) | eral nerve injury, muscle weakness caused by immobilization, joint surgery, pain, deconditioning, muscle spasticity, and re-education of weak or flaccid muscle. Relaxation for chronic pain such as tension headaches, and chronic neck and back pain | ities, good comprehension of simple commands, good concentration, and motor planning skills. Bipolar technique = two active electrodes are applied parallel to muscle fibers at approximately 15 cm, over or near motor points of treated muscles; reference electrode applied between actives or closer to active electrodes. To increase muscular strength of two or more weak muscles: PTA places two active electrodes widely spaced; to increase muscular strength of one weak muscle: PTA places two active electrodes close together; instrument sensitivity must be high for one or two or more weak muscles; PTA to instruct patient to contract muscle isometrically holding for as long as possible (up to 10 seconds) to produce a tall and loud audiovisual signal. As patient's motor recruitment improves, active electrodes must be placed closer together and instrument sensitivity decreased. For relaxation: PTA places two active electrodes closely spaced; instrument sensitivity must be low; PTA instructs patient to relax and to lower audiovisual signal; PTA applies breathing or imagery exercises. As patient is able to relax, instrument sensitivity must be increased and patient should perform functional activities. Treatment time = first 5 minutes and then 10 to 30 minutes. |

MUSCULOSKELETAL INTERVENTIONS

Therapeutic Massage Application

Table 3-24   Application of Therapeutic Massage[9]

Application of massage: (1) When applying therapeutic massage to a specific anatomical region of the patient's body, the patient should be comfortable in a relaxed position. (2) The treatment part should be in a gravity eliminated position or in a position in which the gravity assists the venous flow. (3) The patient's body part must be draped and well supported. (4) The PTA should start with light effleurage and then advance to deep effleurage and other types of stroking necessary in that specific intervention. (5) When using all forms of massage, deep effleurage is followed by pétrissage, then friction, and then tapotement, concluding with vibration and light effleurage. (6) Massage should begin in the proximal segments of the lower or upper extremity and move distally and return to proximal region. (7) On the lower or upper extremity, all effleurage movements must be directed distal to proximal, especially for edema treatment. (8) Therapeutic massage treatment is dependent on the patient's tolerance and specific intervention. (9) As with other physical agents or modalities, therapeutic massage is a passive modality and should be used for a short period of time as an adjunct, not as a substitute, to active interventions such as therapeutic exercises and activities and patient education.

Orthotics

Table 3-25   Orthotics[10]

Orthopedic shoes

For the patient (client) with orthopedic impairments and functional limitations, the orthopedic shoes reduce pressure on sensitive deformed structures and are a foundation for AFOs and more extensive bracing. The most common orthopedic shoes are: (1) The Blucher lace stay (has a separation between anterior margin of the lace stay and the vamp; offers adjustability for edema). (2) The Balmoral lace stay (the lace stay is continuous with the vamp). (3) The Low Quarter Height shoe (below the malleoli); does not restrict foot or ankle motion. (4) The High Quarter height shoe (covers the malleoli); indicated for rigid pes equinus or to increase stability without an AFO. (5) Shoes with reinforcements. (6) Shoes with special soles. (7) Shoes with high heels or low heels.

Foot orthoses: appliances that apply forces to the foot. Can be soft inserts (made of viscoelastic plastics, rubber, rigid plastics, or metal); the Longitudinal arch support (LAS) (corrects for flat foot—pes planus). Examples of LAS are: (1) The Scaphoid pad (made of rubber); used under navicular bone. (2) The UCBL insert (applies medial force to calcaneus and lateral and upward force to medial midfoot). (3) The Thomas heel (corrects for pronated foot—flexible pes valgus). (4) The Metatarsal bar (takes pressure off metatarsal heads). (5) The Rocker bar (improves weight shift on metatarsals); helps in late stance. (6) The shoe lifts (for leg-length discrepancy). (7) The heel wedges (absorb forces at heel contact); alter alignment of calcaneus.

Ankle foot orthoses (AFOs): appliances made of a foundation, ankle control, foot control, and a superstructure. The foundation is made of a shoe and a plastic or metal component. The traditional foundation has a steel stirrup that can be solid stirrup (for maximum stability) or split stirrup (eases donning the orthosis). Types of AFOs: (1) Solid Ankle AFO (limits all foot and ankle motion); used for severe pain and instability; increases stride length and cadence in hemiplegia. (2) Hinged Solid Ankle AFO (similar to Solid Ankle AFO); provides slight sagittal motion for foot flat position in early stance; used for spastic diplegia in children. (3) Bichannel adjustable ankle locks (BiCAALs) is an alternative to Solid Ankle AFO; resists PF and DF. (4) Ypsilon AFO (carbon composite AFO); provides assistance to DF; used for mild to moderate isolated foot drop. (5) Anterior Stop AFO (limits ankle DF); prevents excessive knee flexion or "buckling"; helps in late stance of gait. (6) Posterior Stop AFO (limits ankle PF); prevents knee hyperextension/recurvatum. (7) Posterior Leaf Spring AFO (provides DF assistance); used for foot drop. (8) Steel DF Spring Assist AFO—Klenzak Joint (has DF spring assist in each stirrup); provides DF assistance; used for foot drop—bulkier than posterior leaf. (9) Toe Off AFO (provides DF assistance); used for mild to severe food drop and instability. (10) Spiral AFO (controls but does not eliminate motion in all planes); fits snugly for maximal control; contraindicated for fluctuating edema. (11) Silicone ankle foot orthosis (SAFO) is a contemporary AFO made of silicone for drop foot; provides a flexible dynamic function giving comfort and cosmesis for foot and ankle; good for heel strike with a smooth transition to toe off.

Other types of orthoses are: (1) Floor reaction force orthosis (type of Solid Ankle AFO); resists knee flexion; provides a knee extension moment to control knee flexion in stance. (2) Tone-reducing orthoses: plastic AFOs designed for spastic CP and spastic hemiplegia (apply constant pressure to plantaflexors and invertors); used for equinovarus and moderate spasticity with varus instability; patients achieve better foot and knee control; contraindicated in fixed deformity. (3) Supramalleolar orthosis: used for the ankle to maintain foot in neutral alignment; allows ankle DF/PF; does not offer knee control; used for spastic diplegia. (4) Stabilizing boots AFOs: custom-made AFOs for paraplegia (used by adults); conform to patient's legs and feet; feet angled at 15° PF; legs angled posterior to keep knees extended; patient keeps stability leaning backward; used with crutches or walker.

continues

Types of Musculoskeletal Interventions **183**

Table 3-25 (continued)

Knee ankle foot orthosis (KAFO): appliances made of a shoe, foundation, ankle control, and superstructure. KAFO may include also foot control. KAFO controls for knee flexion/extension and genu valgum and genu varum; used for paralysis or limb deformity. Most common knee flexion or extension control of a KAFO is the drop ring lock (may have the spring-loaded retention buttons to unlock each upright; the pawl lock with bail release for simultaneous locking of uprights); drop ring lock and pawl lock are contraindicated with knee flexion contracture. Sagittal stability of KAFO uses: the leather kneecap; rigid anterior band (made of plastic; can be suprapatellar or pretibial bands; both do not interfere with sitting; easier to don); the electronic stance control mechanism (newer; prevents knee flexion in stance without interfering with knee extension; permits knee flexion in swing). Frontal plane knee control (for genu varum or genu valgum) uses: plastic calf shells (semirigid shell for valgum applies lateral force at the knee; semirigid shell for varum applies medial force at the knee); valgum correction strap (knee cap with a fifth strap buckled around lateral upright; less effective than semirigid shells). Specialized newer KAFO: KAFO with computer controlled knee joint. Craig Scott KAFO: custom-made KAFO for paraplegia (used by adults). It includes shoe reinforced with transverse and longitudinal plates; BiCAAL AFO set in slight DF; pawl lock with bail release; single thigh band. It allows patient to stand with backward lean to prevent untoward hip or trunk flexion. The walkabout orthosis: custom-made pair of KAFOs permitting hip flexion and extension and restricting hip abduction, adduction, and rotation.

Hip knee ankle foot orthosis (HKAFO): KAFO with added pelvic band and hip joints. HKAFO controls for hip abduction, adduction, rotation, and flexion. To reduce internal or external rotation, you can use a strap. To reduce flexion, a drop ring lock can be added.

Trunk hip knee ankle foot orthosis (THKAFO): HKAFO with a metal band to anchor the trunk. THKAFO is not widely used because it is difficult to don, the metal band is uncomfortable, and restricts ambulation in swing to or swing through (when the hip joints are locked). Reciprocating gait orthosis (RGO): custom-made THKAFO. It has the hips joined by one or two metal cables or rods, the knees stabilized with knee locks (offset knee joints or pretibial bands), and the feet with solid AFOs. It is used for bilateral lower extremities and trunk paralysis. The patient can walk with crutches (using four or two point gait) by shifting weight to the right, tucking the pelvis (by extending the upper thorax), pressing on the crutches, and allowing the left leg to swing through. The same but in reverse procedure follows for the right leg to swing.

Standing frames (for standing without crutches; used for children or adults); swivel walker (for standing and twirling without crutches; used for children and adults; similar to standing frames except for the slightly rocking base to enable a swiveling gait); parapodium (for standing and performing activities without crutches; allows sitting; used for children and adults; children can also move from place to place by rotating the upper torso to shift weight causing the frame to rock and rotate).

Corset: used for low back musculoskeletal disorders, sacroiliac support and for SCI (assists with respiration). The corset increases intra–abdominal pressure but reduces frontal movement. The increase in the intra–abdominal pressure reduces stress on the posterior spinal musculature diminishing the load on the lumbar intervertebral disks.

Lumbosacral orthoses (LSOs): control or limit flexion, extension, and lateral control. Examples: LS flexion extension lateral control orthosis (LS FEL) (such as Knight spinal orthosis) that controls flexion, extension, and lateral flexion. Alternate version of LS FEL is used for spondylolisthesis (controls extension). LS FEL for low back pain is controversial. A plastic LS FEL jacket restricts motion in all directions.

Thoracolumbosacral orthoses (TLSOs): limit flexion and extension (and gross spinal movement). TLSO amount of movement varies from one person to another. Examples are TLSO flexion/extension (such as Taylor brace), which may be used for SCI.

Cervical orthoses are: (1) Soft foam rubber collar (may be used for whiplash; gives minimal support). (2) Four poster orthosis (may be used for cervical fracture and SCI; gives moderate support). (3) Halo orthosis or Minerva orthosis (may be used for cervical fracture and SCI; gives maximal support).

Scoliotic curves orthoses are: (1) Cervical thoracic lumbosacral orthosis (CTLSO) such as the Milwaukee (the oldest orthosis for scoliosis) that may be used for all kyphotic and scoliotic curves of 40° or less. (3) TLSO such as Boston that is used for midthoracic or lower scoliosis of 40° or less curves; also used for spondylolisthesis and conditions with severe trunk weakness such as muscular dystrophy. Other TLSOs for scoliosis are: (4) Wilmington (has tight contact and fit; is custom made); (5) The Charleston bending brace and the Providence brace (to wear only at night when the effects of gravity are at minimum; provide overcorrection of spinal curve).

Externally powered orthoses: pneumatic foot control or functional electrical stimulation (FES)—enable patients to ambulate in their residences or in the community (in rare cases). FES uses electrical stimulation (ES) to the quadriceps and gluteus maximus. The peroneal nerves may also use ES (to initiate DF and reflex hip flexion) if the ankles are not supported by bilateral AFOs. To use the FES, the patient (client) needs full passive mobility in all joints and to be able to control the timing and the amount of electrical current to transfer from a chair to the standing position and to walk in different directions.

Types of Musculoskeletal Interventions **185**

Orthotic Interventions

Table 3-26 Orthotic Interventions

Patient education for skin inspection, orthosis care, and donning/doffing the orthosis.

AROM, PROM, and static and dynamic balance and gait training using the orthosis.

Assessments or reassessments are: (1) Assessment of the discrepancy of limb length. (2) Assessment of sensation.

Functional activities using the orthosis. Traditional MMT for muscle function if permitted. In cases of spasticity, you may use functional tests of motor performance (see Part 4, Section 1)

Assessment and reassessment of gait deviations using the orthosis. Examples of common gait deviations and possible causes are: (1) Lateral trunk bend in early stance (caused by: medial upright of the KAFO may be too high; excessive abduction of hip joint of HKAFO; requires a cane; insufficient shoe lift; weak gluteus medius; abduction contracture; hip pain; poor balance; short leg). (2) Circumduction during swing (caused by: the knee may be locked; may have excessive PF; inadequate PF stop; inadequate DF assist; weak hip flexors; extensor synergy; weak dorsiflexors; pes equinus; knee or ankle ankylosis). (3) Hyperextended knee in early stance (caused by: inadequate PF stop or knee lock; pes equinus; weak quads; extensor synergy; short contralateral LE; contralateral knee or hip flexion contracture). (4) Knee instability in early stance (caused by: too much knee flexion; inadequate knee lock; inadequate DF stop; weak quads; knee pain; knee or hip flexion contracture; flexor synergy; short contralateral LE). (5) Foot slap in early stance (caused by: weak DF; inadequate dorsiflexor assist; inadequate plantarflexion stop). (6) Flat foot contact during early stance (caused by: inadequate DF stop; inadequate traction from the sole; requires a cane; poor balance; pes calcaneus). (7) Anterior trunk bending in early stance—leans forward as weight is transferred to LE (caused by: inadequate knee lock; weak quads; hip and knee flexion contracture). (8) Posterior trunk bending in early stance—leans backward as weight is transferred to LE (caused by: inadequate hip lock; knee lock; weak gluteus maximus; knee ankylosis). (9) Hip hiking in swing (caused by: knee lock; inadequate DF stop; inadequate PF stop; short contralateral LE; weak hip flexors; extensor synergy; weak dorsiflexors; pes equinus; knee and ankle ankylosis). (10) Vaulting (exaggerated PF of contralateral LE) in swing (caused by: knee lock; inadequate DF and PF assist; weak hip flexors; pes equinus; extensor spasticity; short contralateral LE; weak dorsiflexors; knee or ankle ankylosis).

Transitibial (Below Knee) Prostheses

Table 3-27   Below Knee Amputation Prostheses[10]

Foot and ankle assembly: nonarticulated feet that are light in weight, durable, attractive, and most popular. Types of nonarticulated feet are: (1) Solid ankle cushion heel (SACH) foot (simple design; least cost; lowest function; permits PF in early stance; absorbs shock; hyperextends in late stance). (2) Stationary attachment flexible endoskeleton (SAFE) foot (good on uneven terrain; permits medial–lateral motion in the rear foot; heavier and more expensive than SACH).

Foot and ankle assembly: articulated feet that have a metal bolt or cable; are shock absorbent; control plantarflexion; have dorsiflexion stop; can loosen over time. Types of articulated feet are: (1) Single axis feet (most common; permits PF, DF, and toe break; does not allow medial–lateral or transverse motion). Single axis feet may use rotators (components placed above the prosthetic foot to absorb shock in the transverse plane; used with active individuals who had transfemoral amputations). (2) Multiple axis feet (move slightly in all planes for maximum contact with irregular walking surface; reduce shearing forces on residual limb; heavier and less durable than single axis or nonarticulated feet). Other types of foot and ankle prosthetic componentry include: (3) Energy storing, dynamic elastic response. (4) Energy storing with multiaxial features. (5) Energy storing with vertical shock pylon. Energy storing and dynamic response feet have internal structures that absorb energy during stance and release energy at toe off. They provide a smoother and more energy efficient gait; are extremely lightweight and durable. Examples of energy storing dynamic response feet are: Flex Foot, Springlite Foot (weights under 11 ounces; has shock absorption and smooth transition to midstance and toe off), Seattle Foot, and Carbon Copy II foot (is energy storing and energy releasing or dynamic feet; can be used to play basketball or to run).

Exoskeletal and endoskeletal shanks (substitution for human leg): Exoskeletal shank is made of wood or rigid plastic. Endoskeletal shank is made of aluminum or rigid plastic pylon covered with foam rubber and a sturdy stocking or similar finish. The pylon permits slight adjustment.

Transtibial socket: plastic receptacle for the amputated foot. Below-Knee amputation (BKA) requires a patellar tendon bearing (PTB) socket (has a prominent indentation over patellar tendon). Newer BKA sockets are hypobaric (with total surface bearing; no indentation). These sockets are custom made through a computer-aided design (CAD) or computer-aided manufacture (CAM). An electronic sensor transmits a detailed map of the limb to a computerized program consisting of socket shaped variations. The prosthetist selects the appropriate shape and transmits it to an electronic carver that creates the model and then the plastic is

continues

Types of Musculoskeletal Interventions   **187**

Table 3-27   (continued)

shaped over the computer generated model. Sockets have "reliefs," which are concavities over sensitive areas such as bony prominences. Sockets can be unlined made of thin thermoplastic with removable liners (polyethylene foam liners). "Buildups" are convexities in the socket over pressure tolerant areas. Transtibial socket usually has a polyethylene foam liner that is removable. Other sockets made of thin thermoplastic in a rigid frame can be unlined. These types of sockets adhere to the skin better than rigid plastic sockets improving prosthetic suspension. Plastic sockets or socket liners should be washed to keep it clean, especially in warm climates.

Suspension: to hold the prosthesis in place—can be supracondylar cuff or suprapatellar suspension. Supracondylar cuff suspension increases medial lateral stability of the prosthesis. Supracondylar/suprapatellar (SC/SP) suspension has a high anterior wall that terminates above the patella, accommodating a short amputated limb. The only problem with SC/SP suspension may be that the anterior wall interferes with kneeling and is not cosmetically appealing in sitting. Modern transtibial prosthesis still use a supracondylar cuff suspension made of leather. It allows the patient (client) to adjust the tightness of the suspension. The suspension cuff may have a fork strap or a waist belt that are indicated for patients (clients) who climb ladders or perform long duration activities when the prosthesis is not supported on the ground. Patients with sensitive skin may need thigh corset suspension; however, prolonged use of a thigh corset suspension may produce pressure atrophy of the thigh, and it is also difficult to don. Another type of suspension may be the vacuum assisted socket suspension that promotes fluid exchange, increases proprioception, reduces moisture, and regulates edema fluctuations.

Transfemoral (Above Knee) Prostheses

Table 3-28   Above Knee Amputation Prostheses[10]

Foot and ankle assembly: the same as transtibial prostheses. SACH foot or single axis foot is used the most.

Knee unit: allows the user to bend the knee. It is made of axis (single axis hinge or polycentric linkage that has better stability); friction mechanism (can have constant or variable friction); extension aid (assists with knee extension in late swing phase of gait; can be external in front of knee axis and internal within the knee unit); and mechanical stabilizers (manual lock; friction brake). The knee unit uses constant friction (remains the same) or variable friction mechanisms (friction changes with high friction in early swing of gait, less friction in mid swing of gait and increase friction again in late swing of gait). The friction can be applied through the clamp sliding (is the least expensive), hydraulically (using oil), or pneumatically (using air). Hydraulic and pneumatic friction units are the best because they allow symmetrical movements. Another type of newer friction knee unit can use computer-programmed electronic sensors that provide almost instant friction adjustments in gait patterns accommodating various terrains and also bicycle riding. Knee extension mechanisms are external aid (made of elastic webbing; most simple; may pull knee in extension while sitting) and internal extension aid (elastic strap or coiled spring; keeps knee flexed when sitting; included in pneumatic/hydraulic units). Stabilizing mechanisms for knee units: manual lock (engaged pin lock prevents knee flexion; most simple; need to disengage pin lock in sitting); friction brake (one version in clamp sliding allows knee flexion to 25°; another version in hydraulic units stabilizes better). Types of newer computer-programmed electronic sensors for the knee unit: Rheo Knee (uses a knee's microprocessor that adjusts resistance during stance; maintains knee stability on uneven terrain; uses a lithium battery) and C-Leg (uses computerized sensors and hydraulic pistons; useful for stepping down out of a vehicle, and descending curbs, ramps, or stairs).

Transfemoral socket: quadrilateral socket (with a horizontal posterior shelf for ischial tuberosity and gluteal muscles) and ischial containment socket. Transfemoral sockets are made of flexible plastic (that provides sensory input from external objects) enclosed in a rigid frame that transmits weight to the ground. Concave "reliefs" are made for pressure sensitive areas and to allow contraction of gluteus maximus and rectus femoris. An alternate socket called ischial containment socket (or contoured adducted trochanter controlled alignment method socket - CAT-CAM) increases the entire transfemoral socket stability. Slight socket flexion allows hip extensors contraction to reduce lumbar lordosis for equal step length. An example of CAT-CAM is the Comfort Flex Socket System (also called the Hanger Comfort Flex Socket) combined with the Otto Bock C-Leg. This newer type of AKA prosthesis uses a microprocessor-controlled hydraulic knee with swing and stance control. It accommodates for uneven surfaces, stairs, slopes, biking, running, dancing, and golfing.

Suspension: total suction (provides maximum control of the prosthesis); partial suction (requires one or more socks or a silicone liner); no suction (has a distal hole; no pressure between inside and outside the socket; requires a pelvic band).

Prosthetics: Levels of Amputation

Table 3-29   Levels of Amputation

Toe disarticulation: amputation at the metatarsal phalangeal joint.

Transmetatarsal: amputation through the midsection of all metatarsals.

Symes ankle disarticulation with attachment of heel pad to distal end of tibia. It may include removal of tibial and fibular flares and both malleoli.

Transtibial amputation: below the knee amputation (BKA). Short BKA: less than 20% of tibial length. Long BKA: more than 50% of tibial length. Standard BKA: between 20% and 50% of tibial length.

Knee disarticulation: amputation through the knee joint (femur is intact).

Transfemoral amputation: above the knee amputation (AKA). Short AKA: less than 35% of femoral length. Long AKA: more than 60% of femoral length. Standard AKA: between 35% and 60% of femoral length.

Hip disarticulation: amputation through the hip joint (pelvis is intact).

Hemipelvectomy: resection of lower half of pelvis.

Hemicorporectomy: amputation of both lower extremities and pelvis (below L4–L5 level).

Prosthetics: Pressure Tolerant and Pressure Sensitive Areas

Table 3-30   Prosthetics: Pressure-Tolerant and Pressure-Sensitive Areas

Pressure Tolerant (Buildup) Areas	Pressure Sensitive (Relief) Areas
BKA:	**BKA:**
Patellar tendon	Fibular head and neck
Proximal and medial tibia (at pes anserinus)	Anterior tibial crest
Tibial and fibular shafts	Tibial condyles
Belly of gastrocnemius	Anterior distal tibia
	Medial and lateral hamstring tendons
AKA:	**AKA:**
Ischial tuberosity	Distolateral end of femur
Gluteals	Pubic symphysis
Lateral sides of residual limb	Perineal area
Distal end (rarely may be sensitive)	Adductor longus tendon

Prosthetic Interventions

Table 3-31   Prosthetic Interventions

Functional interventions: bed mobility; transfers; ADLs; gait training with prosthesis and assistive device (such as crutches, and walker for balance deficits); wheelchair training; mobility without prosthesis (for use at night).

Residual limb care: use of removable rigid dressing and temporary prosthesis (both help with early ambulation); residual limb wrapping (using elastic bandages and figure-of-eight technique); use of shrinker (easier to apply than elastic bandages); prevention of contracture (positioning the patient prone as much as possible during the day and attaching a posterior board to the wheelchair in sitting; to avoid knee flexion, and hip flexion, abduction, and ER).

Patient education: care of residual limb (including desensitizing activities, hygiene, and bandaging of residual limb); care of the uninvolved extremity; proper positioning; exercises; education about edema, pain, and changes in skin color; phantom limb—normal; phantom pain—abnormal and disabling; HEP.

Therapeutic exercises: individualized; AROM; stretching (for hip and knee extensors); strengthening (AKA needs strength in residual hip extensors and abductors mostly; BKA needs strength in residual knee extensors and flexors mostly); balance and coordination training.

Balance and coordination training: can start at parallel bars especially for patients with AKA prosthesis (because it is difficult to control the mechanical knee); static balance training on the amputated side; increasing gradually the prosthetic tolerance (to minimize skin abrasion). Some clinicians prefer not to use parallel bars because patients pull on them. When using parallel bars, encourage the patient to rest the hand on bars and not to grip on it hard. For patients who grip on parallel bars, use a sturdy mat platform table to start balance training with standing posture (equal weight bearing and without excessive lordosis). The PTA should stand near patient's prosthesis to encourage patient to shift weight symmetrical and in stepping movements (may use a mirror for visual feedback); patient to exercise in standing performing hip flexion (causes the knee to bend), hip extension (stabilizes the knee in stance); stepping on a low stool with involved and uninvolved LE (causes to shift weight symmetrically).

Transfer training: start with wheelchair (has armrest) to another w/c transfers (patient to transfer weight to uninvolved LE first, then push on w/c armrests); later practice w/c to mat and back, w/c to sofa (deep upholstered) and back, w/c to low chair and back, w/c to toilet and back, and w/c to automobile and back (patient to sit sideways with both feet out of the car door, then to pivot on the seat and swing the prosthesis into the car).

continues

Table 3-31   (continued)

Gait training: gait is progression from dynamic balance training; use PNF exercises; use rhythmic counting and walking with music to improve gait symmetry and speed; for patient who fatigues fast use an assistive device such as a cane (or two canes) or forearm crutches (careful because the patient may lean on axillary crutches). If the patient is able to ambulate indoors without cane, use the cane when ambulating outdoors (to negotiate curbs and on uneven surfaces). Patients with generalized weakness may need an aluminum walker (for maximum stability). The patient should not lean too far forward on the walker; for BKA prosthesis may use a two-wheeled walker (as opposed to a four legs walker) to increase speed.

Stairs (with rails), ramps, and curbs climbing: patients with BKA prosthesis having Syme's can ascend and descend stairs and inclines with equal step length; patients with unilateral AKA prosthesis ascend by leading with the uninvolved LE and descend by placing the involved LE on the lower step. The techniques are the same for curbs when no rails are available; when stairs, ramps, or curbs are too steep, patient (client) may ascend diagonally or sidestepping with the prosthesis on the downhill side.

Prosthetic gait deviation assessment for BKA: (1) Excessive knee flexion in early stance (causes: socket too far anterior; high shoe heel; insufficient PF; socket excessively flexed; stiff heel cushion; weak quads; knee flexion contracture). (2) Inadequate knee flexion in early stance (causes: socket too far posterior; socket not flexed enough; soft heel cushion; low heel shoe; excessive PF; weak quads; spastic quads). (3) Medial thrust at midstance (cause: excessive foot outset). (4) Lateral thrust at midstance (cause: excessive foot inset). (5) Premature knee flexion in late stance also called "drop-off" (causes: socket too far forward; high shoe heel; insufficient PF; socket flexed too much; DF stop too soft; knee flexion contracture). (6) Delayed knee flexion in late stance (causes: socket too far back; socket not flexed enough; DF stop too stiff; excessive PF; low shoe heel; extensor spasticity).

Prosthetic gait deviation assessment for AKA[10]: (1) Circumduction in swing (causes: prosthesis too long; locked knee unit; socket too small; loose socket; loose friction; inadequate suspension; foot in PF; abduction contracture). (2) Abducted gait in stance (causes: long prosthesis; inadequate lateral wall adduction; high or sharp medial wall; abduction contracture; weak abductors). (3) Lateral trunk bending in stance (causes: short prosthesis; low lateral wall; high or sharp medial wall; weak abductors; hip pain; abduction contracture). (4) Medial or lateral whip at heel off (causes: faulty socket contour; knee bolt rotated externally or internally; foot mal rotated). (5) Vaulting in swing (causes: too long prosthesis; too small socket; inadequate suspension; too little knee flexion). (6) Forward flexion in stance (causes: unstable knee unit; instability). (7) High heel rise in swing (causes: inadequate friction; too little tension in the extension aid). (8) Foot slap at heel contact (cause: stiff heel cushion). (9) Uneven step length (causes: insufficient socket flexion; uncomfortable socket; hip flexion contracture; instability).

Phases of Gait Cycles

Table 3-32   Phases of Gait Cycles—Traditional Versus RLA[9]

Heel strike	Initial contact
Heel strike to foot flat	Loading response
Foot flat to midstance	Midstance
Midstance to heel off	Terminal stance
Toe off	Preswing
Toe off to acceleration	Initial swing
Acceleration to midswing	Midswing
Midswing to deceleration	Terminal swing

Muscle Activation Patterns

Table 3-33   Muscle Activation Patterns[9]

Heel strike: person's heel contacts the ground. Muscles: quadriceps muscles and ankle dorsiflexors muscles (anterior tibialis, extensor hallucis longus, and extensor digitorum longus).

Foot flat: person's sole of the foot makes contact with the ground (immediately after the heel strike). Muscles: gastrocnemius and soleus.

Midstance: person's full body weight is taken by the reference extremity. Muscles: hip and ankle extensor muscles control the forward motion of the trunk; hip abductors stabilize the pelvis.

Heel off: after the midstance when the person's heel leaves the ground. Muscles: ankle plantarflexors have peak activity immediately after the heel off to propel the body forward.

Toe off: person's toe is still in contact with the ground. Muscles: hamstrings and quadriceps contribute to forward propulsion.

Acceleration: starts at the toe off of reference extremity until the midswing of the same reference extremity. Muscles: hip flexor muscles (iliopsoas) help to accelerate the extremity and propel it forward.

continues

Table 3-33 (continued)

Midswing: reference extremity moves directly beneath the person's body. Muscles: hip and knee flexor muscles and ankle dorsiflexors muscles contract to achieve foot clearance of reference extremity.

Deceleration: reference extremity is slowing down with the knee extended in preparation for heel strike. Muscles: hamstrings work hard to decelerate the reference extremity in preparation for the heel strike.

Common Gait Deviations: Stance Phase

Table 3-34   Gait Deviations—Stance Phase

Lateral bending of trunk: weak gluteus medius (Trendelenburg gait).

Backward leaning of trunk: weak gluteus maximus (difficulty walking stairs/ramps).

Forward leaning of trunk: weak quadriceps or hip/knee flexion contracture.

Excessive hip flexion: weak hip extensors or tight hip/knee flexors.

Decreased hip flexion: weak hip flexors or tight hip extensors.

Decreased hip extension: tight hip flexors.

Excessive knee flexion: weak quadriceps or knee flexion contracture (difficulty walking stairs/ramps).

Hyperextension of knee: weak (or tight) quadriceps or contracture of plantarflexors.

Toes contact at heel strike: weak dorsiflexors, tight plantarflexors, shorter leg, or painful heel.

Foot slap (steppage gait): weak dorsiflexors or excessive hip/knee flexion.

Foot flat: weak dorsiflexors (normal for children under 2 years of age).

Excessive dorsiflexion (calcaneus gait): weak plantarflexors.

Excessive plantarflexion (equinus gait): tightness or contracture of plantarflexors.

Varus foot throughout stance: weak peroneal or tight anterior tibialis.

Limited push off: weak plantarflexors or pain in forefoot.

Short stance on involved extremity and uneven gait pattern: pain in ambulation (antalgic gait).

Common Gait Deviations: Swing Phase

Table 3-35   Gait Deviations—Swing Phase

Limited pelvic retraction (forward rotation of pelvis): weak hip flexors and abdominals.

Limited hip and knee flexion: weak hip and knee flexors.

Circumduction: weak hip and knee flexors.

Hip hiking of quadratus lumborum: weak hip and knee flexors.

Excessive hip and knee flexion (steppage gait): shorter leg, tight plantarflexors, or weak dorsiflexors.

Limited knee flexion: tight quadriceps, weak hamstrings, or knee pain.

Excessive knee flexion: tight hamstrings.

Foot drop (equinus gait): weak dorsiflexors or tight plantarflexors.

Varus or inverted foot: weak peroneals or tight anterior tibialis.

Equinovarus: tight posterior tibialis and gastrocnemius and soleus.

Gait Training Points

Table 3-36   Gait Training Points

Key points of control while guarding the patient: patient's shoulder, the opposite pelvis, and the safety belt.

Patient loses balance forward: pull with one hand the patient back by the safety belt, and hold with the other hand the patient's anterior shoulder assisting the patient to regain balance. If balance cannot be regained and the patient is falling forward, the patient must be instructed to remove the assistive devices and reach for the floor while the therapist would retard the patient's forward fall by holding the patient by the safety belt. During the fall, the patient can be instructed to cushion the fall by bending the elbows and turning the head to one side.

Patient loses balance backward: hold with one hand the patient by the safety belt, assisting with the other hand on the patient's posterior shoulder. The therapist's lower extremity is on the patient's involved pelvis to help the patient regain balance. If balance cannot be regained and the patient is falling backward, the patient must be instructed to remove the assistive devices while the therapist would lower the patient toward the floor by holding onto the safety belt.

Canes: widen BOS, improve balance (unload forces on involved LE up to 30%), and reduce forces acting at the stance hip. Canes are not intended for weight–bearing restrictions (such as NWB or PWB). Canes are used in the hand opposite to the affected (involved) lower extremity (reasons: widens BOS with decreased lateral shifting of COM than when used ipsilaterally; approximates a normal reciprocal gait pattern; reduces forces created by the abductor muscles acting at the involved hip in the stance phase—creates gravitational moment at the stance hip). Cane measurement: must be 6 inches from the lateral border of the toes; top of the cane must be at greater trochanter and elbow flexed at about 20° to 30°.

Crutches: improve lateral stability and balance, and decrease weight bearing on

continues

Table 3-36   (continued)

involved LE (patient education not to lean on axillary crutches because of the potential damage of radial nerve and axillary artery). Crutches are awkward in small and crowded areas. Axillary crutches measurement: in standing position from 2 inches (width of 2 fingers) bellow the axilla at 2 inches lateral and 6 inches anterior to the foot (can also subtract 16 inches from patient's height). Elbow must be flexed at about 20° to 30° when using crutches. Forearm crutches measurement: in standing position, distal end at 2 inches lateral and 6 inches anterior to the foot; elbow must be flexed at about 20° to 30°; forearm cuff must be at 1.0 to 1.5 inches bellow the elbow. Gait patterns for crutches: 3-point gait, modified 3-point gait; 4-point gait; 2-point gait; swing to; swing through.

Walkers: widen BOS, decrease weight bearing fully or partially on involved LE, improve balance, and provide lateral and anterior stability. Walkers offer the greatest stability. Walker measurement: the walker handgrip (handle) must be at the greater trochanter, and elbow must be flexed at about 20° to 30°. Nonrolling walkers can use FWB, PWB, or NWB patterns.

Wheelchair Measurements

Table 3-37   Wheelchair Measurements[9]

Taken on a firm surface (sitting or supine); hips, knees, and ankles should be positioned at 90°.

Seat width measurement: measure the widest part of hips and add 2 inches to the measurement. Typical seat width dimensions: standard adult wheelchair = 18 inches; narrow adult or junior wheelchair = 16 inches; extra wide adult wheelchair = 22 inches. Potential problems: extra wide seat width can cause difficulty reaching; narrow seat width can cause lateral pelvis and thighs discomfort.

Seat depth measurement: measure from posterior buttocks on lateral side of the thigh to popliteal fossa and subtract 2 inches from the measurement. Typical seat width dimensions for standard adult, narrow adult, junior, and extra wide adult wheelchairs = 16 inches. Potential problems: too long seat depth can cause circulatory problems to posterior knees, posterior tilt sitting, and kyphotic posture; too short seat depth can cause inadequate thigh support.

Seat height measurement (measured relative to entire wheelchair): 2 inches measurement from the floor to the lowest point on the bottom of the foot plate of the footrest (or first measuring leg length and adding 2 inches to the measurement). Leg length measurement: measure from the bottom of patient's shoe to posterior popliteal fossa and subtract 2 inches. Typical seat height dimensions for standard adult, narrow adult, and extra wide adult wheelchairs = 20 inches; for junior

wheelchair = 18.5 inches. Potential problems: too short leg length can cause
excessive weight on ischial seat and decubitus ulcers; too long leg length can
cause sacral sitting and sliding forward in the wheelchair.

Back height measurement: measure from the seat platform to lower angle of the
patient's scapula, mid scapula, or top of the shoulder, depending on patient's
needs. If a cushion is used, it must be added to the measurement.

Wheelchair's Postural Support System

Table 3-38   Wheelchair's Postural Support System[10]

Solid insert (is a seat support) can be: (1) Padded insert board. (2) Reinforcement
board inside cushion cover. (3) Contoured or flat insert board between cushion
and wheelchair. Benefits of the solid insert: increases stability; decreases possibility of LE's adduction and IR; decreases possibility of posterior pelvic tilt and slipping forward in the seat; improves pelvic position; encourages neutral pelvic tilt
and symmetrical spinal alignment; can promote trunk extension and upper body
stability; increases head and UE function; has low cost. Limitations of the solid
insert: increases seat height; can shift on seat to cause asymmetrical seating.

Solid hook-on seat (is a seat support) can be installed using hardware to hook to the
seat rails. It has adjustable angle and height to be able to change positions of the
seat surface on the wheelchair's frame. Benefits of the solid hook-on seat: creates stable base of support; improves pelvic position; decreases possibility of LE's
adduction and IR, posterior pelvic tilt, and slipping forward in wheelchair (by raising the anterior portion of the solid hook-on seat); encourages neutral pelvic tilt
and symmetrical alignment of the spine. If posterior portion of the solid hook-on
seat is raised, it can facilitate trunk cocontraction. Limitations of the solid hook-on
seat: difficult to remove; adds weight to wheelchair's frame.

Pressure relieving foam (custom or premade contoured seat cushion) can increase
surface contact and improve pressure distribution and relief. It has different
degrees of firmness, and the generic types work well for symmetrical individuals.
Benefits of the pressure relieving foam: increases surface contact; improves distribution of weight; accommodates moderate and severe postural asymmetry; is
low maintenance; allows easier positioning and repositioning of the patient
(client) for the caregiver. Limitations of the pressure relieving foam: is expensive;
can interfere with sliding transfers; can cause a feeling of being locked in
because the movement on the cushion surface is restricted.

Comfort cushion (planar or contoured seat cushion) is made of layered foam, and is
used for postural control and for limited ROM. Benefits of the comfort cushion:

continues

MUSCULOSKELETAL
INTERVENTIONS

Table 3-38 (continued)

promotes neutral pelvic position; increases patient's comfort; creates a stable base of support; does not interfere with sliding transfers; is inexpensive; is lightweight; patient can sit anywhere on the cushion without any discomfort. Limitations of the comfort cushion: does not offer pressure relief; gives minimal support and postural control.

Pressure relieving air cushion (seat cushion) responds to patient's weight and increases surface contact to improve distribution of weight and relief (bony prominences feel like floating). Benefits of the pressure relieving air cushion : is very lightweight; offers pressure relief (moderate to significant); improves moderate to significant postural asymmetry; increases sitting time; prevents decubitus ulcers (especially over bony prominences); improves postural control for specific body segments (using segmented air cushions). Limitations of the pressure relieving air cushion: is expensive; may be unstable for some patients (clients); decreases UE reach distance (because users keep arms closed to the body for stability); may make transfers difficult because the unstable base; the air pressure needs to be monitored carefully; needs continuous maintenance.

Pressure relieving fluid or fluid/foam combination cushion (seat cushion) has generic contour or planar surface contour with fluid filled sack. The bony prominences feel immersed in the fluid (increases surface contact); accommodates limited ROM (by cutting foam base as needed); generic contoured shapes work well with symmetrical individuals. Benefits of the pressure relieving fluid or fluid/foam combination cushion: provides a stable base of support for proper seating alignment; controls postural alignment (using add-on pieces); increases comfort and sitting tolerance (especially for oblique pelvis); improves head and shoulders alignment; can be used for moderate to significant seating needs; increases sitting time; decreases possibility of decubitus ulcers (especially over bony prominences); increases pelvic stability (especially with gel medium fluid); is easier to position and reposition (for caregivers). Limitations of the pressure relieving fluid or fluid/foam combination cushion: is expensive; some maintenance is required; heavier than foam or air; can cause a feeling of being locked in because the movement on the cushion surface is restricted.

Solid insert (back support) maintains pelvic alignment and can accommodate back contour and provide postural control (with special foaming). Benefits of the solid insert: maintains pelvic alignment (when interfaced with seat surface); improves upright seating, trunk, and head alignment; provides some lateral support (with shaped foam); increases trunk control and distal extremities function; can be easily removed; adds minimal weight to the wheelchair. Limitations of the solid insert: may not be stable in the chair; can be easily lost or left behind when folding the wheelchair.

Pita back (back support) is a solid board padded or unpadded that slips in to a pocket in the back upholstery of the wheelchair. It provides mild to moderate support and is used for patients (clients) who need a slight reminder to sit upright. Benefits of the pita back: encourages trunk extension; is lightweight; is easy to put it on and to remove it. Limitations of the pita back: provides only slight degree of support; can be lost or left behind when wheelchair is folded.

Solid hook on (back support) is a very stable back support that can be aligned and angled as necessary. It accommodates for limited ROM; can hold planar, contoured, molded back, or air flotation cushion; can be custom made or manufactured; mounts using permanent (can strengthen the wheelchair frame) or removable hardware. Benefits of the solid hook on support: improves upright sitting; accommodates for limited ROM; accommodates for any degree of deformity; increases UE and head control; improves comfort and pressure relief; maintains trunk and pelvis alignment; resists extensor thrusting; allows additional attachments (such as headrests). Limitations of the solid hook on support: increases wheelchair weight; requires manipulation and removal of hardware to fold the wheelchair.

Head and neck supports (specialized supports) are used for patients with fair, poor, or absent head control. The hardware can be fixed or removable. Benefits of the head and neck supports: improve anterior, posterior, or lateral head and neck control; promote neutral cervical spine and head position; eliminate uncontrolled lateral flexion and rotation (that disturbs trunk and pelvis alignment); assist with respiration, feeding, swallowing, and visual interaction; improve safety during patient's (client's) transportation. Limitations of the head and neck supports: may interfere with head movement; may trigger extensor thrust; may cause skin problems in areas of high pressure.

Lateral trunk support (specialized support) is used for weak or spastic trunk muscles. It can be straight or contoured and the hardware can be fixed or swing away (for transfers). Benefits of the lateral trunk support: improves trunk stability and control; increases pelvic alignment; controls lateral trunk flexion; facilitates UE movement; improves respiration, feeding, and swallowing; increases safety during patient's movement. Limitations of the lateral trunk support: may interfere with trunk movement; increases weight of the wheelchair (chair); may interfere with patient's self propelling using the UE.

Anterior chest support (specialized support) is used for upright trunk posture and shoulder control. It can be maximally or minimally supportive (having additional features such as straps, padded straps, etc.). Benefits of the anterior chest support: eliminates forward lean; discourages shoulder protraction (as in CVA); improves trunk control (and respectively respiration), eating, swallowing and visual interaction; improves UE, shoulder (promotes better head posture), and

continues

Table 3-38   (continued)

head control; improves trunk upright position; stabilizes trunk to free arms and head for movement. Limitations of the anterior chest support: restricts trunk movement; long usage may limit trunk control improvements.

Lateral hip guides (specialized supports) are used for pelvic alignment. Lateral hip guides assist with maintenance of pelvic position on contoured seat. Benefits of the lateral hip guides: improve weight distribution (symmetrical weight bearing) on pelvis; increase sitting time; increase upper and lower body segments alignment; reduce asymmetries in trunk and LEs. Limitations of the lateral hip guides: may interfere with transfers (if not removable); can cause a feeling of being locked in on the seat; increase weight of the wheelchair (chair).

Lateral knee guides (specialized supports) may be built into the cushion contours or fabricated separate (from padded wood or plastic) and attached to the seat or armrest of wheelchair. Lateral knee guides should extend to the end of the knee for maximal control. Benefits of the lateral knee guides: maintain alignment of LE; reduce excessive abduction and ER; assist to maintain pelvic alignment; improve trunk and UE position and function; reduce forward sliding of pelvis on the seat of the wheelchair. Limitations of the lateral knee guides: if they are too high (as needed) may interfere with transfers (if they are not removable); add weight to the wheelchair (chair).

Medial knee block (specialized support) may be built into the cushion contours or fabricated separate (or removable flip down block). Medial knee block must be positioned at distal portion of the limb (between condyles) for maximal control and should never be used to stabilize the pelvis on the seat by pressing it into the groin. Also, it should never be used to prevent patient (client) from sliding off the front of the seat. Benefits of the medial knee block: prevents LE from moving into adduction; prevents pelvic forward rotation (when used with both LEs oriented to one side with one LE adducted and the other LE abducted); maintains broad and stable base of support; decreases spasticity (if wide enough); maintains LE alignment. Limitations of the medial knee block: may interfere with transfers; increases weight of the wheelchair (chair).

Anterior knee block (specialized support) is the most effective way to maintain proper pelvic position on the seat. It needs MD approval if hips are subluxed, dislocated, or not properly formed. Benefits of the anterior knee block: helps to maintain a broad and stable base of support; improves pelvic alignment and functional use of the upper body; may facilitate trunk cocontraction, extension, and improved UE ROM (when used with forward sloped seat); reduces extensor tone; increases stability. Limitations of the anterior knee block: may impose too much pressure at the hips and over the patella; patient (client) may feel restricted.

Wheelchair Training

Table 3-39   Wheelchair Training Elements

Patient (client) and/or caregiver education in wheelchair use, safety, and maintenance

Patient (client) and/or caregiver education in proper alignment and pressure relief
activities (such as arm push-ups, weight shifting by leaning to one side then the
other side)

Patient (client) and/or caregiver education in use of wheelchair's postural supports:
positioning of supports; benefits and limitations of supports; care and maintenance of supports; schedule of use of supports

Manual wheelchair propulsion training (using both UEs, using one UE, and using one
UE and one LE): forward and backward propulsion on flat surfaces and uneven
surfaces; turning by pushing harder with one hand than the other hand and taking
sharp turns (by pulling one wheel backward while pushing the opposite wheel forward); negotiating obstacles (such as curbs and thresholds).

Power wheelchair training: for driving skills and safety; use of switches (on and off
and turns); use of joystick; safe stopping.

Management of wheelchair wheel locks: use of footrests and armrests; transfer
safety with the wheelchair locked; transfers using removable or swing away armrests; transfers using removable or swing away leg rests.

Community mobility using the wheelchair practice: mobility ascending ramps backward (by moving the center of gravity forward; forward lean of the trunk; using
quick and short strokes for propulsion); mobility descending ramps (by gripping
the hand rims loosely; increasing the grip to control the speed of the descent;
or/and descending in advanced wheelie position by keeping the spine against the
wheelchair back for steep ramps; using gloves).

Wheelchair's curb negotiation practice: how to pop up a wheelie (moving into a
wheelie position)—patient places one hand posteriorly on the hand rims and pulls
the hand rims forward abruptly and forcefully; patient trunk and head are moved
forward to keep the wheelchair from tipping backwards; how to maintain balance
in the wheelie position—the wheelchair tips further back when the wheels are
pushed forward; the wheelchair tips into upright position when the wheels are
pulled back; patient to come up onto balance on the rear wheels with the front
casters off the ground.

Wheelchair curb ascent practice: patient (client) places front casters up on the curb;
patient (client) pushes rear wheels up the curb; patient (client) uses momentum to
assist.

MUSCULOSKELETAL
INTERVENTIONS

continues

Types of Musculoskeletal Interventions   **201**

Table 3-39 (continued)

Wheelchair curb descent practice: patient (client) can descend backwards with forward head and trunk lean; patient (client) pushes rear wheels up the curb; patient (client) can descend forward in wheelie position.

Wheelchair ascending and descending stairs practice: using the wheelchair; assisted on buttocks bringing wheelchair behind; advanced techniques.

Patient (client) education and practice in how to fall safely techniques and how to return to wheelchair.

Patient (client) practice in how to transfer into a car (by placing the wheelchair inside the car by pulling wheelchair behind the car seat or using a wheelchair lift).

Routine maintenance of the wheelchair: normal cleaning and upkeep; power chair battery maintenance.

Musculoskeletal Intervention Patterns

APTA's Guide to Physical Therapist Practice[11]—APTA's Musculoskeletal Intervention Patterns

Table 3-40   Therapeutic Exercises[11]

1. Strength, power, and endurance training for head, neck, limb, pelvic floor, trunk, and ventilatory muscles (such as active assistive, active, and resistive exercises, including concentric, dynamic, isotonic, eccentric, isokinetics, isometric, and plyometric; aquatic programs; standardized, programmatic, complementary exercise approaches task-specific performance training).
2. Flexibility exercises (such as muscle lengthening; range of motion; stretching).
3. Relaxation exercises (such as breathing strategies; movement strategies; relaxation techniques; standardized, programmatic, complementary exercise approaches).
4. Balance, coordination, and agility training (such as developmental activities training; motor function training and retraining such as motor control and motor learning; neuromuscular education and reeducation; perceptual training; posture awareness training; standardized, programmatic, complementary exercise approaches task-specific performance training).
5. Body mechanics and postural stabilization (such as body mechanics training; posture awareness training; postural control training; postural stabilization activities).
6. Gait and locomotion training (such as developmental activities training; gait training; implement and device training; perceptual training; standardized, programmatic, complementary exercise approaches wheelchair training).

Table 3-41   Functional Training in Self Care and Home Management, Including ADL and IADL[11]

1. ADL training (such as bathing; bed mobility and transfer training; developmental activities; dressing; eating; grooming; toileting).
2. Devices and equipment use and training (such as assistive and adaptive device and equipment training during ADL and IADL; orthotic, protective, or supportive device or equipment training during ADL and IADL; prosthetic device or equipment training during ADL and IADL).
3. Functional training programs (such as back schools; simulated environments and tasks; task adaptation).
4. IADL training (such as caring for dependents; home maintenance; household chores; shopping; structured play for infants and children; yard work).

5. Injury prevention or reduction (such as injury prevention education during self-care and home management; injury prevention or reduction with use of devices and equipment; safety awareness training during self care and home management).

Table 3-42   Prescription, Application, and as Appropriate, Fabrication of Devices and Equipment (Assistive, Adaptive, Orthotic, Protective, Supportive, and Prosthetic)[11]

1. Adaptive devices (such as environmental controls; raised toilet seats; seating systems).
2. Assistive devices (such as canes; crutches; long-handled reachers; power devices; static and dynamic splints; walkers; wheelchairs).
3. Orthotic devices (such as braces; casts; shoe inserts; splints).
4. Prosthetic devices (such as lower extremity and upper extremity).
5. Protective devices (such as braces; cushions; helmets; protective taping).
6. Supportive devices (such as compression garments; corsets; elastic wraps; neck collars; serial casts; slings; supportive taping).

Table 3-43   Functional Training in Work (Job/School/Play), Community, and Leisure Integration or Reintegration Including IADL, Work Hardening, and Work Conditioning[11]

1. Devices and equipment use and training (such as assistive and adaptive device and equipment training during IADL; orthotic, protective, or supportive device or equipment training during IADL; prosthetic device or equipment training during IADL).
2. Functional training programs (such as back schools; simulated environments and tasks; task adaptation).
3. IADL training (such as community service training involving instruments; school and play activities training including tools and instruments; work training with tools).
4. Injury prevention or reduction (such as injury prevention education during work at job, school or play, community, and leisure integration or reintegration; injury prevention or reduction with use of devices and equipment; safety awareness training during work at job, school or play, community, and leisure integration and reintegration).
5. Leisure and play activities and training.

Table 3-44 Manual Therapy Techniques (Excludes Joint Mobilization)[11]

1. Manual traction
2. PROM
3. Massage (such as connective tissue massage; therapeutic massage)
4. Soft tissue mobilization
5. Manual lymphatic drainage

Table 3-45 Physical Agents and Mechanical Modalities[11]

1. Physical agents (such as cryotherapy—cold pack, ice massage, vapocoolant spray; hydrotherapy—pools, whirlpool tanks, contrast baths, and pulsatile lavage; sound agents—phonophoresis and ultrasound; thermotherapy—dry heat, hot packs, paraffin baths; light—infrared and laser).
2. Mechanical modalities (such as compression therapies—taping, contact casting, compression garments, total contact casting, and vasopneumatic compression devices; gravity-assisted compression devices—standing frame and tilt table; traction devices—intermittent, positional, and sustained; mechanical motion devices—CPM).

Table 3-46 Electrotherapeutic Modalities[11]

1. Biofeedback
2. Electrical muscle stimulation (such as EMS, FES, NMES, TENS, HVPC).
3. Electrotherapeutic delivery of medications (such as iontophoresis).

Table 3-47 Patient/Client Related Instruction[11]

Instruction, education, and training of patients/clients and caregivers regarding current condition (pathology; pathophysiology—disease, disorder, or condition; impairments, functional limitations, or disabilities); enhancement of performance; health, wellness, and fitness; plan of care; risk factors (for pathology; pathophysiology—disease, disorder, or condition; impairments, functional limitations, or disabilities); transitions across settings; transitions to new roles.

Arthritic Disorders and Intervention Patterns

Table 3-48   Arthritic Disorders and Intervention Patterns

Arthritic Disorders	Interventions
Degenerative joint disease (DJD) or degenerative osteoarthritis: degeneration of articular cartilage with hypertrophy of the subchondral bone and joint capsule of weight bearing joints.	Pain management and control of inflammation (physical agents and modalities); joint protection and function (splints, orthotics, gait training with assistive devices, and task modifications); increase flexibility and strength (ROM, stretching, and strengthening exercises); patient education about joint protection. Precaution: resistive exercises.[12]
Rheumatoid arthritis: systemic disease with symmetric pattern of dysfunction in synovial tissues and articular cartilages of the joints of the hands, wrists, elbows, shoulders, knees, ankles, and feet. Also affected MCP and PIP joints (pannus formation and ulnar drift). DIP joints are spared.	Pain management and control of inflammation (physical agents and modalities); prevention of deformities and maintenance of ROM (splints and orthotic devices for ADLs); gait training with assistive devices and task modifications; increase flexibility, strength, and endurance using ROM exercises, stretching exercises (HS, finger flexors, or biceps brachii), and strengthening exercises; patient education for joint protection and disease progression. For JRA, see Part VIII.
Systemic lupus erythematosus (SLE): progressive systemic inflammatory disease characterized by inflammation and damage of connective tissue anywhere in the body. Most common areas include skin, joints, nervous system, kidneys, lungs, and other organs. SLE presents with butterfly rash across nose, cheeks, and other exposed areas of the body.	Pain management (physical agents and modalities); increase strength (aquatic therapy); decrease chronic fatigue (activity pacing and energy conservation); joint protection (gait training with assistive devices); patient education for postural awareness and daily walking.

MUSCULOSKELETAL INTERVENTIONS

continues

Table 3-48   (continued)

Arthritic Disorders	Interventions
Ankylosing spondylitis (called Marie Strumpell Bechterew, or rheumatoid spondylitis): progressive inflammatory disorder that initially affects the spine and the sacroiliac joints. Later, other joints away from the spine as well as organs (eyes, heart, lungs, and kidneys) can be affected. Posture is affected resulting in kyphosis deformity of CS/TS and a decrease in lumbar lordosis.	Maintenance of proper posture: deep breathing and stretching exercises (back extension exercises); task modifications and ergonomic modifications (workplace); patient education for posture awareness and proper sleeping patterns (on firm mattress without pillows). Exercise programs are customized for the individual patient (swimming is preferred).
Psoriatic arthritis: chronic, erosive inflammatory disorder associated with psoriasis. Erosive degeneration occurs in the joints of the digits (ends finger or toes) as well as the spine.	Joint protection and maintenance of joint mobility (splints and orthotics; gait training using assistive devices; stretching exercises); patient education for joint protection.
Gout: chronic genetic disease of uric acid metabolism that occurs as an acute, episodic form of arthritis. It is observed at the knee and great toe of the foot causing severe to excruciating pain.	Pain management and stress reduction (TENS and EMG biofeedback for relaxation); joint protection and maintenance of joint mobility (braces and orthotics; gait training with assistive devices); patient education about the disease, relaxation and stress management to control pain, general fitness exercises, and joint protection; HEP for stretching and strengthening exercises (aquatic exercises are also recommended).
Fibromyalgia: nonspecific rheumatoid disorder characterized by general musculoskeletal pain localized to all muscles. Myofascial pain syndrome is localized to one or a few muscles.	Pain management and promotion of relaxation (TENS, MHP, massage, whirlpool, breathing exercises, EMG biofeedback for relaxation); flexibility improvement using a progressive graded exercise

Fibromyalgia causes chronic pain with diffuse aching or burning in the muscles, stiffness, fatigue, disturbed sleep patterns, and depression.

program (walking, biking, stationary bicycle, swimming, low-impact aerobics, or water aerobics).

Bursitis and Intervention Patterns

Table 3-49   Tendonitis and Bursitis and Intervention Patterns

Tendonitis and Bursitis	Interventions
Rotator cuff tendonitis (RCT) also called pitcher's shoulder, shoulder impingement syndrome, swimmer's shoulder, and tennis shoulder: progressive overuse disorder caused mostly by sports. It results from mechanical impingement of distal attachment of rotator cuff on anterior acromion or coracoacromial ligament with repetitive overhead activities.	Pain management and joint protection: using physical agents and modalities such as ice massage, ice pack, MHP, ES, US, phonophoresis, and iontophoresis. Patient education: no shoulder flexion or abduction between 60 and 120 degrees (painful arch); joint protection; modification of ADLs. Improve flexibility: using stretching exercises (post. capsule). Increase strength: using Codman's pendulum exercises (in the beginning), AAROM; first strengthen scapular stabilizers and then rotator cuff muscles.
Lateral epicondylitis (tennis elbow), medial epicondylitis (golfer's elbow), and medial valgus stress overload (MVSO). Tennis elbow is chronic inflammation of ECRB tendon. Golfer's elbow is chronic inflammation of FCU tendon. MVSO is inflammation of medial ulnar ligament and capsule from repetitive overuse. All are caused by sports or occupations or cumulative trauma from work injuries.	Acute: RICE, US, ES, phonophoresis, iontophoresis, gentle AROM, splint protection (bracing with counterforce brace for tennis elbow), patient education (to avoid repetitive motions and prevention), and stretching exercises. Subacute: progress with PREs as tolerated and pain free; gradual return to function training; task modifications if needed. For MVSO, avoid exercises in valgus position of elbow.

MUSCULOSKELETAL INTERVENTIONS

continues

Musculoskeletal Intervention Patterns   **209**

Table 3-49   (continued)

Tendonitis and Bursitis	Interventions
DeQuervain's tenosynovitis: inflammation of EPB and abductor pollicis longus tendons at the first dorsal compartment of the hand from repetitive microtrauma.	Acute: RICE, US, phonophoresis, iontophoresis, ES, splint protection, activity modification, friction massage, stretching exercises, and patient education for activity modifications.
Anterior tibial periostitis (shin splints) and medial tibial stress syndrome (MTSS): overuse conditions caused by abnormal biomechanical alignment, poor conditioning, or improper training methods. Muscles involved can be anterior tibialis and EHL (for anterior compartment) or posterior tibialis for posterior and medial compartment (MTSS).	Pain management and edema control (physical agents and modalities); activity modifications (orthotics, patient education for proper training methods and prevention of recurrence); flexibility improvement (stretching exercises); strengthening exercises (dorsiflexors and evertors for anterior tibial periostitis and plantarflexors and invertors for MTSS).
Subacromial/subdeltoid bursitis and trochanteric bursitis: caused by trauma, chronic overuse, inflammatory arthritis (such as RA) or biomechanical/gait abnormalities (for trochanteric bursitis). Athletes are prone to shoulder bursitis from overuse when the arm is at or above shoulder level. Also, hip bursitis is seen in runners or athletes who participate in running-oriented sports such as soccer or football.	Acute: RICE; joint protection (splint or brace); reduction of pain and inflammation (physical agents and modalities); promotion of functional activities (strengthening exercises); patient education for proper usage and recurrence prevention. Shoulder bursitis: use Codman's pendulum exercises and AAROM exercises in acute stage. Trochanteric bursitis: US is effective, and stretching exercises for ITB tightness.[12]
Carpal tunnel syndrome (CTS): tenosynovitis or inflamed tendons producing a compression syndrome of the median nerve (due to inflammation of tendons). Caused by occupations	Nonoperative: Pain management and relief of aggravating factors (physical agents and modalities; patient education for job/task modifications; joint protection and support (resting

(carpenters, factory workers, or food processing workers) or during pregnancy. Patients may have thenar muscles atrophy and in extreme cases Ape hand deformity.

splints or night splints in 0° to 20° extension); return to function training (ROM, stretching and strengthening exercises). Postoperative: edema management (physical agents and modalities; soft tissue mobilization of scar tissue); return to function (ROM exercises; ADLs; strengthening exercises of hand such as gripping exercises and UE exercises); desensitization of tissues; patient education about CTS, scar tissue massage, and job/task modifications to prevent recurrence.

Strains, Sprains, Dislocations, and Fractures and Intervention Patterns

Table 3-50   Strains, Sprains, Dislocations, and Fractures and Intervention Patterns

Strains, Sprains, Dislocations, and Fractures	Interventions
Strains: injuries to muscles and tendon from direct trauma, overstretch, or excessive muscular contraction. Three grades: 1—mild injury; 2—moderate injury; 3—severe injury. Common strain: rotator cuff tears (RCT); hip strain (of HS, iliopsoas, adductors, and rectus femoris); HS strain: most common in runners; lumbar spine strain (from sudden violent contraction or fast stretch of combined ext./rot.). RCT is degenerative strain, occurring over time with impingement at the acromion from	Nonoperative: Small tears: pain management (RICE; physical agents and modalities); patient education for ADLs modifications (no overhead activities for RCT) and recurrence prevention; stretching exercises (shoulder flex. and abd. for RCT); strengthening exercises (postacute). Hip strain main goals: patient education to avoid in acute-phase full knee extension combined with forward flexion; gait training with crutches to limit HS irritation. For adductor longus strain to avoid early aggressive

MUSCULOSKELETAL INTERVENTIONS

continues

Table 3-50 (continued)

Strains, Sprains, Dislocations, and Fractures	Interventions
repetitive use and trauma or falling on to an outstretched hand.	stretching. Large tears may need surgery. For HS strain: acute—PRICE; gentle PROM/ AAROM; subacute—AROM; aquatic exercises and strength (submaximal isometrics). Postoperative (RCT): Codman's pendulum, shoulder isometrics, AAROM, strength exercises, and gradual return to function training.
Sprains: injuries to ligaments from direct or indirect trauma. Three grades: 1—mild; 2—moderate; 3—severe (may need surgery). Common sprains: (1) AC joint sprain (from direct fall on acromion or indirect from a fall on outstretched arm); (2) MCP or IP joint sprain; (3) Skier's thumb (rupture of ulnar collateral ligament of MCP from hyperextension of thumb in skiing); (4) Knee sprains: ACL (most commonly sprained), PCL, MCL, LCL; (5) Ankle sprains: lateral ligaments (ATF, CF, PTF) or medial ligament (deltoid ligament; rare); meniscal tear (sudden trauma or gradual degeneration); (6) Lumbar spine sprain (from sudden violent force or repeated stress).	Nonoperative: RICE; physical agents and modalities; NWB or WBAT; braces, splints and orthotics for immobilization and weight bearing reduction; isometrics; CPM machine, PROM, AAROM, AROM; isotonic exercises; CKC exercises; isokinetic and isotonic exercises; general conditioning program (especially for LS); cycling and stair climbing activities; proprioception, balance, and coordination; patient education to prevent recurrence (especially for LS for lifting and sitting). Return to prior level of function training. Postoperative: follows similar with nonoperative, except for WB status and post–op precautions (such as for ACL reconstruction—no knee extension in final 40° extension and no OKC knee extension with resistance placed distally). Meniscal repair: no NWB and no knee flexion from 90° to 100° for 4 to 6 weeks; no squats for 3 to 6 months.

Glenohumeral subluxation (partial dislocation); glenohumeral dislocation: at shoulder joint in abduction, extension, and ER (for anterior dislocation); abduction, flexion, and IR (for posterior dislocation). Anterior dislocations are more common; posterior are rare. Common types: (1) Bankart lesion is an avulsion of capsule and anterior labrum from the glenoid rim with disruption of medial scapular periosteum; (2) Perthes lesion is similar to Bankart except the medial scapular periosteum remains intact; (3) Hill-Sachs lesion is a compression fracture from impaction of posterolateral humeral head against anterior/inferior glenoid rim (may result in a loose body).

Nonoperative: immobilization (braces, orthotics, slings); physical agents and modalities; strengthening exercises of uninvolved joints and general conditioning; patient education for precautions (for anterior lesion—no shoulder abduction and ER) and activity modifications; Codman's pendulum; active assistive stretching exercises (flexion); strengthening exercises (isometrics, T-band) of rotator cuff (concentrate on infraspinatus and teres minor), scapular stabilizers and anterior shoulder muscles; precautions when starting isotonic resistive exercises; proprioceptive exercises CKC exercises. Postoperative: similar with nonoperative, but varies considering the procedure and the patient.

Fractures (Fx): (1) Scapular and clavicular Fx (from direct or indirect trauma); (2) Proximal humerus Fx (of humeral head, lesser or greater tuberosity or humeral shaft); (3) Supracondylar Fx (transverse fracture distal one third of humerus often in children); (4) Intercondylar Fx (of articular surface of elbow); (5) Radial head Fx (from a fall on outstretched arm); (6) Olecranon Fx (from a fall on olecranon); (7) Elbow Fx; (8) Colles' Fx (from a fall onto an outstretched arm; distal radius displaced dorsal = dinner fork deformity); (9) Smith's Fx (from a fall onto an outstretched arm with elbow supinated; distal radius displaced ventral); (10) Scaphoid Fx (from fall

Nonoperative: pain management and swelling reduction (physical agents and modalities; in UEs may use compression pump for lymphedema); immobilization (casts, splints, orthotics, or slings); mobility training (transfers; gait training with assistive devices and NWB/PWB or TTWB; balance training); patient education on signs of circulatory problems (especially in wrist Fx.) and to prevent recurrence and for safety; functional use of extremity (ROM exercises; adaptive equipment); functional activities of nonimmobilized joints; restoration of motion post immobilization (ROM exercises); strengthening exercises after immobilization. Postopera-

continues

Table 3-50   (continued)

Strains, Sprains, Dislocations and Fractures	Interventions
onto an outstretched arm in younger person); (11) Boxer's Fx (neck of fifth metacarpal); (12) Bennet's Fx (proximal to first metacarpal); (13) Mallet Finger (avulsion Fx or tendon injury of extensor tendon = DIP joint flexion contracture); (14) Patellar Fx; (15) Hip Fx (most common in geriatric; untreated can cause avascular necrosis of hip); (16) Pelvis and acetabulum Fx; (17) Ankle Fx (uni/bi/tri/malleolar); (18) Distal tibia Fx; (19) Calcaneal Fx (from a fall from a height); (20) Talus Fx (from a fall from a height and landing on foot on crouched position).	tive: mobility training (transfers; gait training with assistive devices and NWB/PWB or TTWB as per MD/DO; balance training); Patient education for surgical complications or precautions, to prevent recurrence and for safety; functional use of extremity (ROM exercises; ADLs; strengthening exercises using isometrics first and then isotonics; CKC exercises first and then OKC exercises); functional activities of nonimmobilized joints.

Thoracic Outlet Syndrome, Adhesive Capsulitis, Low-Back Disorders, Plantar Fasciitis, and Arthroplasties and Intervention Patterns

Table 3-51 Thoracic Outlet Syndrome, Adhesive Capsulitis, Low-Back Disorders, Plantar Fasciitis, and Arthroplasties and Intervention Patterns

Thoracic Outlet Syndrome, Adhesive Capsulitis, Low-Back Disorders, Plantar Fasciitis, and Arthroplasties	Interventions
Thoracic outlet syndrome (TOS): compression of the neurovascular bundle (brachial plexus, subclavian artery/vein, vagus and phrenic nerves, sympathetic trunk) in thoracic outlet, between bony and soft tissue structures. Compression occurs when the size or shape of the thoracic outlet is altered. Causes of TOS: poor or strenuous posture, trauma, or constant muscle tension in shoulder girdle (caused by drooping shoulder and forward head postures, carrying heavy loads, or osteoporosis); and repetitive overhead movements such as in athletes (swimmers, tennis and volleyball players, or baseball pitchers) or occupations (electricians and painters).	Pain management: Physical agents and modalities; patient education for task modifications (work, play, or sleep) and avoidance of repetitive movements; postural retraining including postural awareness and correction; stretching exercises of anterior scalenes and pectoralis minor; strengthening exercises including scapular stabilization such as scapular retraction and seated rowing exercises with T-band or tubing.[5] The PT may need to create a personalized intervention program specific to the patient's symptoms. Vascular or neurologic TOS may need surgery.
Adhesive capsulitis (frozen shoulder): restriction in shoulder ROM secondary to inflammation and fibrosis of shoulder capsule usually following injury or repetitive microtrauma. It has capsular pattern of limitation	Early acute stage: cryotherapy; thermotherapy; US; TENS; EMG biofeedback for muscle relaxation; Codman's pendulum; AAROM with wand and pulleys in pain free mode; isometric exercises. Subacute stage: restora-

continues

MUSCULOSKELETAL INTERVENTIONS

Table 3-51 (continued)

Thoracic Outlet Syndrome, Adhesive Capsulitis, Low-Back Disorders, Plantar Fasciitis, and Arthroplasties	Interventions
such as ER, abduction and flexion, and least restricted in IR. It is primary idiopathic (occurs spontaneously) and secondary (posttrauma or immobilization).	tion of normal scapular motion (stretching exercises; scapular stabilization strengthening exercises); recovery of function (strengthening exercises using isotonic first and then PREs for deltoid, rotator cuff, and upper arm muscles); postural reeducation to avoid shoulder protraction and kyphotic postures.
Lumbar stenosis: narrowing of spinal canal secondary to osteoarthritis. Produces pain (from nerve root compression) in LS extension. Lumbar spondylolysis: bony defect in the lumbar vertebrae (can be a fracture of pars interarticularis). Lumbar spondylolisthesis: one superior vertebrae slipping over inferior vertebrae (usually at L4–L5 and L5–S1). Causes of spondylolisthesis: congenital, mechanical (or isthmic is most common), trauma (young patients need cast), or degenerative.	Precaution for all: No extension exercises (produces increased symptoms). Interventions depend on symptoms. Stenosis: William's flexion exercises; postural reeducation; patient education for lifting techniques, sitting, and sleeping; physical conditioning. Nonoperative spondylolisthesis: pain management and decrease swelling (using physical agents and modalities); joint protection (lumbar corset, orthoses); abdominal muscle strengthening (lumbar stabilization exercises; curl ups); tasks or activities modifications.[12] Postoperative (for patients with radicular symptoms or high grade slippage): patient education for precautions (no lumbar extension); LEs circulation (ankle pumps); orthosis; gait training; ROM exercises; strengthening exercises (UEs and LEs); LS strengthening exercises (after bone healing); return to function training.

Lumbar disk: herniated nucleus pulposus (HNP). Causes: disc protrusion (nucleus bulges against intact annulus), extruded disc (nucleus extends through annulus but nuclear material is confined by the posterior longitudinal ligament), or sequestrated disc (nucleus is free within spinal canal). Patients have radicular signs: posterior thigh pain and numbness going down the knee and pain in buttocks radiating down to legs. Patients may have peripheralization (repeated forward flexion causes symptoms to radiate down the legs); centralization (repeated movements or positions cause symptoms to move away from the legs toward lumbar spine midline).

Nonoperative: pain modulation (physical agents and modalities; lumbar traction—patient prone for posterior HNP); joint protection (corset or orthosis); increase flexibility (stretching exercises either in flexion or extension, depending on centralization); patient education about HNP, proper body mechanics, and posture; increase strength (William's flexion or McKenzie extension exercises depending on centralization); increase cardiovascular fitness; tasks modifications (work, play, or school); postural reeducation; return to function training (ADLs; balance training). Postoperative: patient education for postoperative precautions (no bending, lifting, or trunk rotation; no sitting for more than one hour at a time; proper posture); bed mobility and transfers (log-roll technique); gait training with walker or crutches; LEs circulation (ankle pumps); isometrics (ensure proper breathing; avoid Valsalva); CKC exercises; ROM and strengthening exercises; general conditioning; return to function training.

Scoliosis: lateral curvature of cervical, thoracic, or lumbar spine. Causes: idiopathic or neuromuscular. Structural: irreversible lateral curvature of spine with fixed vertebral rotation (forward flexion more than 25° causes a hump). Nonstructural: reversible (forward flexion more than 25° decreases the curvature). Most

Nonoperative: stretching exercises (tight muscles on concave side); strengthening exercises (all muscles on convex side); bracing (TLSO and/or Milwaukee for curves less than 40°); shoe lift (for mild scoliosis); postural reeducation (postural awareness); breathing exercises; aquatic therapy. Postoperative:

continues

Table 3-51 (continued)

Thoracic Outlet Syndrome, Adhesive Capsulitis, Low-Back Disorders, Plantar Fasciitis, and Arthroplasties	Interventions
common nonstructural: "S" curve (right thoracic, left lumbar curve) in adolescent females. Surgery is indicated when curve is in excess of 40°.	postop brace (TLSO); effective cough and pulmonary hygiene post–op; gait training; activity limitation up to several months.
Plantar fasciitis: chronic inflammation of plantar aponeurosis (with or without calcaneal heel spur). Causes: biomechanical (abnormal inward twisting or rolling of foot); high arches, flat feet, tight calf muscles, or tight tendons at the back of the heel; excessive pronation (most common); repetitive activities (prolonged walking on hard or irregular surfaces or running).	Increase proper mechanical alignment (eliminate the causes); physical agents and modalities (for pain and swelling); stretching exercises (calf stretching and toe extension stretching exercises); friction massage; patient education regarding selection of footwear; orthotic fitting; strengthening exercises after pain and swelling subsided (of intrinsic and extrinsic muscles of foot); general body conditioning (best is in the pool to decrease WB).
Total hip arthroplasty (THA) or total hip replacement (THR): replacement of femoral head and acetabulum with prostheses. Can be cemented or noncemented (noncemented femoral stem can cause persistent thigh pain and antalgic gait for up to 2 years postoperative). Hemiarthroplasty: replacement of femoral head with a bipolar prosthesis. Indications for THA: osteoarthritis, RA, fracture, pain, reduced ambulation, and reduced ADLs.	Patient education for THA precautions (do not lie on surgical site; do not cross legs; do not sit on low surfaces that hips are higher than 90°; use a raised toilet seat; do not bend down to pick up objects from floor; do not turn your toes in/out; anterolateral THA—no ER; posterolateral THA—no IR); LEs circulation (ankle pumps); isometrics (proper breathing; avoid Valsalva); bed mobility and transfers; gait training with assistive devices (PWB or TTWB or WBAT as per MD/DO); AROM exercises (knee flexion and uninvolved LE exercises for

SLR and isometrics); balance exercises (single-leg standing; balance board); proprioceptive training; aquatic therapy (cardiovascular program with WB restrictions); return to function training.

Total knee arthroplasty (TKA) or total knee replacement (TKR): replacement of degenerated articular surfaces of tibia, femur, and/or patella with metal, plastic, or a combination prosthesis. Can be cemented (may loosen in time with active patients) or noncemented (longer WB restrictions to allow the surrounding bone to grow into prosthesis). Indications for TKA: osteoarthritis, RA, pain, and reduced function.

CPM; LEs circulation (ankle pumps); isometrics (proper breathing); bed mobility and transfers; gait training with assistive device (PWB, WBAT as per MD/DO); patellar mobilization; ROM exercises (AAROM exercises such as SLRs; SAQ exercises); isotonic exercises (knee extension exercises); stationary bike; treadmill; CKC exercises; balance training (balance board); proprioceptive training; endurance training; aquatic therapy (cardiovascular program with WB restrictions); return to function training.

Total shoulder replacement (TSA): replacement of a fractured or necrotic proximal humerus with prosthesis. Indications for TSA: osteoarthritis, avascular necrosis, osteoporosis, and RA. Sometimes patients need a rotator cuff repair with TSA (longer immobility and rehab).

Shoulder sling; gentle AAROM exercises; isometrics (for rotator cuff repair—no deltoid exercises); strengthening exercises of wrist, hand, elbow; Codman's Pendulum; scapular ROM exercises; scapular stabilization exercises; HEP (wand, pulleys, or cane exercises); light PREs (by week 6 postoperative without rotator cuff repair); return to function training (by 6 months postoperative without rotator cuff repair).

Phases of Tissue Healing and Clinical Interventions

Tissue Healing and Interventions

Table 3-52   Tissue Healing and Interventions

Tissue Healng and Clinical Signs	Interventions
Inflammatory phase (begins immediately after injury; lasts 2 to 4 days). Signs: pain (dolor), heat (calor), redness (rubor), swelling (tumor), and loss of function (functio laesa).	Rest the area (immobilize and protect the affected area; exercise the unaffected areas; NWB or PWB; PROM if applicable; CPM postoperative); ice (apply ice or cold); compression (taping, bracing, or orthotics); elevation (elevate the part); decrease pain (use physical agents and modalities for pain management and swelling); patient education (educate about avoidance of activities and how to protect the area).
Fibroblastic phase (begins immediately after the inflammatory phase at approximately fifth day; lasts up to 3 weeks). Signs: lessening of inflammation; may still have pain and weakness.	Protect the area (bracing or orthotics; progressive WB such as PWB or WBAT); decrease pain (physical agents and modalities for pain management and swelling); increase ROM and function (use scar mobilization techniques; PROM, AAROM, AROM; isometric exercises; stretching exercises (start with light stretching because tissue is delicate in the beginning); CKC if pain and swelling subsided; ADLs); patient education (educate the patient how to protect the affected area; to avoid excessive motion for tissue irritation/destruction).
Remodeling phase (lasts from 3 weeks to 3 months). Signs: inflammation is resolved. Caution: if scar tissue is irritated or stressed, the fibroblastic activity continues; patient may present with pain, swelling, stiffness, and muscle guarding.	Increase strength and function to normal (restore stability, mobility, joint arthrokinematics, gradual return to work/school/hobbies); patient education (to avoid future injury).

SECTION 3-6

Bones

Human Skeleton

Bones makes up the framework of the human body. The human skeleton has 206 bones with 80 of the trunk (axial skeleton) and 126 of the limbs (appendicular skeleton). (Figure 3-58)

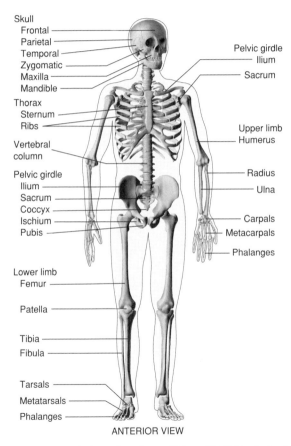

Skull
  Frontal
  Parietal
  Temporal
  Zygomatic
  Maxilla
  Mandible
Thorax
  Sternum
  Ribs
Vertebral column
Pelvic girdle
  Ilium
  Sacrum
  Coccyx
  Ischium
  Pubis
Lower limb
  Femur
  Patella
  Tibia
  Fibula
  Tarsals
  Metatarsals
  Phalanges

Pelvic girdle
  Ilium
  Sacrum
Upper limb
  Humerus
  Radius
  Ulna
  Carpals
  Metacarpals
  Phalanges

ANTERIOR VIEW

Figure 3-58   The Human Skeleton. From Human Biology: Fifth Edition by Daniel Chiras, 2005, page 217, Figure 12.2 called The Human Skeleton

MUSCULOSKELETAL INTERVENTIONS

Carpal Bones

Table 3-53 Carpal Bones

Proximal Raw	scaphoid (navicular); lunate; triquetrum; pisiform
Distal Raw	trapezium; trapezoid; capitate; hamate

Tarsal Bones

Table 3-54 Tarsal Bones

Calcaneus; cuboid; first metatarsal; talus; navicular; first cuneiform (medial cuneiform); second cuneiform (intermediate cuneiform); third cuneiform (lateral cuneiform)

Muscles: Function, Nerve, Origin, Insertion, and Palpation

MUSCULOSKELETAL INTERVENTIONS

See Figure 3-59.

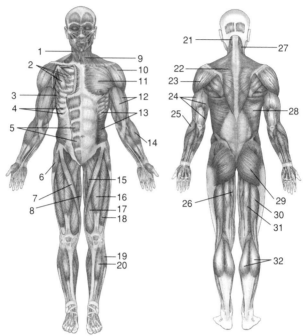

1. Sternocleidomastoid	13. External abdominal	24. Triceps brachii
2. Pectoralis minor	oblique	25. Extensor carpi
3. Serratus anterior	14. Brachioradialis	radialis longus
4. External intercostals	15. Adductor longus	26. Adductor magnus
5. Rectus abdominis	16. Rectus femoris	27. Splenius
6. Tensor fasciae latae	17. Vastus medialis	28. Latissimus dorsi
7. Sartorius	18. Vastus lateralis	29. Gluteus maximus
8. Gracilis	19. Peroneus longus	30. Biceps femoris
9. Platysma	20. Tibialis anterior	31. Semitendinosus
10. Deltoid	21. Levaor scapulae	32. Gastrocnemius
11. Pectoralis major	22. Trapezius	
12. Biceps brachii	23. Deltoid	

Figure 3-59 Anterior and Posterior Superficial Muscles. From Anatomy and Physiology: Understanding the Human Body by Robert Clark, page 159, Figure 10.3 called The anterior [left] and posterior [right] superficial muscles

Pelvis and Hip Muscles

See Table 3-55.

Knee Muscles

See Table 3-56.

Ankle/Foot Muscles

See Table 3-57.

Shoulder Muscles

See Table 3-58.

Rotator Cuff Muscles

See Table3-59.

Elbow and Forearm Muscles

See Table 3-60.

Wrist, Hand, and Finger Muscles

See Table 3-61.

Neck, Trunk, and Back Muscles

See Table 3-62.

MUSCULOSKELETAL INTERVENTIONS

Table 3-55 Pelvis and Hip Muscles[13]

Muscle	Function	Nerve	Origin	Insertion	Palpation
Iliopsoas	Hip flexion adduction, external rotation	Femoral nerve (L2–L3)	Iliac fossa, Anterior, and lateral surfaces of T12–L5	Lesser trochanter of the femur	Psoas major can be palpated distal to inguinal ligament on medial side of sartorius
Tensor fascia latae (helps knee to extend)	Combined hip flexion, abduction, internal rotation	Superior gluteal nerve (L4–L5)	ASIS	Through the iliotibial tract to the lateral condyle of the tibia	Iliotibial tract can be palpated at its insertion into the lateral tibial tubercle of the knee
Sartorius	Hip flexion, abduction, external rotation	Femoral nerve (two branches; L2–L3)	ASIS	Proximal part of the medial surface of the shaft of the tibia (Pes Anserinus)	Palpated at its origin, slightly inferior to the ASIS

Muscle	Function	Nerve	Origin	Insertion	Palpation
Gluteus maximus (sciatic nerve lies underneath)	Hip extension, hyperextension, external rotation	Inferior gluteal nerve (L1–L5; S1–S2)	Posterior sacrum and ilium	Posterior femur distal to greater trochanter and to iliotibial band	Palpated in prone, when buttocks are squeezed together, or when extending hip and flexing knee
Gluteus medius (with gluteus minimus and TFL abducts the thigh at the hip joint)	Hip abduction	Superior gluteal nerve (L4–S1)	Outer surface of ilium	Greater trochanter of femur (lateral surface)	Origin can be palpated slightly below iliac crest in side-lying with leg to be palpated raised in a few degrees of abduction
Gluteus minimus	Hip abduction, Internal rotation	Superior gluteal nerve (L4–S1)	Lateral ilium	Greater trochanter of femur (anterior border)	Cannot be palpated
Adductor magnus	Hip adduction	Superior gluteal nerve (L4–S1)	Outer surface of the ilium	Entire linea aspera and adductor tubercle	Can be palpated only as a group

continues

Table 3-55 (continued)					
Muscle	Function	Nerve	Origin	Insertion	Palpation
Adductor brevis	Hip adduction	Obturator nerve (L3–L4)	Outer surface of inferior ramus of pubis	Proximal part of linea aspera and pectineal line	Cannot be palpated individually, only as a group
Adductor longus	Hip adduction	Obturator nerve (L3–L4)	Outer surface of inferior ramus of pubis	Middle one third of linea aspera	Cannot be palpated individually, only as a group
Piriformis (muscle spasm can cause tenderness of sciatic nerve)	Hip external rotation	Nerves originating from S1 and S2 nerve root segments	Sacrum	Greater trochanter of femur (superior border)	Cannot be palpated

Table 3-56 Knee Muscles[13]

Muscle	Function	Nerve	Origin	Insertion	Palpation
Rectus femoris (powerful knee joint stabilizer)	Hip flexion, knee extension	Femoral nerve (L2–L4)	AIIS	Quadriceps tendon into tibial tubercle	Palpated as part of the quadriceps femoris group. For atrophy, measure the circumference of each thigh at 3 inches above mid patella.
Vastus medialis	Knee extension	Femoral nerve (L2–L4)	Linea aspera	Quadriceps tendon into tibial tubercle	Palpated as part of quadriceps femoris group
Vastus lateralis	Knee extension	Femoral Nerve (L2–L4)	Linea aspera	Quadriceps tendon into tibial tubercle	Palpated as part of quadriceps femoris group
Vastus intermedius	Knee extension	Femoral nerve (L2–L4)	Anterior femur	Quadriceps tendon into tibial tubercle	Palpated as part of quadriceps femoris group

continues

MUSCULOSKELETAL INTERVENTIONS

Muscles: Function, Nerve, Origin, Insertion, and Palpation **231**

Table 3-56 (continued)

Muscle	Function	Nerve	Origin	Insertion	Palpation
Biceps femoris	Knee flexion, hip extension	Sciatic nerve for long head (S1–S3); common peroneal nerve for short head (L5–S2)	Long head: ischial tuberosity; short head: lateral lip of linea aspera of femur	Common tendon of the two heads inserts at the head of the fibula	Palpated near its insertion into head of fibula when flexing knee
Semimembranosus	Knee flexion, hip extension	Tibial portion of sciatic nerve (L5–S2)	Ischial tuberosity	Medial condyle of tibia posterior surface	Hamstrings group palpated from common origin on ischium to insertion
Semitendinosus	Knee flexion, hip extension	Sciatic nerve (L5–S2)	Ischial tuberosity	Anteromedial surface of the shaft of tibia (pes anserinus)	Hamstrings group palpated from common origin on ischium to insertion

Table 3-57 Ankle/Foot Muscles[13]

Muscle	Function	Nerve	Origin	Insertion	Palpation
Gastrocnemius	Ankle plantarflexion, knee flexion	Tibial nerve (S1–S2)	Medial and lateral condyles of femur	Through Achilles tendon into calcaneus	Gastrocnemius and soleus to be observed in action asking patient to walk on his or her toes
Soleus	Ankle plantarflexion	Tibial nerve (S1–S2)	Posterior fibula and tibia	Through Achilles tendon into calcaneus	Gastrocnemius and soleus to be observed in action asking patient to walk on his or her toes
Tibialis anterior	Ankle dorsiflexion, foot inversion	Deep peroneal nerve (L4–S1)	Lateral tibia and interosseous membrane	First cuneiform and metatarsal	Palpated medially at the dorsum of foot at its insertion onto the first metatarsal and

continues

MUSCULOSKELETAL INTERVENTIONS

Table 3-57 (continued)

Muscle	Function	Nerve	Origin	Insertion	Palpation
					the first cuneiform bones
Tibialis posterior (supports medial longitudinal arch of foot)	Foot inversion, Ankle plantarflexion	Tibial nerve (L5–S1)	Interosseous membrane, adjacent tibia, and fibula	Navicular and most tarsals and metatarsals	Tendon palpated behind and inferior to medial malleolus
Peroneus longus (supports lateral longitudinal arch of foot)	Foot eversion, ankle plantarflexion	Superficial peroneal nerve (L4–S1)	Lateral proximal fibula and interosseous membrane	Plantar surface of the first cuneiform and metatarsal	Tendon palpated with peroneus brevis tendon behind lateral malleolus
Peroneus brevis	Foot eversion, ankle plantarflexion	Superficial peroneal nerve (L4–S1)	Lateral two thirds of the lateral surface of fibula	Plantar surface of the fifth metatarsal bone	Tendon palpated with peroneus longus tendon behind lateral malleolus

Muscle	Function	Nerve	Origin	Insertion	Palpation
Extensor digitorum longus (EDL)	Extension of the four lesser toes, ankle dorsiflexion, foot eversion	Deep peroneal nerve (L4–S1)	Anterior surface of shaft of fibula	Distal phalanx of the four lesser toes	EDL tendon palpated lateral to EHL when toes are extended
Extensor hallucis longus (EHL)	Extension of the great toe, ankle dorsiflexion, foot inversion	Deep peroneal Nerve (L4–S1)	Fibula and interosseous membrane	Distal phalanx of the great toe	EHL tendon palpated lateral to tibialis anterior when the big toe extends
Flexor digitorum longus (FDL)	Flexion of the four lesser toes, ankle plantarflexion, foot inversion	Tibial nerve (L5–S1)	Posterior tibia	Distal phalanx of the four lesser toes	FDL tendon palpated immediately behind the posterior tibialis, just above the medial malleolus, when toes are flexed
Flexor hallucis longus (FHL) Maintains medial longitudinal arch of foot	Flexion of the great toe, ankle plantarflexion, foot inversion	Tibial nerve (L5–S1)	Posterior fibula and interosseous membrane	Distal phalanx of the great toe	Cannot be palpated

MUSCULOSKELETAL INTERVENTIONS

Table 3-58 Shoulder Muscles[13]

Muscle	Function	Nerve	Origin	Insertion	Palpation
Upper trapezius	Scapular elevation, upward rotation	Spinal accessory nerve—CN XI (C3–C4)	Occipital protuberance, nuchal ligament	Outer half of the clavicle, acromion process	Palpated with middle and lower trapezius from origin through clavicle, acromion, spine of scapula; for lower angle continue to spinous processes of lower thoracic vertebrae (T12)
Middle trapezius (pulls scapula medially)	Retraction of shoulder girdle	Spinal accessory nerve—CN XI (C3–C4)	Spinous processes of C7–T3	Superior lip of spine of scapula	The same as above
Lower trapezius (pulls scapula downward)	Scapular depression, upward rotation	Spinal accessory nerve—CN XI (C3–C4)	Spinous processes of middle and lower thoracic vertebrae	Base of spine of scapula	The same as above

Muscle (Function)	Function	Nerve	Origin	Insertion	Palpation
Serratus anterior (prevents winging of scapula)	Scapular protraction, upward rotation	Long thoracic nerve (C5–C7)	Lateral surface of the upper eight ribs	Anterior surface of vertebral border of scapula	Palpated at medial wall of axilla, over the ribs
Rhomboid major and minor (raises medial border of scapula)	Scapular retraction, downward rotation	Dorsal scapular nerve (C5)	Nuchal ligament and spinous processes of C7 and T5	Vertebral border of scapula between the spine and the inferior angle	Palpated under the overlying trapezius; patient must have arm in the back in IR pushing hand posteriorly into PTA's hand
Levator scapulae (raises medial border of scapula)	Scapular elevation, downward rotation	C3 and C4 nerves, and dorsal scapular nerve (C5)	Transverse processes of C1–C4	Vertebral border of scapula between superior angle and base of spine	Cannot be palpated
Deltoid (anterior, middle, and posterior)	Shoulder abduction, flexion, extension, hyperextension, internal rotation,	Axillary nerve (C5–C6)	Anterior at lateral third of the clavicle; middle at acromion process of	Anterior, middle, and posterior at deltoid tuberosity of humerus	Palpated from acromion to deltoid tuberosity of humerus

continues

MUSCULOSKELETAL
INTERVENTIONS

Muscles: Function, Nerve, Origin, Insertion, and Palpation **237**

Table 3-58 (continued)

Muscle	Function	Nerve	Origin	Insertion	Palpation
	external rotation, horizontal adduction		scapula; posterior at inferior lip of spine of scapula		
Pectoralis major and minor (rotates scapula forward and downward)	Major: shoulder flexion to about 90° internal rotation, adduction, horizontal adduction. Minor: scapular rotation.	Major: lateral and medial pectoral nerves (C5–T1) Minor: medial pectoral nerve (C8–T1)	Major: clavicular head at medial third of clavicle; sternal head at anterior surface of sternum, and costal cartilage of first six ribs. Minor: third, fourth, and fifth rib	Major: both heads at lateral lip of bicipital groove of humerus (crest of greater tubercle). Minor: medial border of coracoid process	Major: palpated bilaterally mostly toward the medial portion; breast tissue overlies the pectoralis major. Minor: cannot be palpated.
Latissimus dorsi (assists rotating scapula downward)	Shoulder extension, adduction, internal rotation, hyperextension	Thoracodorsal Nerve (C6–C8)	Spinous process of T7–L5, sacrum and iliac crest, and lower three ribs	Bicipital groove of humerus (floor and medial lip)	Palpated easier along the posterior wall of the axilla when patient abducts the arm

| Teres major | Shoulder extension, adduction, internal rotation | Subscapular nerve (C5–C6) | Axillary border of scapula near inferior angle | Medial lip of bicipital groove of humerus (crest of lesser tubercle) | Palpated on lateral border of scapula just below the axilla |

MUSCULOSKELETAL INTERVENTIONS

Table 3-59 Rotator Cuff Muscles[13]

Muscle	Function	Nerve	Origin	Insertion	Palpation
Supraspinatus (assists deltoid in abduction)	Shoulder abduction	Suprascapular nerve (C5–C6)	Supraspinous fossa of scapula	Greater tuberosity of humerus	Palpated as a group at greater tuberosity of humerus when patient has shoulder extended passively
Infraspinatus	Shoulder external rotation, horizontal abduction	Suprascapular nerve (C5–C6)	Infraspinous fossa of scapula	Greater tuberosity of humerus	The same as above
Teres Minor	Shoulder external rotation, horizontal abduction	Axillary nerve (C5–C6)	Axillary border of scapula	Greater tuberosity of humerus	The same as above
Subscapularis	Shoulder internal rotation, abduction	Subscapular nerve (C5–C6)	Subscapular fossa of scapula	Greater tuberosity of humerus	Cannot be palpated

Table 3-60 Elbow and Forearm Muscles[13]

Muscle	Function	Nerve	Origin	Insertion	Palpation
Biceps brachii (is the main supinator)	Elbow flexion, forearm supination	Musculocutaneous nerve (C5–C6)	Short head: coracoid process of scapula. Long head: supraglenoid tubercle of scapula.	Bicipital tuberosity of radius	Palpated distally toward insertion when patient flexes the elbow
Triceps brachii	Elbow extension	Radial nerve (C7–C8)	Long head: infraglenoid tubercle of the scapula. Lateral head: lateral/posterior surfaces of proximal humerus Medial head: medial/posterior surfaces of distal humerus.	Olecranon process of ulna	Palpated from infraglenoid tubercle to just before olecranon process; patient must be leaning on a table with the arm slightly abducted and the hand on the table (as if a crutch supported arm)

continues

MUSCULOSKELETAL
INTERVENTIONS

Table 3-60 (continued)

Muscle	Function	Nerve	Origin	Insertion	Palpation
Brachialis	Elbow flexion	Musculocuta-neous nerve (C5–C6)	Distal part of ante-rior surface of humerus	Ulnar tuberosity and coronoid process of ulna	Cannot be pal-pated
Brachioradialis (assists rotat-ing forearm to mid prone)	Elbow flexion	Radial nerve (C5–C6)	Lateral supra-condylar ridge of humerus	Styloid process of radius	Palpated on anterolateral aspect of arm, when patient has elbow flexed at 90° and is making a fist pushing up under the edge of a table
Supinator	Forearm supina-tion	Radial nerve (C6)	Lateral epicondyle of humerus and the adjacent ulna	Anterior surface of proximal radius	Cannot be pal-pated

Pronator teres	Forearm pronation, elbow flexion	Median nerve (C6–C7)	Medial epicondyle of humerus, coronoid process of ulna	Lateral surface of radius at its midpoint	Palpated as the common tendon of wrist flexor and pronator muscle group, at the medial epicondyle of humerus

Table 3-61 Wrist, Hand, and Finger Muscles[13]

Muscle	Function	Nerve	Origin	Insertion	Palpation
Flexor carpi ulnaris (FCU)	Wrist flexion, ulnar deviation	Ulnar nerve (C8–T1)	Medial epicondyle of humerus	Pisiform and base of the fifth metacarpal	FCU tendon palpated proximal to pisiform on ulnar side of palmaris longus when patient flexes wrist against resistance
Flexor carpi radialis (FCR)	Wrist flexion, radial deviation	Median nerve (C6–C7)	Medial epicondyle of humerus	Base of the second and third metacarpal (palmar surface)	FCR tendon palpated radial to palmaris longus when patient flexes wrist and radially deviates hand
Extensor carpi ulnaris (ECU)	Wrist extension, ulnar deviation	Radial nerve (C6–C8)	Lateral epicondyle of humerus	Base of fifth metacarpal	Palpated starting at ulnar styloid process and going toward ECU insertion

	Function	Nerve	Origin	Insertion	Palpation
Extensor carpi radialis longus (ECRL)	Wrist radial deviation, extension	Radial nerve (C6–C7)	Supracondylar ridge of humerus	Base of second metacarpal	Palpated on radial side of dorsal radial tubercle, when patient clenches fist
Extensor carpi radialis brevis (ECRB)	Wrist extension	Radial nerve (C6–C7)	Lateral epicondyle of humerus	Base of third metacarpal	Palpated on radial side of dorsal radial tubercle, when patient clenches fist
Flexor digitorum superficialis (FDS)	Finger flexion of proximal interphalangeal (PIP) and metacarpophalangeal (MCP) joints	Median nerve (C7, C8, T1)	Lateral epicondyle of humerus, coronoid process, and radius	Sides of middle phalanx of the four fingers	Can be isolated for a specific finger to be tested by holding the non-tested fingers in extension, and asking patient to flex the PIP joint of tested finger

continues

MUSCULOSKELETAL INTERVENTIONS

Table 3-61 (continued)

Muscle	Function	Nerve	Origin	Insertion	Palpation
Flexor digitorum profundus (FDP)	Flexion of all three joints of fingers	Median and ulnar nerves (C8–T1)	Upper three fourths of the ulna	Distal phalanx of the four fingers	Can be isolated for a specific finger to be tested by stabilizing MCP and IP joints of tested finger in extension, asking the patient to flex only DIP of tested finger
Extensor digitorum (extensor digitorum communis)	Extension of all three joints of fingers (MP, PIP, DIP)	Radial nerve (C6–C8)	Lateral epicondyle of humerus	Base of distal phalanx of fingers 2–5	Palpated between carpus and MCP joints when fingers are extended

Muscle	Function	Nerve	Origin	Insertion	Palpation
Extensor digiti minimi (EDM)	<u>Extension of all joints of the fifth finger</u> (MP, PIP, DIP)	Radial nerve—deep branch (C6–C8)	Lateral epicondyle of humerus	Base of distal phalanx of the fourth finger	Palpated as a slight indentation lateral to the ulnar styloid process when patient's palm is resting on the table and patient raises little finger
Flexor pollicis longus (FPL)	<u>Flexion of all joints of the thumb</u> (IP, MP, CMC)	Median nerve (C8–T1)	Anterior surface of radius	Distal phalanx of thumb	Palpated on palmar side of thumb asking patient to flex and extend thumb
Extensor pollicis longus (EPL)	<u>Extension of all joints of the thumb</u> (IP, MP)	Radial nerve (C6–C8)	Middle posterior ulna and interosseous membrane	Base of distal phalanx of thumb, dorsal surface	Palpated on dorsal side of thumb asking patient to extend and flex the thumb

continues

Table 3-61 (continued)

Muscle	Function	Nerve	Origin	Insertion	Palpation
Abductor pollicis longus (APL)	Abduction of the thumb	Radial nerve (C6–C7)	Posterior radius, interosseous membrane, and middle ulna	Base of the first metacarpal	Palpated on radial palmar side of thumb
Dorsal interossei	Abduction of the fingers at the MCP joint	Ulnar nerve (C8–T1)	Adjacent metacarpals	Base of proximal phalanx	Cannot be palpated, except for the first that is palpable at base of proximal phalanx of first finger
Palmar interossei	Adduction of the fingers at the MCP joint	Ulnar nerve (C8–T1)	Respective metacarpals	Base of proximal phalanx as originated	Cannot be palpated
Adductor pollicis	Adduction of the thumb	Ulnar nerve (C8–T1)	Capitate, base of the second metacarpal, palmar surface of the third metacarpal	Base of proximal phalanx of thumb	Palpated (with difficulty) on palmar side of web space of thumb

Opponens pollicis	Opposition of the thumb	Median nerve (C6, C7)	Trapezium bone and flexor retinaculum	First metacarpal	Palpated along radial shaft of first metacarpal; it is lateral to abductor pollicis brevis
Abductor pollicis brevis	Abduction of the saddle joint of the thumb	Median nerve (C6, C7)	Transverse carpal ligament, tuberosity of scaphoid, and ridge of trapezium	Radial side of base of proximal phalanx of thumb	Palpated in center of thenar eminence, medial to opponens pollicis
Flexor digiti minimi	Flexion of CMC and MCP joints of the fifth finger	Ulnar nerve (C8–T1)	Hook of hamate and flexor retinaculum	Base of proximal phalanx of the fourth finger	Palpated on palmar surface of little finger when flexing little finger

continues

MUSCULOSKELETAL INTERVENTIONS

Table 3-61 (continued)

Muscle	Function	Nerve	Origin	Insertion	Palpation
Opponens digiti minimi	Opposition of the fifth finger	Ulnar nerve (C8–T1)	Hamate bone and flexor retinaculum	Fifth metacarpal	Palpated on hypothenar eminence on radial side of the fifth metacarpal
Abductor digiti minimi	Abduction of MCP joint of the fifth finger	Ulnar nerve (C8–T1)	Pisiform bone, tendon of flexor carpi ulnaris	Proximal phalanx of little finger	Palpated on the ulnar border of the hand

Table 3-62   Neck, Trunk, and Back Muscles[13]

Muscle	Function	Nerve	Origin	Insertion	Palpation
Sternocleido-mastoid	Cervical flexion and rotation to the opposite side	Accessory nerve—CN XI (C2, C3)	Sternum and clavicle	Mastoid process	Palpated from manubrium and clavicle to mastoid
Scalene (anterior, medius, posterior)	Bilaterally assisting in neck flexion and unilateral neck lateral flexion	Lower cervical nerve	Transverse processes of cervical vertebrae	First and second ribs	
Rectus abdominis	Trunk flexion and compression of the abdomen	Seventh through twelfth intercostal nerves (T7–T12)	Pubis	Cartilage of the fifth, sixth, and seventh ribs	Palpated at midline of thorax over linea alba when patient is performing a sit-up

continues

MUSCULOSKELETAL INTERVENTIONS

Table 3-62 (continued)

Muscle	Function	Nerve	Origin	Insertion	Palpation
External oblique	Bilateral trunk forward flexion, unilateral lateral flexion and rotation to the opposite side	Eighth through twelfth intercostal nerves, iliohypogastric and ilioinguinal nerves	Lower eight ribs laterally	Iliac crest and linea alba.	Palpated distally until reaching anterior superior iliac spine; fibers run from out to in, as if both hands were inserted in the pockets
Internal oblique	Bilateral trunk forward flexion, unilateral lateral flexion and rotation to the same side	Eighth through twelfth intercostal nerves, iliohypogastric and ilioinguinal nerves	Inguinal ligament, iliac crest, thoracolumbar fascia	Cartilages of the 10–12 ribs and the linea alba	Palpated on lateral part of anterior abdominal wall distal to the rib cage; fibers run from in to out as if both hands were taken out of the pockets

Muscle	Function	Nerve	Origin	Insertion	Palpation
Quadratus Lumborum (fixes twelfth rib during inspiration, depresses twelfth rib during forced expiration)	Lateral bending of the trunk (to the same side)	Twelfth thoracic (T12) and first lumbar (L1) nerves	Iliac crest	Transverse processes of L2, L5, and twelfth rib	Cannot be palpated
Erector spinae: sacrospinalis, iliocostalis, longissimus dorsi and spinalis dorsi	Head and vertebral column bilateral extension, unilateral lateral flexion	Spinal nerves	Spinous processes, transverse processes, and ribs from occiput to sacrum and ilium	Spinous processes, transverse processes, and ribs from occiput to sacrum and ilium	Palpated on both sides of vertebral column by asking patient to extend the spine while prone

MUSCULOSKELETAL INTERVENTIONS

Thenar and Hypothenar Muscles

Table 3-63 Thenar and Hypothenar Muscles[13]

Thenar muscles	Abductor pollicis brevis; opponens pollicis; flexor pollicis brevis
	Thenar area innervation: median nerve
Hypothenar muscles	Abductor digiti minimi; opponens digiti; flexor digiti minimi
	Hypothenar area innervation: ulnar nerve

References

1. Norkin, CC, White DJ. *Measurement of Joint Motion: A Guide to Goniometry*, 3rd ed. Philadelphia: F.A. Davis Company; 2003.

2. Hislop, HJ, Mongomery, J. *Daniels and Worthingham's Muscle Testing: Techniques of Manual Examination*. Philadelphia: W.B. Saunders Company; 2002.

3. Magee, DJ. *Orthopedic Physical Assessment*, 4th ed. Philadelphia: Saunders; 1997.

4. Gulick, D. *Ortho Notes: Clinical Examination Pocket Guide*. Philadelphia: F.A. Davis Company; 2005.

5. Rothstein, JM, Roy, SH, Wolf, SL, Scalzitti, DA. *The Rehabilitation Specialist's Handbook*, 3rd ed. Philadelphia: F.A. Davis Company; 2005.

6. Kisner, C, Colby, LA. *Therapeutic Exercise: Foundations and Techniques*. Philadelphia: F. A. Davis Company; 2002.

7. Tan, KC. *Practical Manual of Physical Medicine and Rehabilitation: Diagnostics, Therapeutics, and Basic Problems*. St. Louis: Mosby-Year Book, Inc.; 1998.

8. Hecox, B, Tsega, AM, Weisberg, J, Sanko J. *Integrating Physical Agents in Rehabilitation*, 2nd ed. Upper Saddle River, NJ: Pearson Education Inc.; 2006.

9. Dreeben, O. *Introduction to Physical Therapy for Physical Therapist Assistants*. Sudbury, MA: Jones and Bartlett Publishers; 2007.

10. O'Sullivan, SB, Schmitz, TJ. *Physical Rehabilitation: Fifth Edition*. Philadelphia: F.A. Davis Company; 2007.

11. The American Physical Therapy Association. *Guide to Physical Therapist Practice: Second Edition*. Alexandria, VA: APTA; 2001; revised 2003.

12. Pauls, JA, Reed KL. *Quick Reference to Physical Therapy*. Gaithersburg, MD: Aspen Publishers, Inc.; 1996.
13. Moore, KL. *Clinically Oriented Anatomy: Third Edition*. Baltimore, MD: Williams and Wilkins; 1992.

MUSCULOSKELETAL
INTERVENTIONS

Part IV

Neurologic Interventions

NEUROLOGIC
INTERVENTIONS

Neurologic Data Collection

Patient's Arousal Levels

Table 4-1 Patient's Arousal Levels[1]

Arousal Level	Description
Alert	Patient is aware of his or her environment, paying attention to the therapist and able to cooperate with treatment.
Coma	Patient is totally unresponsive to stimuli and cannot be awakened. Patient is not able to express himself or herself. Patient can be monitored with the Glasgow Coma Scale (includes three activities: eye opening; best motor response; verbal response).
Lethargic	Patient is drowsy and ready to sleep. Patient has difficulty concentrating on tasks and needs stimulation to keep awake.
Obtunded	Patient has diminished arousal and awareness to his or her environment. Patient may require repeated stimulation to notice the therapist.
Stupor (Semi Coma)	Patient has decreased responsiveness to his or her environment and cannot interact with the therapist. Patient needs noxious (unpleasant) stimulation to be aroused.

Memory and Amnesia Terms

Table 4-2 Memory and Amnesia Terms[2]

Memory: mental registration, retention and recollection of past experiences, knowledge, ideas, and sensations.

Short-term (immediate) memory: immediate recollection of experiences, knowledge, ideas, and sensations that occurred in the immediate past (seconds to minutes). The capacity of short-term memory is approximately seven items.

Long-term memory: recollection of experiences, knowledge, ideas, and sensations that occurred in the distant past (days, months, years). The capacity of long-term memory is unlimited.

Amnesia: significant loss of memory. It can be caused by CVA, seizure, trauma, alcoholism, intoxication, senility, or an unknown cause.

Anterograde (post-traumatic) amnesia: amnesia for events that occurred after the onset of amnesia. It involves amnesia of new learned material that was acquired after the causative event. It is more common.

Retrograde amnesia: amnesia for events that occurred prior to the onset of amnesia. It involves amnesia of prior learned material that was acquired prior to the causative event. It is less common.

Ranchos Los Amigos Levels of Cognitive Functioning

Table 4-3   LOCF

I. No response: patient is unresponsive to any stimuli.

II. Generalized response: patient responds inconsistently and non-purposefully to stimuli. Responses such as total body movements or vocalization may be the same regardless of the stimulus.

III. Localized Response: patient responds inconsistently but purposely to stimuli. Patient may follow uncomplicated commands such as squeezing the hand or closing the eyes.

IV. Confused—Agitated: patient is in a high level of activity. Patient exhibits bizarre, non-purposeful behavior relative to stimuli and environment. Patient is unable to cooperate directly with the treatment. Patient's cognitive deficits are: (1) Very limited gross attention span; (2) Confabulation; (3) Incoherent and inappropriate verbalization; (4) Impairment in short- and long-term memory; (5) Unable to discriminate among persons or objects.

V. Confused—Inappropriate: patient is able to respond somewhat consistently to simple commands. Patient responds in a non-purposeful, random, or fragmented way to complex or unstructured activities. Patient exhibits gross attention span in regard to the environment but is highly distractible and cannot focus. Patient is able to perform learned tasks with structure. Patient's cognitive deficits are difficulty with complex and unstructured activities, inability to learn new information, inability to focus on a specific task, impaired memory, confabulation, and inappropriate verbalization.

VI. Confused—Appropriate: patient appears to demonstrate goal-directed and appropriate behavior but is dependent on external input or instruction. Patient consistently follows simple commands and demonstrates carryover for relearned tasks (such as self-care activities). Patient's cognitive deficit is related to incorrect responses due to memory problems. Past memories have more depth and detail than more recent ones.

VII. Automatic—Appropriate: patient appears to demonstrate appropriate behavior. Patient is oriented to environment. Patient performs daily routines automatically mostly in a robot-like manner. Patient demonstrates carryover for new learning activities but at times has difficulty remembering them. Patient is able to initiate social and recreational activities but needs organization. Patient's cognitive deficits are minimal confusion and impaired judgment.

VIII. Purposeful—Appropriate: patient recalls and integrates past and recent events. Patient is oriented and reactive to environment. Patient demonstrates independent carryover for new learning. Patient's cognitive deficits are: (1)

Decreased abstract reasoning; (2) Decreased tolerance to stress; (3) Judgment difficulties in emergency or unusual situations; (4) Decreased premorbid abilities.

Terms of Cognitive-Perceptual Deficits

Table 4-4   Cognitive-Perceptual Deficits[1]

Agnosia: inability to recognize familiar objects with one sensory modality, but able to recognize the same object with another sensory modality.

Anosognosia: denial, neglect, and lack of awareness of the presence or severity of a person's own neurologic dysfunction (such as paralysis in stroke).

Apraxia: inability to produce purposeful movements, although there is no sensory or motor loss. Patient has intact sensation, strength, coordination, and comprehension.

Ideational apraxia: inability to produce purposeful movements on his or her own or on command.

Ideomotor apraxia: inability to produce purposeful movements on command but can produce them on his or her own.

Figure–Ground discrimination deficit: inability to pick out an object from the background on which it is embedded.

Form constancy deficit: inability to pick out an object from an array of similarly shaped objects.

Homonymous hemianopsia: blindness in the outer half of the visual field of one eye and the inner half of the visual field of the other eye. Patient cannot receive information from either the right or the left of the visual environment.

Position in space deficit: inability to determine and interpret spatial concepts such as up or down, in or out, in front or behind, or under or over.

Somatognosia: inability to identify own or other person's body parts and the relationship of one body part to another. Somatognosia is impairment in body scheme.

Spatial-relation deficit: inability to perceive the relationship between self and one or more objects.

Right/left discrimination deficit: inability to identify the right and left sides of one's own body or that of the examiner.

Topographical orientation deficit: inability to understand and remember the relationship of one place to another.

Unilateral neglect: inability to register and integrate visual stimuli and perceptions from one side of the environment (usually the left side). Patient ignores stimuli occurring in that side of personal space. It is not attributed to any sensory problem.

Speech and Communication Functions and Impairments

Table 4-5   Speech and Communication Functions and Impairments

Speech and Communication Functions	Impairments
Expressive function: assessment of fluency of speech and speech production	(1) Broca's aphasia (nonfluent, expressive, or motor aphasia): speech is interrupted, uncoordinated, difficult to produce, and with awkward articulation. It is the result of a lesion involving the third frontal convolution of the left hemisphere. (2) Verbal apraxia: inability to volitionally articulate as a result of a lesion in the cortical dominant hemisphere. (3) Dysarthria: speech production difficulty caused by motor impairments related to respiration, phonation, articulation, and jaw and tongue movements. It is the result of a lesion in the CNS and PNS.
Receptive function: assessment of comprehension	(1) Wernicke's aphasia (fluent or receptive aphasia): auditory comprehension is impaired while speech is spontaneous and flowing smoothly. It is the result of a lesion in the posterior first temporal gyrus of the left hemisphere. (2) Global aphasia: severe aphasia with impairments in comprehension and speech production.

Sensory Function—Sensory Receptors

Table 4-6   Sensory Receptors: Function and Testing

Sensory Receptors	Function and Testing
Barognosis (combined cortical sensations)	Function: ability to recognize different gradations of weight in similar size or shape objects. Testing: the PTA places different weights with the same size (shape), one at a time, in the patient's tested hand. The patient with eyes closed is asked to indicate if the weight is "heavier" or "lighter" than the previous one (or comparing bilaterally).

Graphesthesia (combined cortical sensations)	Function: ability to recognize numbers, letters, or symbols traced on the skin. Testing: the PTA traces with a pencil numbers, letters, or symbols on patient's tested hand. The patient with eyes closed is asked to identify the figures drawn on the skin.
Kinesthesia (deep sensations)	Function: sensation and awareness of active or passive movement. Testing: the PTA moves the patient's limb. Patient with eyes closed is asked to identify the direction of movement (up or down, in or out) while the limb is in motion. Patient with eyes closed may also duplicate the movement with the opposite limb.
Pain (superficial sensations)	Function: ability to recognize sharp or dull sensation in response to sharp or dull stimuli. Testing: the PTA applies a disposable safety pin or a paper clip to patient's skin. Patient with eyes closed is asked to indicate when the stimulus is felt.
Proprioception (deep sensations)	Function: position sense and the awareness of the joints at rest. Testing: the PTA positions the patient's limb. Patient with eyes closed is asked to identify the limb's position (up or down, in or out).
Stereognosis (combined cortical sensations)	Function: ability to recognize by touch or manipulation the shape of familiar objects. Testing: the PTA gives the patient one object (such as a coin, a key, or a pencil). Patient with eyes closed is asked to name the object.
Touch (superficial sensations)	Function: ability to differentiate between touch and non-touch in response to slight touch or no touch. Testing: the PTA applies a cotton ball (or a piece of tissue) to patient's tested skin. Patient with eyes closed must respond to PTA ("yes" or "no") to indicate when the stimulus was applied.
Two-point discrimination (combined cortical sensations)	Function: ability to differentiate between one or two blunt points applied to the skin simultaneously (the smallest distance between two stimuli). Testing: the PTA applies simultaneously two stimuli (the rounded part of two paper clips) to patient's tested skin. Patient with eyes closed is asked to differentiate between one or two stimuli. When two stimuli are perceived by the patient, the PTA needs to measure the distance between the stimuli. Consideration must be given to acute perception of stimuli in the distal UEs as compared with LEs.

Sensory Function—Dermatomes

Table 4-7 Dermatomes*

Dermatomes represent sensory distribution of the cutaneous nerves corresponding to the spinal segments providing their innervation. As a sensory assessment, dermatomes are evaluated first as superficial sensations, before deep or combined (cortical) sensations. Dermatome testing is performed in a distal to proximal direction. It is generally not necessary to test every segment of each dermatome; testing general body areas is sufficient.

Upper-extremity dermatomes: C1—top of the head; C2—temple, forehead, occiput; C3—neck, posterior cheek; C4—superior part of chest above axilla (clavicle area); C5—lateral aspect of the arm, deltoid muscle region; C6—anterior arm, lateral side of hand to thumb, and index finger; C7—lateral arm and forearm to index, long, and ring fingers; C8—middle arm and forearm to long, ring, and little fingers.

Trunk dermatomes: T1—medial side of forearm to base of little finger; T2—axillary region; T4—nipple level; T6—xiphoid process level; T10—umbilicus level; T12—anterior superior iliac crest level.

Lower-extremity dermatomes: L1—lower abdomen and groin region; L2—anterolateral thigh (back and front of thigh to knee); L3—anteromedial thigh, leg, upper buttock; L4—medial buttock, lateral thigh, medial leg, dorsum of foot, large toe; L5—posterior lateral thigh, lateral leg, dorsum of foot, medial half of sole, first to third toes; S1—lateral plantar surface of foot, posterior thigh and leg; S2—posterior thigh and leg; S3—groin, medial thigh to knee; S4–S5—perineum, genitals, lower sacrum

*For the dermatome chart, see Figure 4-1 (pages 286–287)

Motor Function—Tonal Abnormalities

Table 4-8 Hypertonia and Hypotonia

Clonus: cyclical, spasmodic fluctuation of muscle contraction and relaxation in response to a repeated stretch of a spastic muscle. Usually spastic muscles react to a large and quick stretch by increasing their resistance. Clonus is common in plantarflexors and jaw and wrist muscles of upper motor neuron (UMN) lesions.

Cogwheel rigidity: condition when tremor coexists with rigidity. It is common in Parkinson's disease (PD). When moving the patient's extremity passively, it feels like a cogwheel (by letting go, then increasing the resistance to movement).

Decerebrate rigidity: condition when it is a sustained contraction and posturing of the trunk and extremities in full extension. It indicates a grave condition with a lesion in the brain stem between the superior colliculi and the vestibular nuclei.

Decorticate rigidity: condition when it is a sustained contraction and posturing of the trunk and lower extremities in extension and upper extremities in flexion. It is less grave than decerebrate rigidity with a lesion in the corticospinal tract at diencephalon (above superior colliculus).

Dystonia: prolonged involuntary muscular contractions causing repetitively twisting or writhing of body parts and fluctuations in muscle tone (with increased or decreased muscular tone). It can be found in CNS lesions (commonly in basal ganglia), neurodegenerative disorders (Wilson's disease or PD), or metabolic disorders (amino acid or lipid). Dystonia can also be found in torticollis, and the primary idiopathic dystonia can be inherited.

Flaccidity: decreased or absent muscular tone (hypotonia). The extremities are easily moved passively (floppy) without any resistance. It is common in lower motor neuron (LMN) lesions affecting the anterior horn cell or peripheral nerve and in UMN lesion of cerebellum or pyramidal tract.

Lead-pipe rigidity: constant rigidity. It is not dependent on the velocity of passive movement.

Rigidity: Resistance to passive movement involving agonist and antagonist muscles. It characterized by stiffness and inability to bend or be bent. It is caused by a lesion in basal ganglia. It is common in PD.

Spasticity: increased tone or resistance of muscles. It causes stiff and awkward movements. It is a result of an UMN lesion.

Motor Function—Myotatic Reflexes (Stretch Reflexes)

Table 4-9   Stretch Reflexes

Nerve Root	Site and Testing
C5–C6	Biceps: patient sitting with arm flexed and supported. Tap over the biceps tendon in the cubital fossa. Normal response: elbow flexion.
C7–C8	Triceps: patient sitting with arm supported in abduction and elbow flexed. Tap over the triceps tendon (above olecranon). Normal response: elbow extension.
L2–L4	Quadriceps (patellar): patient sitting with knee flexed (and foot unsupported). Tap over quadriceps tendon between the patella and tibial tuberosity. Normal response: knee extension.
L5–S2	Hamstrings: patient prone with knee half flexed and supported. Tap over hamstrings tendon at the knee. Normal response: knee flexion.
S1–S2	Achilles (ankle): patient prone with foot over the end of the table. Tap tendon above its insertion on the calcaneus. Normal response: foot plantarflexion.

Motor Function—Grading Scale for Muscle Stretch Reflex

Table 4-10   Grading Scale for Muscle Stretch Reflex

0 Absent: No visible muscle contraction.

1+ Hyporeflexia: Slight muscle contraction with little or no joint movement.

2+ Normal: Slight muscle contraction with slight joint movement.

3+ Hyperreflexia: Brisk (visible) muscle contraction with moderate joint movement.

4+ and 5+ Abnormal: Strong muscle contraction. Patient (client) can have clonus and/or the reflex can spread to the contralateral side.

Motor Function—Babinski's Reflex

Table 4-11 Babinski's Reflex

Babinski's reflex testing: normal response is the dorsiflexion of the great toe when the lateral border of the sole of the foot is stimulated (stroked).

Babinski's reflex testing: abnormal response is the extension of the great toe, and fanning of the other toes, when the lateral border of the sole of the foot is stimulated (stroked). Abnormal response indicates a lesion of the corticospinal (pyramidal) tract. It is a normal reflex in infants under the age of 6 months.

Motor Function—Cranial Nerves Functions and Impairments

Table 4-12   Cranial Nerves: Functions and Impairments

Cranial Nerves (CNs)	Functions and Impairments
CN I—olfactory (sensory)	Function: smell. Impairment: anosmia (loss of the sense of smell).
CN II—optic (sensory)	Function: vision and pupillary reflexes. Impairments: blindness and absence of pupillary reflexes (when shining the light in the eye).
CN III—oculomotor (motor and sensory). Muscles: medial, superior and inferior rectus; inferior oblique; levator palpebrae superioris.	Function: elevates upper eye lids; constricts pupil; moves eyes up/down. Impairments: ophthalmoplegia (paralysis of ocular muscles with eye deviation); severe ptosis (difficulty raising the eyelids); mydriasis (abnormal pupil dilation).

CN IV—trochlear (motor and sensory).
Muscle: superior oblique.

Function: depresses the adducted eye. Impairments: weakness in depression of ipsilateral adducted eye; diplopia (double vision).

CN V—trigeminal (motor and sensory).
Muscles: masseter; temporalis; pterygoids; mylohyoid; tensor tympani; palatini; anterior belly of digastric.

Function: sensation from face, cornea, and muscles of mastication. Impairments: loss of facial sensation and corneal reflex; weakness and atrophy of muscles of mastication; deviation of open jaw to ipsilateral side.

CN VI—abducent (motor and sensory).
Muscle: lateral rectus.

Function: abduction of the eye. Impairments: diplopia; convergent strabismus (the eye deviates by turning inward); paralysis of ipsilateral eye muscle.

CN VII—facial (motor and sensory). Muscles: buccinator; stapedius; stylohyoid; platysma; occipitalis; posterior belly of digastric.

Function: facial expression; articulation; winking; food and drink ingestion; nasal and lacrimal secretions; salivary secretions; taste. Impairments: paralysis of ipsilateral upper and lower facial muscles; loss of lacrimation; dry mouth and decreased salivation; loss of taste ipsilateral in the anterior two thirds of the tongue.

CN VIII—vestibulocochlear (sensory).

Function: hearing; equilibrium. Impairments: nerve deafness; dysequilibrium; vertigo (sensation of having objects moving around the person); nystagmus (involuntary cyclical movements of the eyes).

CN IX—glossopharyngeal (motor and sensory).
Muscles: stylopharyngeus; superior pharyngeal constrictor.

Function: elevates the pharynx; salivary secretions; taste; sensations in the root of the tongue, tonsils, uvula, and soft palate. Impairments: Minimal dysphagia (difficulty swallowing); partial dry mouth; loss of taste ipsilateral in the posterior third of the tongue; loss of gag reflex; anesthesia in the tonsillar region.

CN X—Vagus (motor and sensory).
Muscles: palate; pharyngeal constrictors; laryngeal intrinsics.

Function: taste; swallowing; phonation; slowing of the heart rate; constriction of bronchioles; increased peristalsis; digestive secretions; sensations to auditory meatus; sensation to pharynx and larynx; visceral sensations. Impairments: dysphagia; hoarseness; paralysis of soft palate with deviation of velum and uvula to the con-

continues

Table 4-12 (Continued)

Cranial Nerves (CNs)	Functions and Impairments
	tralateral side; anesthesia of pharynx and larynx on the ipsilateral side; anesthesia of ipsilateral auditory meatus.
CN XI—spinal accessory (motor and sensory). Muscles: SCM; trapezius.	Function: swallowing; phonation; movements of head and shoulder. Impairments: muscular weakness in shrugging the shoulders on the ipsilateral side; muscular weakness in turning the head to the opposite side.
CN XII—hypoglossal (motor and sensory). Muscles: styloglossus; hyoglossus; genioglossus; tongue intrinsics.	Function: movements of the tongue. Impairments: atrophy of the ipsilateral muscles of the tongue; tongue deviation to the ipsilateral side on protrusion.

Motor Function—Cerebellar Dysfunction Characteristics

Table 4-13 Cerebellar Dysfunction Characteristics

Cerebellar Dysfunctions	Characteristics
Ataxia: uncoordinated movements. It is a combination of cerebellar and sensory dysfunction.	Can be observed on the patient's gait, posture, and patterns of movement such as dysmetria and movement decomposition.
Dysarthria: speech articulation dysfunction. It is also called scanning speech.	The speech is hesitant, slow, with inappropriate pauses and lengthened syllables. The melodic quality of speech is distorted. Patient demonstrates normal words selection and grammar.
Dysdiadochokinesia: impaired ability to perform rapid alternating movements.	Patient is unable to perform rapid forearm supination and pronation. As speed increases, patient's movements become irregular with rhythm and range deficits.
Dysmetria: inability to judge the distance or range of a movement.	Patient is unable to reach an object by either overestimating or underestimating the distance where the object is located.
Hypotonia: decrease in muscle tone due to cerebellar dysfunction.	Patient demonstrates reduced resistance to passive movement. Patient's muscles are soft and flaccid.

Intention (kinetic) tremor: involuntary oscillatory movement of a limb during voluntary motion. Intention tremor is absent at rest.	Patient demonstrates involuntary tremor when trying to reach a target. The tremor increases when the limb is close to the target or when the movement speed increases.
Movement decomposition (dyssynergia): inability to perform a smooth movement at once.	When asked to complete a movement, the patient performs a series of component parts of the movement.
Postural (static) tremor: involuntary oscillatory movement of the body during standing (static) posture.	Patient demonstrates involuntary postural tremor back and forth when trying to maintain a standing posture. It may also be observed in a limb held against gravity.

Motor Function—Basal Ganglia Dysfunction Characteristics

Table 4-14   Basal Ganglia Dysfunction Characteristics

Basal Ganglia Dysfunctions	Characteristics
Akinesia: inability to initiate movement	Patient is unable to start any movement. Patient needs a large amount of concentration and effort to start any limb movement. Akinesia can be found in late stages of parkinsonism.
Athetosis: slow, involuntary, twisting movements	Patient demonstrates slow and involuntary twisting or writhing in the upper extremities (mostly hands), neck, tongue, face, and trunk. These movements can be present in combination with spasticity. Athetosis can be found in the athetoid type of cerebral palsy.
Bradykinesia: slow or decreased movement	Patient demonstrates a slow, shuffling gait, difficulty initiating the movement, or difficulty changing the direction of movement. Patient also may demonstrate decreased arm swing in gait and difficulty stopping when the movement started. Bradykinesia can be found in PD.
Chorea: involuntary, rapid, irregular, and jerky movements	Patient demonstrates involuntary, rapid, jerky movements of the extremities or facial muscles. Chronic (hereditary) chorea is characteristic of Huntington's disease.

continues

Table 4-14 (continued)

Basal Ganglia Dysfunctions	Characteristics
Resting tremor: involuntary, rhythmic, oscillatory movement at rest	Patient demonstrates involuntary tremor in the hands in the form of "pill-rolling" movements (as a pill is rolled between the thumb and the first two fingers). Patient also may have involuntary pronation and supination of forearm and jaw tremor. Resting tremor is characteristic of PD.
Rigidity: increased muscular tone (see table 4-8)	Patient demonstrates stiffness and inability to bend or be bent. Cogwheel rigidity: alternate giving and increased resistance to passive movement. Lead-pipe rigidity: constant resistance to movement. Both are observed in basal ganglia disorders.

Motor Function—Characteristics of Upper Motor Neuron and Lower Motor Neuron Lesions

Table 4-15   UMN Versus LMN

UMN Characteristics (CNS Lesions)	LMN Characteristics (CNS and PNS Lesions)
Diagnostics: SCI; CVA; TBI; CP; MS; hydrocephalus	Diagnostics: polio; tumor; trauma; muscular dystrophy; Guillain-Barré; Bell's palsy; trigeminal neuralgia
Hypertonicity (dependent on velocity); spasticity (especially in the antigravity muscles); contractures; abnormal posturing; deformity	Hypotonicity; flaccidity; proximal weakness (myopathy); distal weakness (neuropathy)
Involuntary muscle spasms in the flexor or extensor muscles	Fibrillation potentials (spontaneous depolarization of muscle fibers not visible through the skin); fasciculations (visible, spontaneous twitching of muscle groups)
Paralysis: paresis	Paralysis
Disuse atrophy (variable)	Neurogenic atrophy (rapid and severe)
Hyperreflexia; clonus; positive Babinski	Hyporeflexia with diminished or absent deep tendon reflexes; floppy limbs
Dyssynergic patterns of voluntary movements	Weak or absent voluntary movements

Motor Function—Coordination Tests and Scoring

Table 4-16   Coordination Tests and Scoring

Gross motor coordination tests: finger to nose; finger to therapist's finger; finger to
    finger; forearm supination and pronation; clapping; alternately touch nose to
    finger; heel on shin; foot tapping; alternately heel to knee; alternately heel to toe
Fine motor coordination tests: thumb to finger opposition; grasp and release test;
    standardized tests
Scoring: 0 (zero) = unable; 1 (one) = severe impairment; 2 (two) = moderate impair-
    ment; 3 (three) = minimal impairment; 4 (four) = normal performance

NEUROLOGIC INTERVENTIONS

Motor Function—Balance Tests and Scoring

Table 4-17   Balance Tests and Scoring

Standing static balance test (eyes open to eyes closed): patient is standing in double
    limb stance; patient is standing in single limb stance.
Romberg static balance test (eyes open to eyes closed): patient is standing with feet
    in normal stance position; can detect ataxia.
Sharpened Romberg static balance test (eyes open to eyes closed): patient is stand-
    ing in a tandem heel to toe position. It is more sensitive than Romberg static bal-
    ance test.
Dynamic balance tests: patient is standing, walking, turning, and stopping; tandem
    walking (placing the heel of one foot directly in front of the toe of the opposite
    foot); walking sideways, backward, and cross-stepping.
Functional balance tests: (1) Berg Balance Scale (measures skill on 14 functional
    activities); (2) Functional reach test (patient stands without support and reaches
    forward as far as possible with shoulder at 90° flexion, elbow extended and hand
    fisted without losing balance); (3) Tinetti mobility test (measures skill on six func-
    tional activities such as sitting balance, standing on one leg, turning, ambulation,
    stepping over obstacles); (4) Timed get up and go test.
Scoring: (1) Normal = patient maintains steady static balance without support, and
    dynamically can shift weight in all directions; (2) Good = patient maintains static
    balance without support, and dynamically can pick objects off floor; (3) Fair =
    patient maintains static balance with handhold, and dynamically maintains bal-
    ance while turning head and trunk; (4) Poor = in static balance patient requires
    handhold and support, and dynamically is unable to accept any challenge or to
    move without loss of balance.

Functional Balance Test—Berg Balance Scale

Table 4-18   Berg Balance Scale[1]*

Sitting to Standing
Patient instruction: Please stand up. Try not to use your hands for support.
( ) 4 able to stand without using hands and stabilizes independently
( ) 3 able to stand independently using hands
( ) 2 able to stand using hands after several tries
( ) 1 needs minimal aid to stand or stabilize
( ) 0 needs moderate to maximal assist to stand

2. Standing Unsupported
Patient instruction: Please stand for 2 minutes without holding.
( ) 4 able to stand safely 2 minutes
( ) 3 able to stand 2 minutes without supervision
( ) 2 able to stand 30 seconds unsupported
( ) 1 needs several tries to stand unsupported 30 seconds
( ) 0 unable to stand 30 seconds without support

3. Sitting with Back Unsupported but Feet Supported on Floor or on a Stool
Patient instruction: Please sit with arms folded for 2 minutes.
( ) 4 able to sit safely and securely 2 minutes
( ) 3 able to sit 2 minutes with supervision
( ) 2 able to sit 30 seconds
( ) 1 able to sit 10 seconds
( ) 0 unable to sit without support 10 seconds

4. Standing to Sit
Patient instruction: Please sit down.
( ) 4 sits safely with minimal use of hands
( ) 3 controls descent by using hands
( ) 2 uses back of legs against chair to control descent
( ) 1 sits independently, but has uncontrolled descent
( ) 0 needs assistance to sit

5. Transfers
PTA arranges chairs for a pivot transfer. PTA can use either two chairs (one with armrests and one without armrests) or a bed/mat and a chair (with armrests). Patient is asked to transfer one way toward a seat without armrests and one way toward a seat with arms.

* See copy in the Appendices—to be used for patient's records.

( ) 4 able to transfer safely with minor use of hands
( ) 3 able to transfer safely with definite need of hands
( ) 2 able to transfer with verbal cuing and/or supervision
( ) 1 needs one person to assist
( ) 0 needs two people to assist or supervise to be safe

6. Standing Unsupported with Eyes Closed
Patient instruction: Please close your eyes and stand still for 10 seconds.
( ) 4 able to stand 10 seconds safely
( ) 3 able to stand 10 seconds with supervision
( ) 2 able to stand 3 seconds
( ) 1 unable to keep eyes closed for 3 seconds but stands safely
( ) 0 needs help to keep from falling

7. Standing Unsupported with Feet Together
Patient instruction: Place your feet together and stand without holding.
( ) 4 able to place feet together independently and stand safely 1 minute
( ) 3 able to place feet together independently and stand with supervision for 1 minute
( ) 2 able to place feet together independently but unable to hold for 30 seconds
( ) 1 needs help to assume the position but can stand for 15 seconds, feet together
( ) 0 needs help to assume the position and unable to stand for 15 seconds

8. Reaching Forward with Outstretched Arm While Standing
Patient instruction: Please lift arm to 90°. Stretch out your fingers and reach forward as far as you can.
PTA places a ruler at the tips of the outstretched fingers—patient should not touch the ruler when reaching. Distance recorded by the PTA is from the patient's finger-tips (with the patient in the most forward position). The patient should use both hands when possible to avoid trunk rotation.
( ) 4 can reach forward confidently 20–30 cm (10 inches)
( ) 3 can reach forward safely 12 cm (5 inches)
( ) 2 can reach forward safely 5 cm (2 inches)
( ) 1 reaches forward but needs supervision
( ) 0 loses balance when trying, requires external support

9. Pick Up Object from the Floor from a Standing Position
Patient instruction: Please pick up the shoe (or slipper) which is placed in front of your feet.
( ) 4 able to pick up the shoe safely and easily
( ) 3 able to pick up the shoe but needs supervision

continues

Neurologic Data Collection

Table 4-18   (continued)

( ) 2 unable to pick up the shoe, but reaches 2–5 cm (1–2 inches) from the shoe and keeps balance independently

( ) 1 unable to pick up and needs supervision while trying

( ) 0 unable to try and needs assistance to keep from losing balance (or falling)

10. Turning to Look Behind over Your Left and Right Shoulders While Standing

Patient instruction: Please turn and look directly behind you over toward the left shoulder. Repeat to the right.

PTA, standing in back of the patient, may pick up an object to look at directly encouraging the patient to turn around.

( ) 4 looks behind from both sides and weight shifts well

( ) 3 looks behind one side only, other side shows less weight shift

( ) 2 turns sideways only but maintains balance

( ) 1 needs close supervision or verbal cuing

( ) 0 needs assistance while turning

11. Turn 360°

Patient instruction: Please turn completely around in a full circle, pause, and then turn a full circle in the other direction.

( ) 4 able to turn 360° safely in 4 seconds or less

( ) 3 able to turn 360° safely, one side only, 4 seconds or less

( ) 2 able to turn 360° safely, but slowly

( ) 1 needs close supervision or verbal cuing

( ) 0 needs assistance while turning

12. Place Alternate Foot on Step or Stool While Standing Unsupported

Patient instruction: Please place each foot alternately on the step stool. Continue until each foot has touched the step stool 4 times.

( ) 4 able to stand independently and safely and complete 8 steps in 20 seconds

( ) 3 able to stand independently and complete 8 steps in more than 20 seconds

( ) 2 able to complete 4 steps without aid with supervision

( ) 1 able to complete more than 2 steps but needs minimal assistance

( ) 0 needs assistance to keep from falling (or is unable to try)

13. Standing Unsupported One Foot in Front

PTA needs to demonstrate the action to the patient.

Patient instruction: Please place one foot directly in front of the other. If you feel that you cannot place your foot directly in front, try and step far enough ahead that the heel of your forward foot is ahead of the toes of your other foot.

To score 3 points (at number 3), the length of the step should exceed the length of the other foot and the width of the stance should approximate the patient's normal stance width.

( ) 4 able to place foot tandem independently and hold 30 seconds
( ) 3 able to place foot ahead of the other independently and hold 30 seconds
( ) 2 able to take a small step independently and hold 30 seconds
( ) 1 needs help to step but can hold 15 seconds
( ) 0 loses balance while stepping or standing

14. Standing on One Leg

Patient instruction: Please stand on one leg as long as you can without holding.

( ) 4 able to lift leg independently and hold longer than 10 seconds
( ) 3 able to lift leg independently and hold 5–10 seconds
( ) 2 able to lift leg independently and hold 2 seconds (or longer)
( ) 1 tries to lift leg but unable to hold 3 seconds. Patient remains standing independently
( ) 0 unable to try or needs assistance to prevent fall

Maximum total score = 56

Functional Balance Test—Timed Get Up and Go Test and Normatives

Table 4-19   Timed Get Up and Go Test[3]

Place a chair (approximately 17 inches in height) against a wall or a firm object to prevent it from sliding backward (for patient's safety). Place a cone on the floor exactly 8 feet away. The distance to place the cone must be measured from the edge of the chair to the back of the cone. Ensure at least 4 feet clearance beyond the cone to allow for turning room. PTA needs a stopwatch.

Starting position: patient is seated in the chair with hands on thighs and feet on the floor.

Testing: patient is instructed that on the signal "go" he or she will rise from the chair, walk "as quickly as possible" around the cone, and return to a seated position in the chair. While rising from the chair, the patient is permitted to push off of thighs or chair. The patient is told that he or she will be timed and should therefore walk as quickly as possible but not to run. PTA demonstrates the action to the patient. Patient is allowed one practice trial followed by two test trials.

Scoring: PTA begins the timer when the "go" signal is given (even if the patient has not begun to move) and stops the time at the exact instant that the patient's but-

continues

Table 4-19 (continued)

tocks contacts the chair after the walk segment. The scores of both test trials must be recorded but the faster of the two trials must be recorded on the assessment form. Results from this test may be compared with age-related normative values.

Assistive device used in testing: it is permitted if required. The type of assistive device needs to be included in the assessment form. If an assistive device was used, the result of the test (the score) cannot be compared with age-related normatives.

Table 4-20   Normatives for Timed Get Up and Go Test[3]

Patient Age	60–64	65–69	70–74	75–79	80–84	85–89	90–94
Normal Range of Scores for Men (in sec)	5.6–3.8	5.9–4.3	6.2–4.4	7.2–4.6	7.6–5.2	8.9–5.5	10.0–6.2
Normal Range of Scores for Women (in sec)	6.0–4.4	6.4–4.8	7.1–4.9	7.4–5.2	8.7–5.7	9.6–6.2	11.5–7.3

Normal range of scores is defined as the middle 50% of each age group. Scores above the range would be considered "above average" for the age group, and those below the range would be "below average."

Motor Deficits of the Cerebral Vascular Accident: Abnormal Synergy Patterns

Table 4-21   CVA Synergy Patterns

Upper-extremity flexion synergy: scapular retraction and elevation or hyperextension; shoulder abduction and external rotation; elbow flexion (strong component); forearm supination; wrist and finger flexion.

Upper-extremity extension synergy: scapular protraction; shoulder adduction (strong component) and internal rotation; elbow extension; forearm pronation (strong component); wrist and finger flexion.

Lower-extremity flexion synergy: hip flexion (strong component), abduction, and external rotation; knee flexion; ankle dorsiflexion and inversion; toe dorsiflexion.

Lower-extremity extension synergy: hip extension, adduction (strong component), and internal rotation; knee extension (strong component); ankle plantarflexion (strong component) and inversion; toe plantarflexion.

Brunnstrom's Spasticity Patterns

Table 4-22   Brunnstrom's Spasticity Patterns

Head rotation to the unaffected side and lateral flexion to the affected (hemi) side
Shoulder adduction and internal rotation
Scapula retraction and depression
Elbow flexion and forearm pronation (can also be supination)
Wrist flexion and ulnar deviation, and fingers/thumb flexion and adduction
Pelvis elevation and backward rotation
Hip extension, adduction, and internal rotation
Knee extension and foot plantarflexion and inversion
Toes flexion and adduction

Motor Deficits of the Cerebral Vascular Accident: Brunnstrom's Stages of Recovery

Table 4-23   Brunnstrom's Six Stages of Recovery

Stage 1—patient starting to recover from hemiplegia. Patient exhibits: flaccidity; hyporeflexia; no voluntary movement of the affected upper and lower extremities.

Stage 2—patient exhibits the following: beginning of spasticity; hyperreflexia; strong synergy patterns of the affected upper and lower extremities; minimal voluntary movement of the affected areas (including upper and lower extremities).

Stage 3—patient exhibits the following: severe spasticity; voluntary movement of the affected upper and lower extremities only in synergy patterns.

Stage 4—patient exhibits the following: spasticity begins to decrease; synergy begins to decrease; beginning of voluntary movement without synergy.

Stage 5—patient has the capability to progress in the recovery process. If progress continues, patient exhibits the following: minimal synergy patterns; more complicated learned movement (motor) patterns without synergy; coordination deficits.

Stage 6—patient has the capability to progress to normal. If progress continues, patient exhibits no spasticity, and motor control and coordination are restored to normal.

Cerebral Vascular Accident—Gait Deficits

Table 4-24 CVA Gait Deficits

Hip: retraction (caused by trunk and limb spasticity); hiking (caused by weak abdominals); Trendelenburg limp (caused by weak abductors); circumduction (caused by hamstrings spasticity, foot drop and/or decreased ROM in hip/knee flexion); scissoring (caused by adductors spasticity); poor proprioception; exaggerated hip flexion (because of the flexor synergy).

Knee: increased flexion in stance (caused by hamstrings spasticity and/or weak quadriceps); hyperextension in stance (caused by plantarflexion contracture and/or weak quadriceps); inadequate knee flexion (caused by inadequate hip flexion and/or spastic quadriceps); inadequate knee extension (caused by spastic hamstrings); poor proprioception.

Ankle and foot: equinus gait when the heel does not touch the ground (caused by spasticity or contracture of gastrocnemius and soleus); foot drop (paralysis of dorsiflexors); unequal step length (caused by spastic toe flexors and pain on flexed toes); equinovarus (caused by spastic posterior tibialis and/or gastrocnemius and soleus); exaggerated dorsiflexion (caused by flexor synergy).

Traumatic Spinal Cord Injury Functional Capabilities and Assistance

Table 4-25 SCI Functional Capabilities and Assistance

Most distal nerve root segments innervated: C1, C2, C3 levels. Requirements: full-time attendant; mechanical ventilator or phrenic nerve stimulator during the day; environmental control units to activate light switches, call buttons, and electrical appliances, to turn pages of books, and for speaker phone. Patient function and assistance: totally dependent on assistance with ADLs and transfers; independent using an electric wheelchair (with an electrically controlled reclining back) that has a portable mechanical ventilator, and a microswitch or sip-and-puff controls; has wheelchair and bed skills. Key muscles: face and neck muscles and cranial innervation. Available movements: talking, sipping, blowing, and mastication.

Most distal nerve root segment innervated: C4 level. Requirements: full-time attendant; power tilt-in-space wheelchair (for pressure relief); arm supports (orthotics, flexor hinge hand splint) and adapted eating equipment for a small degree of self-feeding; environmental control units to activate light switches, call buttons, and electrical appliances, to turn pages of books, and for speaker phone. Patient function and assistance: totally dependent on assistance with ADLs, transfers, coughing, glossopharyngeal breathing, and skin inspection; can use head or mouth stick (or sip-and-puff, or hand splint) for typing on the computer keyboard, and is able to play table games (such as cards or checkers), paint or draw; independent with power wheelchair with head, mouth, chin or sip-and-puff controls; has wheelchair and bed skills. Key muscles: diaphragm and trapezius. Available movements: respiration and elevation of scapula.

Most distal nerve root segment innervated: C5 level. Requirements: part-time attendant; equipment set up; mobile arm supports, deltoid aid, and adapted utensils and splints for self-feeding; adapted equipment for limited self-care activities such as grooming and washing; hand splints or typing sticks for typing on the computer keyboard; power tilt-in space wheelchair for pressure relief; sliding board. Patient function and assistance: dependent on some assistance and set up for ADLs, dressing, transfers with sliding board and overhead swivel bar, skin inspection, and coughing with manual pressure to diaphragm; can drive a van with hand controls; has bed and wheelchair skills; independent with manual wheelchair with handrim projections and power wheelchair with arm controls; can self-feed, and can do pressure relief. Key muscles: biceps, brachialis, brachioradialis, deltoid, infraspinatus, rhomboids, and supinator. Available movements: elbow flexion and supination, shoulder abduction to 90° and external rotation, and limited shoulder flexion.

Most distal nerve root segment innervated: C6 level. Requirements: side rails on the bed; universal cuff and adapted utensils for self-feeding; adaptive equipment for dressing and grooming (button hook, zipper pulls); adaptive equipment for bowel and bladder and self-care (in the shower); hand controls and U-shaped cuff for steering wheels; adaptive equipment for self-preparation of occasional light meals. Patient function and assistance: dependent on very little assistance for ADLs; can independently with adaptive equipment self-feed, dress (uses also momentum), perform self-care and bowel and bladder care, transfer (with sliding board), do skin inspection, cough (with pressure to abdomen), drive, prepare light meals, and play wheelchair sports; cannot tie shoes; has bed and wheelchair skills; can use the manual wheelchair with handrim projections all the time, and the power wheelchair for long distances and in the community. Key muscles: ECR, infraspinatus, latissimus dorsi, pectoralis major (clavicular portion), pronator teres, serratus anterior, and teres minor. Available movements: shoulder flexion, adduction, extension, and internal rotation, abduction and upward rotation of scapula, forearm pronation, and wrist extension (tenodesis grasp).

Most distal nerve root segment innervated: C7 level. Requirements: adaptive equipment for dressing (button hook), and self-care (shower chair, hand held shower nozzle, and bathroom handles); bowel and bladder care adaptive equipment (digi-

continues

Table 4-25   (continued)

tal stimulator, raised toilet seat, urinary drainage device); sliding board; wheelchair accessible kitchen; hand controls for the car; adaptive kitchen tools. Patient function and assistance: independent with ADLs, self-feeding, dressing, self-care, transfers (with or without sliding board), bowel and bladder care, manual coughing, light housekeeping, and driving; is able to get in and out of the car; has bed and wheelchair skills; independent with manual wheelchair with friction surface handrims. Key muscles: EPL, EPB, FCR, triceps, and extrinsic finger extensors. Available movements: elbow extension, finger extension, and wrist flexion.

Most distal nerve root segments innervated: C8 to T1 levels. Requirements: some adaptive equipment for self-care (tub seat, grab bars); adaptive equipment for housekeeping; hand controls for the car. Patient function and assistance: independent with ADLs, light housekeeping, meal preparation, transfers, and driving; can work (in a free-architectural barriers environment); has bed and wheelchair skills; independent with a manual wheelchair with standard handrims. Key muscles: FCU, FPL, FPB, and intrinsic and extrinsic muscles of finger flexors. Available movements: all movements of the muscles of the upper extremities, fine coordination, and strong grasp.

Most distal nerve root segments innervated: T4 to T6 levels. Requirements: standing table or standing frame; bilateral KAFOs. Patient function and assistance: independent with bed skills, ADLs, wheelchair skills, transfers, and routine housekeeping; can negotiate curbs and perform the "wheelie" in a manual wheelchair; can participate in wheelchair sports; can perform physiological standing at a standing table (standing frame) using KAFOs. Some patients may ambulate for short distance with KAFOs. Key muscles: long muscles of the back (sacrospinalis and semispinalis) and the top half of intercostal muscles. Available movements: stronger trunk control musculature, pectoral muscles improvement (for lifting), and increased respiratory reserve musculature.

Most distal nerve root segments innervated: T9 to T12 levels. Requirements: bilateral KAFOs, crutches or walker. Patient function and assistance: independent with household ambulation using bilateral KAFOs and crutches (or walker); uses wheelchair only for energy conservation. Key muscles: intercostals and lower abdominals. Available movements: improvement with trunk control and endurance.

Most distal nerve root segments innervated: L2, L3, L4 levels. Requirements: bilateral KAFOs and crutches. Patient function and assistance: able to perform independently functional ambulation using bilateral KAFOs and crutches; uses wheelchair only for energy conservation. Key muscles: iliopsoas, quadratus lumborum, rectus femoris, gracilis, and sartorius. Available movements: hip adduction and flexion, and knee extension.

Most distal nerve root segments innervated: L4, L5 levels. Requirements: bilateral KAFOs and crutches (or canes). Patient function and assistance: able to perform independently functional ambulation using bilateral KAFOs and crutches (or canes); uses wheelchair only for convenience and energy conservation. Key muscles: extensor digitorum, lower back musculature, quadriceps, medial hamstrings (weak), and anterior and posterior tibialis. Available movements: very good trunk control, hip flexion and knee extension, and weak knee flexion.

Mechanisms of Injury for the Traumatic Spinal Cord Injury

Table 4-26   Mechanisms of Injury: Traumatic SCI

Flexion injury: is the most common mechanism of injury causing high percentages of lumbar or cervical SCI at levels T12 to L2 and C4 to C7. Flexion injuries can cause the following: fractures of the anterior vertebral body, spinal processes, pedicles, and laminae; tearing of the posterior spinal ligaments; disk disruptions; dislocation of the anterior vertebral body.

Flexion—Rotation injury can cause the following: fractures of the posterior pedicles, laminae, and articular facets; dislocations or subluxations of faucet joints; tearing of the posterior and interspinous ligaments.

Compression injury can cause the following: concave fractures of the spinal end-plates; comminuted fractures; teardrop fractures; ruptures of the intervertebral disk.

Hyperextension injury can cause the following: fractures of the spinous processes, faucets, and laminae; avulsion fractures of anterior aspect of vertebrae; tearing of the anterior longitudinal ligament; disk rupture.

*Spinal areas of greatest frequency of injury: C5–C7 and T12–L2

Spinal Cord Injury Syndromes

Table 4-27   SCI Syndromes

Anterior cord syndrome (ACS) can produce the following: loss of motor function below the level of lesion (caused by damage to the corticospinal tract); loss of the sense of pain and temperature below the level of lesion (caused by damage to the spinothalamic tract); preservation of the proprioception, kinesthesia, and vibratory sense below the level of lesion. ACS can be caused by flexion injury of cervical region with damage of the anterior spinal cord and/or anterior spinal artery.

continues

Table 4-27 (continued)

Brown-Sequard Syndrome can produce the following: ipsilateral loss of sensation of the dermatome corresponding to the level of lesion; contralateral loss of the sense of pain and temperature of several dermatomes below the level of lesion; ipsilateral loss of motor function (characterized by decreased DTRs, clonus, and positive Babinski), proprioception, kinesthesia, and vibratory sense. Brown-Sequard can be caused by hemisection of the spinal cord with damage on one side of spinal cord (from gunshots or stabbing attacks).

Cauda Equina injury (also called a lower motor neuron injury) can produce most of the time an incomplete lesion with a potential for regeneration.

Central cord syndrome (CCS) can produce the following: severe motor loss of the upper extremities; less severe motor loss of the lower extremities; mild and varying degrees of sensory impairments; preservation of sacral tracts, and bowel, bladder, and sexual functions. Patients may be able to ambulate with some distal upper-extremity weakness (especially after surgeries to relieve cervical compression). CCS can be caused by hyperextension injury of the cervical spine (from motor vehicle accidents) or congenital narrowing of the spinal canal.

Posterior cord syndrome (PCS) can produce the following: loss of proprioception, two point discrimination, and stereognosis below the level of lesion; preservation of motor function, sense of pain, and light touch. PCS can be caused by tabes dorsalis due to late stage syphilis. PCS is very rare.

Sacral sparing can produce the following: incomplete lesion with varying innervation from the intact sacral segments; preserved perianal sensation; preserved contraction of the external anal sphincter.

Classification of Spinal Cord Injury

Table 4-28   SCI Classification

The American Spinal Injury Association[4] classifies SCI injuries as the following: (1) Tetraplegia (complete paralysis of all upper and lower extremities, and trunk including the respiratory muscles due to lesion of the cervical spinal cord); (2) Paraplegia (complete paralysis of both lower extremities and part of the trunk due to lesion of the thoracic or lumbar spinal cord or cauda equina).

SCI is also classified by the American Spinal Injury Association as the following: (1) Complete with no sensory or motor function in the lowest sacral segments (S4 and S5); (2) Incomplete with sensory function but not motor function preserved below the neurologic level (including sacral segments S4 and S5); (3) Incomplete with motor function preserved below the neurologic level, and more than half of key muscles below the neurological level have a muscle grade less than 3; (4) Incomplete with motor function preserved below the neurological level, and at least half of key muscles below the neurological level have a muscle grade of 3 or more; (5) Normal with normal motor and sensory functions.

Neurologic level of lesion is referred to the most caudal segment of the spinal cord with normal motor and sensory function on the right and left sides of the body. Motor or sensory level of lesion is referred to the most caudal segment of spinal cord with bilateral motor and sensory normal function. Motor level is determined by MMT testing of a key muscle (on right or left) at myotome adjacent to the suspected level of impairment. Sensory level is determined by testing light touch and pin prick (on right or left) at key dermatome.

See Figure 4-1.

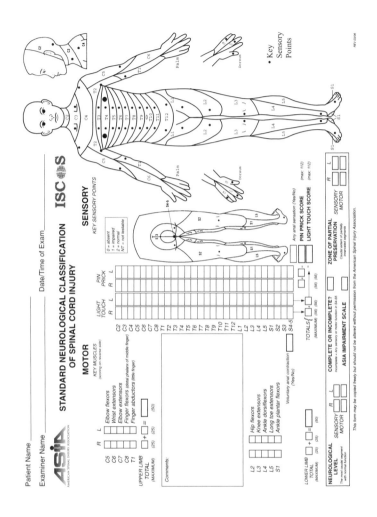

MUSCLE GRADING

0   total paralysis

1   palpable or visible contraction

2   active movement, full range of motion, gravity eliminated

3   active movement, full range of motion, against gravity

4   active movement, full range of motion, against gravity and provides some resistance

5   active movement, full range of motion, against gravity and provides normal resistance

5* muscle able to exert, in examiner's judgement, sufficient resistance to be considered normal if identifiable inhibiting factors were not present

NT not testable. Patient unable to reliably exert effort or muscle unavailable for testing due to factors such as immobilization, pain on effort or contracture.

ASIA IMPAIRMENT SCALE

☐ **A = Complete:** No motor or sensory function is preserved in the sacral segments S4-S5.

☐ **B = Incomplete:** Sensory but not motor function is preserved below the neurological level and includes the sacral segments S4-S5.

☐ **C = Incomplete:** Motor function is preserved below the neurological level, and more than half of key muscles below the neurological level have a muscle grade less than 3.

☐ **D = Incomplete:** Motor function is preserved below the neurological level, and at least half of key muscles below the neurological level have a muscle grade of 3 or more.

☐ **E = Normal:** Motor and sensory function are normal.

CLINICAL SYNDROMES (OPTIONAL)

☐ Central Cord
☐ Brown-Sequard
☐ Anterior Cord
☐ Conus Medullaris
☐ Cauda Equina

STEPS IN CLASSIFICATION

The following order is recommended in determining the classification of individuals with SCI.

1. Determine sensory levels for right and left sides.

2. Determine motor levels for right and left sides.
    Note: in regions where there is no myotome to test, the motor level is presumed to be the same as the sensory level.

3. Determine the single neurological level.
    This is the lowest segment where motor and sensory function is normal on both sides, and is the most cephalad of the sensory and motor levels determined in steps 1 and 2.

4. Determine whether the injury is Complete or Incomplete. (sacral sparing).
    *If voluntary anal contraction = **No** AND all S4-5 sensory scores = **0** AND any anal sensation = **No**, then injury is COMPLETE. Otherwise injury is incomplete.*

5. Determine ASIA Impairment Scale (AIS) Grade:

    Is injury Complete? If YES, AIS=A Record ZPP
    (For ZPP record lowest dermatome or myotome on each side with some (non-zero score) preservation)

    NO ↓   YES

    Is injury motor incomplete?   If NO. AIS=B
    (Yes/voluntary anal contraction OR motor function more than three levels below the motor level on a given side.)

    NO ↓   YES

    Are at least half of the key muscles below the (single) neurological level graded 3 or better?

    NO ↓   YES
    AIS=C   AIS=D

    If sensation and motor function is normal in all segments, AIS=E
    Note: AIS E is used to follow up testing when an individual with a documented SCI has recovered normal function. If at initial testing no deficits are found, the individual is neurologically intact; the ASIA Impairment Scale does not apply.

Figure 4-1 Standard Neurological Classification of Spinal Cord Injury. Reproduced with permission of the American Spinal Injury Association (2006).

Multiple Sclerosis Categories

Table 4-29   MS Categories

Relapsing-Remitting MS: the most common type of MS; patient experiences periods of relapses with acute worsening of the disease and periods of remission with partial or complete disappearance of the disease.

Progressive-Relapsing MS: commonly seen in patients who develop the disease after 40 years of age; the progressive type of disease starting with acute and clear signs and symptoms, and progressing to relapses (that may or may not have recovery or remission periods).

Secondary-Progressive MS: the disease starts as a relapsing-remitting MS that progresses with or without relapses and remissions.

Primary-Progressive MS: a rare form of MS with late onset (after age 40), that progresses constantly without periods of remission.

SECTION 4-2

Clinical Impairments and Functional Limitations of Neurologic Conditions

Clinical Impairments and Functional Limitations of Cerebral Vascular Accidents

Table 4-30   CVA Impairments and Functional Limitations*

Sensory deficits: impaired sensation in the contralateral upper and lower extremity; impaired proprioception; loss of superficial touch and pain and temperature; numbness; thalamic pain syndrome (continuous and severe pain contralaterally; pain can be triggered by noise, bright lights, or light touch); homonymous hemianopsia. Left hemisphere lesion (R hemi) has right-side hemisensory loss. Right hemisphere lesion (L hemi) has left-side hemisensory loss.

Motor deficits: flaccidity and hyporeflexia (immediately after CVA; does not last long); spasticity (on the opposite side of the lesion); hyperreflexia (such as clonus and positive Babinski); synergies; primitive reflex patterns (STNR, ATNR, STLR, TLR); associated reactions (Souques—elevation of hemi UE elicits fingers' extension and abduction; Raimiste—resistance to abduction or adduction in UE or LE elicits abduction or adduction in both opposite UE/LE); paresis or weakness (in MCA stroke, UE is more affected than LE; in ACA stroke, LE is more affected than UE); incoordination and balance deficits; apraxia (ideomotor and ideational). Left hemisphere lesion (R hemi) has difficulty planning and sequencing movements; apraxia (ideational or ideomotor). Right hemisphere lesion (L hemi) has difficulty sustaining a movement.

Gait deficits: Trendelenburg gait (weak abductors); scissoring (spastic adductors); insufficient pelvic rotation during swing; circumduction (weak hip flexors during swing); backward leaning of trunk; exaggerated hip flexion synergy; excessive knee flexion during stance (weak knee extensors); knee in hyperextension as a compensation for weak knee extensors or spastic quads; foot drop; equinus gait (heel does not touch down); varus foot (weight is borne on the lateral side of the foot); unequal step length (hemi leg does not advance through the end of stance into toe off); decreased cadence and uneven timing.

Communication deficits: Broca's or expressive aphasia (speech is impaired; left temporal lobe lesion); Wernicke's or receptive aphasia (auditory comprehension is impaired); global aphasia (speech and comprehension are impaired); dysarthria (motor speech deficit caused by impairments of respiration, articulation, phonation, or sensory feedback). Left hemisphere lesion (R hemi) has the following: speech and language impairments for the dominant hemisphere (right-handed patients); nonfluent or Broca's aphasia; fluent or Wernicke's aphasia; global aphasia; memory impairments related to language.

Perceptual deficits: unilateral neglect (ignores stimuli from the left side); anosognosia (denial of dysfunction); somatoagnosia (cannot comprehend relationship of one body part to another); right and left discrimination (cannot identify right and left sides of body); Pusher syndrome (lateral lean toward the hemiplegic side). Right hemisphere lesion (L hemi) has the following: visual perceptual impairments; left-side unilateral neglect; agnosia; visual-spatial impairments; disturbances of body image and body scheme; memory impairments related to spatial–perceptual information.

General cognitive deficits: attention (deficits in areas of sustained attention, divided attention, selective attention, and alternating attention); memory (short- and long-term memory); confabulation (use of inappropriate words or fabricated stories); perseveration (continued repetition of words, thoughts, or acts unrelated to current activity); impulsiveness; poor planning; inflexibility; impaired judgment; dementia (general decline in higher brain functions such as in judgment, memory, consciousness, communication, and behavior). Left hemisphere lesion (R hemi) cognitive deficits—patient may be: slow; hesitant; cautious; insecure; fearful; aware of impairments; disorganized in problem solving; anxious about his or her poor performance; having difficulty with processing delays; having difficulty with expression of positive emotions; having memory impairments typically related to language; having difficulty processing verbal cues and verbal commands. Right hemisphere lesion (L hemi) cognitive deficits—patient may be: impulsive; indifferent; quick; having poor judgment; underestimating the problems; overestimating the abilities; difficulty grasping the overall organization or pattern, problem solving, and synthesizing information; unaware of impairments; unable to self-correct; at risk for safety; having rigidity of thought; difficulty with abstract reasoning; difficulty with perception of emotions and expression of negative emotions; difficulty processing visual cues; having memory impairments related to spatial–perceptual information.

Affective deficits: emotional lability (pathological crying and laughing; changing easily and quickly from laughing to crying); irritability; agitation; increased frustration; depression (is not psychological but a direct impairment of CVA).

Bladder and bowel deficits: urinary incontinence (due to bladder hyperreflexia or hyporeflexia); bowel incontinence; diarrhea; constipation; bowel impaction.

Indirect impairments: deep venous thrombosis (DVT); pressure sores (decubitus ulcers); decreased ROM; contracture; deformity; shoulder subluxation and pain; RSD; deconditioning.

---

*This is a basic guide; the PTA should consider the PT's initial examination and evaluation.

Clinical Impairments and Functional Limitations of Parkinson's Disease

Table 4-31   PD Impairments and Functional Limitations

Rigidity: cogwheel rigidity (jerky resistance to passive movement); lead-pipe rigidity (constant, uniform resistance to passive movement)

Akinesia (difficulty initiating movement); bradykinesia (difficulty maintaining movement; slowness); hypokinesia (movements reduced in speed, amplitude, and range); freezing episodes (sudden stop during movement); micrographia (abnormally small handwriting)

Resting tremor: pill-rolling tremor (hand tremor at rest); postural tremor (tremor in sitting or standing against gravity)

Postural instability (weak trunk extensor muscles cause a flexed, stooped posture with increased neck, trunk, hips, and knees flexion); back pain (as a result of stooped posture)

Communication and swallowing deficits: dysarthria (decreased voice volume, monotone speech, distorted articulation, and uncontrolled rate of speech); mutism (not speaking or speaking in whispers); sialorrhea (excessive drooling due to increased salivation and decreased swallowing); dysphagia (impaired swallowing; can cause choking or aspiration pneumonia)

Gait deficits: loss of reciprocal arm swing and decreased stride length; festinating gait (progressive increase in speed with shortening of stride); propulsive festinating gait (increase in speed forward; most common); retropulsive festinating gait (increase in speed backward; less common); plantarflexion contracture gait (with narrow base of support)

Visual deficits: blurred vision; difficulty reading (cannot be corrected by glasses); decreased blinking (can produce irritation of the eyes)

Cognitive deficits: bradyphrenia (slowing of thought processes); deficits in learning new skills; deficits in reasoning, abstract thinking, memory, and judgment; dementia (may occur in patients with PD who are 80 years or older)

Indirect impairments: fatigue (weakness and lethargy); masked face (infrequent blinking and lack of facial expression); kyphosis (caused by contractures in hip and knee flexors, hip rotators, adductors, plantarflexors, neck flexors, shoulder adductors, internal rotators, and elbow flexors); scoliosis (caused by leaning to one side); orthostatic hypotension (caused by Levodopa side effects); pulmonary deficits (airway obstruction due to decreased respiratory movements; may be caused by kyphosis)

Clinical Impairments and Functional Limitations of Multiple Sclerosis

Table 4-32   MS Impairments and Functional Limitations

Motor deficits: UMN deficits—spasticity (can be mild to severe); paresis; brisk DTRs; clonus; positive Babinski; involuntary spasm of flexor and extensor musculature; exaggerated cutaneous reflexes; flexion/extension synergy patterns.

Other motor deficits: slow and stiff movements; weak musculature; balance and coordination deficits such as asthenia, ataxia, dysmetria, dyssynergia, dysdiadochokinesia, dizziness, intention tremor, and trunk musculature weakness (all with cerebellar involvement); fatigue; difficulty walking; staggering gait with loss of balance; dysarthria (slurred or unarticulated speech); dysphonia (harsh or hoarse speech); dysphagia (difficulty swallowing).

Sensory deficits: paresthesia (pins and needles or numbness); acute, intense, or burning pain (such as trigeminal neuralgia and headache); Lhermitte's sign for MS symptoms (flexion of the neck produces a sudden, electric shock running down the spine and lower extremities); chronic pain; optic neuritis (inflammation of optic nerve); scotoma (dark spot in the center of the visual field); nystagmus; lateral gaze palsy (incomplete eye adduction); diplopia (double vision).

Cognitive and affective deficits: impaired memory, attention, and concentration; decreased problem solving and judgment; depression; anxiety; emotional lability; euphoria; bipolar affective disorder (alternative periods of depression and mania).

ANS deficits: bowel deficits (such as constipation, bowel impaction, incontinence, or diarrhea); bladder deficits (such as incontinence, urinary frequency and urgency, urinary hesitancy, excessive and frequent urination at night); sexual deficits (such as impotence, vaginal dryness, or loss of libido).

Clinical Impairments and Functional Limitations of Traumatic Brain Injury

Table 4-33   TBI Impairments and Functional Limitations

Motor deficits: hemiparesis; quadriparesis (tetraparesis); abnormal DTRs; clonus; positive Babinski; ataxia, hypotonia, coordination and balance deficits (with cerebellar involvement; patient may have bilateral deficits); flaccidity; spasticity; hypertonicity; rigidity (can be decorticate and/or decerebrate rigidity); muscular atrophy, decreased muscular power and/or endurance; abnormal synergy patterns.

continues

Table 4-33 (continued)

Sensory deficits: sharp and dull discrimination; temperature; light touch; pressure; kinesthesia; proprioception; stereognosis; barognosis; tactile localization; dysphagia.

Perceptual deficits: homonymous hemianopsia; somatognosia; right and left discrimination; anosognosia; figure ground discrimination; position in space deficit; agnosia; apraxia (ideomotor or ideational).

Integumentary deficits: postures that aggravate or relieve pain; pressure areas.

Arousal, mentation, and cognition deficits: anterograde (post-traumatic) amnesia; retrograde amnesia; emotional lability; decreased level of consciousness (coma, vegetative state, or persistent vegetative state); attention deficits; memory loss; altered orientation; impaired safety awareness; decreased problem solving, reasoning, and judgment; perseveration; disinhibition; impulsiveness; aggressiveness; irritability; apathy; sexual inappropriateness; egocentricity.

Speech and communication deficits: Broca's or Wernicke's aphasia; global aphasia; dysarthria; impaired reading comprehension; impaired written expression.

Clinical Impairments and Functional Limitations of Traumatic Spinal Cord Injury

Table 4-34   SCI Impairments and Functional Limitations

Areflexia (spinal shock) occurs immediately after injury. Areflexia is characterized by absence of motor function, appearance of flaccidity, loss of sensation, and reflex activity below the level of lesion, delayed plantar reflex, loss of DTRs, and loss of bulbocavernous and cremasteric reflexes. It can last from several days to several weeks. Areflexia is resolved when bulbocavernous reflex is returned.

Motor and sensory impairments are dependent on the type of clinical syndrome and the level of lesion. Motor impairments can be the following: hypotonia; flaccidity; spasticity; decreased muscular strength, power, and endurance; hypertonia; muscular substitution; gait and balance deficits; functional deficits; community and work dysfunctions. Sensory impairments can be the following: loss or decreased superficial, deep, and combined sensations; pain (traumatic pain after traumatic injury; nerve root pain caused by damage to nerve roots; spinal cord dysesthesia with painful sensations below level of lesion; musculoskeletal pain above the level of lesion most commonly in the shoulder).

Autonomic dysreflexia (hyperreflexia) can occur mostly in lesions above T6 of patients having tetraplegia and high level paraplegia. It is a medical emergency.

PTA needs to do the following: bring patient to a sitting position; call EMS or a nurse (in hospital/SNF); examine bladder drainage system (catheter) for internal/external blockage; release the clamped catheter; examine for bowel impaction. Symptoms are: HTN; bradycardia; headache; profuse sweating; increased spasticity; restlessness; constricted pupils, flushing above the level of lesion; blurred vision; constriction below the level of lesion; nasal congestion; piloerection (goose bumps). Causes may be: bladder distension due to urinary retention (most common); bladder infection or irritation; kidney stones; kidney dysfunction; bowel distension; pressure sores; noxious cutaneous stimuli; environmental temperature changes.

Postural hypotension (orthostatic hypotension) is a decrease in blood pressure while trying to assume an erect position. The cause is prolonged immobilization especially with cervical and upper thoracic SCI. Symptoms include dizziness and/or feeling of fainting. A related problem of postural hypotension for SCI is pitting edema of feet, ankles, and legs.

SNS deficit is impaired temperature control due to damage of spinal cord. Because of hypothalamic dysfunction, the patient looses the ability to sweat or shiver. Symptoms include the following: diaphoresis (excessive sweating as a compensatory mechanism); spotty areas of localized sweating below the level of lesion; body temperature dependent on the environmental temperature.

Respiratory deficit is dependent on the level of lesion and the residual respiratory muscle function. Respiratory impairment is life threatening to the patient with SCI. The effects of respiratory deficit can cause decreased ability to cough, altered breathing pattern, and patient's vulnerability to increased secretions, atelectasis (collapsed lungs), and pulmonary infections.

Bladder and bowel deficits can cause the following: urinary tract infections (UTIs); reflexive or spastic bladder (can empty only to a certain fullness pressure) occurring in UMN lesions at T11–T12 levels or above; flaccid or nonreflexive bladder (can empty only by compressing the lower abdomen) occurring in LMN lesions at T12 level or below; reflexive or spastic bowel occurring with UMN lesions; flaccid or nonreflexive bowel occurring with LMN lesions.

Sexual deficits can cause the following: decreased erectile capacity mostly with LMN and complete SCI lesions; decreased ejaculation mostly with UMN lesion, higher level cord lesions, and complete SCI lesions; decreased female sexual response in LMN lesions (and intact response in UMN lesions); unimpaired fertility. Patients with UMN and incomplete SCI lesions have greater erectile capacity than LMN and complete lesions. Patients with LMN, lower level cord, and complete lesions have a higher incidence of ejaculation as UMN, higher cord level, and incomplete lesions.

continues

Table 4-34 (continued)

Indirect impairments: atelectasis and pneumonia (patients with paralyzed or weak muscles of inspiration); decubitus ulcers; DVT; contractures (most common: hip flexion, adduction and internal rotation contractures; shoulder flexion/extension, internal rotation and adduction contractures); heterotopic ossification (abnormal bone formation in the tendons, connective tissue between muscle, aponeurosis, or peripheral part of the muscle; commonly can affect areas closed to hips and knees); osteoporosis (below level of lesion); renal calculi.

Clinical Impairments and Functional Limitations of Guillain-Barré Syndrome (Polyneuritis)

Table 4-35   Guillain-Barré Impairments and Functional Limitations

Motor deficits: paresis or paralysis (symmetrical distribution; progresses from lower extremities to upper extremities, and from distal to proximal; can produce tetraplegia with respiratory failure); flaccidity (LMN lesion; demyelination of cranial and peripheral nerves); decreased muscular strength, power, and endurance.

Sensory deficits: paresthesia (tingling and burning sensations); anesthesia (of distal extremities in a long gloves and stocking pattern); hyperesthesia; pain (muscular ache; burning pain).

Functional deficits: impaired gait and balance; decreased ADLs; decreased home or work management and integration in the community.

Autonomic deficits: tachycardia; blood pressure fluctuations; arrhythmia.

Clinical Impairments and Functional Limitations of Amyotrophic Lateral Sclerosis

Table 4-36   ALS Impairments and Functional Limitations

Motor deficits: muscular weakness; hyporeflexia; hypotonicity; atrophy; fasciculations; muscle cramps; spasticity; hyperreflexia; cervical extensor weakness; dysarthria; anarthria (loss of motor power to speak distinctly); dysphagia; sialorrhea (excess secretion of saliva).

Sensory deficits: spared for the most part; some patients may have paresthesia or focal pain in the limbs.

Functional deficits: decreased walking ability; decreased ADLs; deconditioning; impaired postural control and balance; decreased home or work management and integration in the community.

Respiratory deficits: respiratory muscle weakness; dyspnea on exertion first and then at rest; fatigue; recurrent sighing; morning headache due to hypoxia; difficulty sleeping in supine position; weak cough.

Cognitive deficits: depression; anxiety; dementia (frontotemporal dementia).

Types of Neurologic Interventions

Motor Function Interventions—Postural Strategies to Regain Balance

Table 4-37 Balance Strategies

Stepping strategy: patient is taking rapid steps (forward, backward, or to the side) to realign the center of mass within the base of support.

Ankle strategy: patient is maintaining balance by using the ankle musculature (dorsiflexors and plantarflexors). Patient is shifting the center of mass forward (using plantarflexors) and backward (using dorsiflexors) while keeping lower extremities relatively rigid. Ankle strategy can be used with patients who exhibit decreased ankle ROM and strength.

Hip strategy: patient is maintaining balance by using the hip and lower trunk musculature. Patient is shifting the center of mass backward (using hip flexors, quadriceps, abdominals, and neck flexors) and forward (using neck, trunk, and hip extensors). Hip strategy can be used with patients who exhibit decreased hip ROM and strength.

Motor Function Interventions—Developmental Motor Skills (Essential Functional Skills)

Table 4-38 Developmental Motor Skills[1]

Mobility: ability to move from one position to another. Examples include rolling; supine to side lying and back; side lying to sit and back; sitting to standing and back.

Stability (or static postural control): ability to maintain static postural stability and orientation. It is also, the same as static balance (or equilibrium) the ability to maintain the center of mass over the base of support without any motion. Examples include prone on elbows; half kneeling; kneeling; quadruped; plantigrade; standing.

Controlled mobility (or dynamic postural control): ability to maintain dynamic postural stability and orientation. It is also, the same as dynamic balance (or equilibrium) the ability to maintain the center of mass over the base of support during motion. Examples include weight shifting while the body is in motion; reaching while the body is in motion.

Skill: ability to consistently perform coordinated movement sequences while interacting with others or for functional activities in home, community, and work. Patients with skill deficits have poorly coordinated movements, and lack of control, precision, and consistency. Examples include reaching and manipulation using upper extremities; walking and talking.

Motor Function Interventions—Restore Movement and Functional Mobility (Using Developmental Sequence Postures)

Table 4-39   Interventions Using the Developmental Sequence Postures[1]

Quadruped posture: places weightbearing through shoulders, elbows, wrists, knees, and hips; improves control of the upper trunk, lower trunk, upper and lower extremities, neck, and head; increases strength in shoulders and hip stabilizers; decreases extensor tone at the knees; increases ROM in extension at the wrists and fingers; produces a wide base of support and a low center of gravity.

Prone on elbows posture: places weightbearing through shoulders and elbows; improves control of the upper trunk, upper extremity, neck, and head; increases strength in shoulder stabilizers musculature; increases ROM in hip extensors; produces a wide base of support and a low center of gravity.

Kneeling and half kneeling posture: places weightbearing through knees and hips, and ankles (in half kneeling); improves control of the upper/lower trunk, lower extremity, head, and neck; increases strength in hip stabilizers; decreases extensor tone at the knees; improves balance reactions; produces a narrow base of support and a high center of gravity in kneeling; produces a wide base of support and a high center of gravity in half kneeling.

Modified plantigrade posture: places weightbearing through joints in the upper and lower extremities; improves control of the head, neck, upper and lower trunk, and upper and lower extremities; improves balance reactions; increases ROM in extension at the wrists and fingers; is a functional posture; produces a wide base of support and a high center of gravity.

Bridging posture: places weightbearing through feet and ankles; improves control of the lower extremities (if bilateral) and trunk; increases strength in hip stabilizers; is a lead-up activity for bed mobility; produces a wide base of support and a low center of gravity.

Standing posture: places weightbearing through lower extremities; improves control of the head, neck, upper and lower trunk, and lower extremities; improves balance reactions; is a functional posture; produces narrow base of support and high center of gravity.

Sitting posture: places weightbearing through upper extremities; improves control of the head, neck, upper and lower trunk, and lower extremities; improves balance reactions; is a functional posture; produces a medium base of support and center of gravity.

Motor Function Interventions—Basic Motor Learning Strategies

Table 4-40 Basic Motor Learning Strategies[1]

In the cognitive ("what to do" decision) stage of learning the skill, the PTA can explain the purpose of the skill; demonstrate the skill accentuating the correct performance; ask the patient to explain the task, its components, and its requirements; point out the similarities of the learned task to other tasks; uses knowledge of performance feedback by focusing on errors as they become consistent (does not concentrate on large numbers of random errors); use knowledge of results feedback by focusing on successful performance; for feedback, ask patient to watch the correct movement; ask patient to evaluate his or her performance; use feedback after each trial in the early learning; use variable feedback later; organize the initial practice of the task; stress controlled movement; provide adequate rest periods; use manual guidance (physically assisting the learner to perform the task; does not overuse it in later stages); break complex tasks into simple components; use repeated practice of the same task; use serial or random practice (when a variety of tasks are practiced randomly across trials) of related skills; use mental practice; avoid stressors and mental fatigue; structure the environment by reducing extraneous stimuli and distractors; emphasize a closed environment before open environment.

In the associated ("how to do" decision) stage of learning the skill, the PTA can use knowledge of performance feedback by focusing on errors as they become consistent (does not concentrate on large numbers of random errors); use knowledge of results feedback by focusing on successful performance and stressing the relevance of the task with function; emphasize proprioceptive feedback (patient's own feeling of the movement); assist learner to improve self-evaluation and decision-making skills; encourage patient to self-assess achievements; use variable feedback (summed feedback is feedback use after a set number of trials; faded feedback is feedback given at first after every trial and then less frequently; bandwidth feedback is feedback given when performance is outside a given error range); avoid excessive augmented feedback; encourage consistency of performance; focus on variable practice order of related skills; progress toward open environment; change the environment; prepare the learner for home, community, and work environment.

In the autonomous ("how to succeed" decision) stage of learning the skill, the PTA can assess need for conscious attention and automaticity of movements; select appropriate feedback (learner demonstrates appropriate self-evaluation and decision-making skills; when errors are evident, use occasional knowledge of per-

continues

formance feedback or knowledge of results feedback); organize practice (stress consistency in variable environments; practice in open environments; use massed practice when the rest time is much less than the practice time); structure environment (vary environments; help patient to be ready for home, community, and work environments; focus on competitive aspects of the task).

Neurologic Facilitation Techniques

Table 4-41 Facilitation Interventions[1]

Agonist Reversals (AR): slow, resisted concentric contraction of agonist muscles moving through the range, followed by a holding contraction in the range position and then an eccentric contraction while moving slowly back to the initial starting position. AR is a proprioceptive neuromuscular facilitation (PNF) technique.

Approximation (AP): compression of joint surfaces to facilitate extensor muscular contractions and provide joint stability. It can be applied manually, during upright positions, in weightbearing positions, in PNF extensor patterns. AP can be applied mechanically using weights, belts or weighted vests, or bouncing while sitting on a Swiss ball. AP can also be applied to shoulders or pelvis in upright weightbearing positions such as in sitting, standing, or kneeling. AP is contraindicated in inflamed joints. AP is a PNF technique.

Contract Relax (CR): strong, isotonic contraction (rotation) of the antagonists (restricting muscles) in a limited ROM, and followed by an isometric contraction holding 5 to 8 seconds. Next, voluntary relaxation takes place, followed by active contraction of the agonist muscles into the newly acquired ROM. CR is a PNF technique.

Hold Relax (HR): strong, isometric contraction of the antagonists (restricting muscles) in the limited ROM, followed by a voluntary relaxation and PROM of the agonists into the newly gained range. HR is a PNF technique.

Hold Relax Active Contraction (HRAC): strong, isometric contraction of the antagonists (restricting muscles) in the limited ROM, followed by a voluntary relaxation and AROM of the agonists into the newly gained range. HRAC is a PNF technique.

Joint traction (JT): manual distraction (or mechanical distraction using ankle or wrist cuffs) to facilitate joint motion and enhance joint awareness. JT can be used in PNF flexor extremity patterns with pulling movements. JT is contraindicated in hypermobile or unstable joints. JT is a proprioceptive facilitation technique.

Manual Contacts (MCs): manual contacts with deep pressure (grip) over the muscles to facilitate muscular contraction. MCs are applied in the opposite direction of desired motion. MCs guide the direction of movement; provide sensory awareness; and are cues to movement. MC is a proprioceptive facilitation technique.

Maximal Resistance (MR): maximum resistance tolerated by the patient applied in PNF patterns to stronger muscles to create an overflow pattern of the weaker muscles. The overflow is the spread of muscular response from the stronger muscles to the weaker ones. MR is a PNF technique.

Muscle positioning (MP): in midrange for greatest muscular tension; in short ranges for weak contractile force; in lengthened range for strong muscular contraction that is enhanced by the stretch mechanism. MP is a PNF technique.

Quick Stretch (QS): short stretch applied to a weak muscle in lengthened range using the diagonal PNF patterns to facilitate the agonist muscular contraction. An example of QS is tapping over the muscle belly or the tendon. QS is a proprioceptive facilitation technique.

Repeated Contractions (RCs): repeated isotonic contractions with quick stretches and resistance performed through the range or part of the range at a point of weakness. RC is a PNF technique.

Resistance: resistance applied to weak muscle. Resistance can be manual (graded); body weight and gravity using upright positions; mechanical (weights, cuffs, vests); isokinetic. Resistance is a proprioceptive facilitation technique.

Resisted Progression (RP): stretching, approximation, and tracking light resistance applied manually (or using T-band) to the patient's pelvis during locomotion. It should not disrupt patient's coordination, momentum, and velocity. Indications for RP are improved timing and control of lower trunk or pelvis during locomotion; increased endurance. RP is a PNF technique.

Rhythmic Initiation (RI): voluntary muscular relaxation, followed by passive movements, active assisted and active resistive movements (using light resistance), and finally active movements. Indications for RI: spasticity, rigidity (as in PD), difficulty initiating movement (as in PD), aphasia, and inability to relax. RI is a PNF technique.

Rhythmic Stabilization (RS): alternating resisted isometric contractions of first the agonist and then the antagonist muscles without any motion allowed. Indications for RS are to increase muscular strength and coordination. RS is a PNF technique.

Slow Reversals (SRs): isotonic contractions first of the agonist muscles and then the antagonist muscles using graded resistance. The resistance is applied first to the stronger muscles, progressing to the weaker muscles. At the end, the limb is moved through full ROM. SR is a PNF technique.

Timing for Emphasis (TE): resistive (strong) isometric contractions causing overflow from strong to weak muscles within a synergistic pattern. Motion is allowed only in the weaker muscles. TE is a PNF technique.

PNF Diagonal Patterns

Table 4-42 Description and Performance of PNF Terminal Positions (Shoulder, Forearm, Wrist, Fingers, Hip, Knee, Ankle)*

UE D1 Extension: Extension, Abduction, Internal Rotation (Scapular Depression, Abduction, and Downward Rotation); Pronation; Ulnar Extension of Wrist; and Abduction and Extension of Fingers including Thumb Abduction.

UE D1 Flexion: Flexion, Adduction, External Rotation (Scapular Elevation, Abduction, and Upward Rotation); Supination; Wrist Radial Flexion; and Fingers Flexion and Adduction including Thumb Adduction.

UE D2 Extension: Extension, Adduction, Internal Rotation (Scapular Depression, Abduction, and Downward Rotation); Pronation; Ulnar Extension of Wrist, and Flexion and Adduction of Fingers including Thumb Opposition.

UE D2 Flexion: Flexion, Abduction, External Rotation (Scapular Elevation, Adduction, and Upward Rotation); Supination; Radial Extension of Wrist; and Fingers Abduction and Extension including Thumb Extension.

LE D1 Extension: Extension, Abduction, Internal Rotation (Posterior Rotation of Pelvis); Knee Extension; and Ankle Plantarflexion and Eversion

LE D1 Flexion: Flexion, Adduction, External Rotation (Anterior Rotation of Pelvis); Knee Flexion; and Ankle Dorsiflexion and Inversion.

LE D2 Extension: Extension, Adduction, External Rotation (Depression of Pelvis); Knee Extension; and Ankle Plantarflexion and Inversion.

LE D2 Flexion: Flexion, Abduction, Internal Rotation (Elevation of Pelvis); Knee Flexion; and Ankle Plantarflexion (or Ankle Dorsiflexion) and Eversion.

*For PNF AROM figures, see Part III.

Neurologic Inhibition Techniques

Table 4-43 Inhibition Interventions[1]

Firm manual contacts (FMCs): applied to midline abdomen; back; palms; lips; soles of feet. Indications: patients with paresthesia or peripheral nerve injury; TBI. FMC is a sensory stimulation technique producing inhibition.

Inhibitory Pressure (IP): deep maintained pressure to tendons; prolonged positioning in extreme lengthened range (prolonged weightbearing quadruped or kneeling; prolonged weightbearing on extended wrists, arms or fingers; modified plantigrade positioning; pressure over calcaneus to decrease plantarflexion tone; tactile deep maintained pressure over acupressure points to decrease pain; firm maintained pressure using cones in the hands or inhibitory splints or casts for lower leg or wrists). IP inhibits muscular tone. IP can also be used in combination with relaxation techniques (deep breathing or relaxing environment). IP is a sensory stimulation technique producing inhibition.

Neutral Warmth (NW): wrapping body or body parts using Ace wraps or towel wrap; applying snug fitting clothes such as gloves, socks, and/or tights; using tepid baths; using air splints. NW is indicated to decrease muscular tone, reduce pain, and produce relaxation and a calming effect. Indications for NW: patients with increased sympathetic activity; patients with high arousal levels; spasticity. Precaution for NW: do not overheat (can increase tone). NW is a sensory stimulation technique producing inhibition.

Prolonged Icing (PI): immersion in cold water or ice chips; ice towel wraps or ice packs; ice massage. PI is indicated to decrease muscular tone, reduce muscular spasms, and decrease metabolism of the tissue. Precaution of PI: monitor patient carefully for SNS effects such as increased arousal, fight or flight response, or protective withdrawal mechanism. PI is a sensory stimulation technique producing inhibition.

Prolonged Stretch (PS): slow, maintained stretch applied at maximum available lengthened range to inhibit muscular contraction and tone. PS can be applied: using positioning, inhibitory splinting, and/or casting; using traction; using mechanical low load weights. PS is a proprioceptive facilitation technique producing inhibition.

Rhythmic Rotation (RRo): relaxation achieved with slow, repeated rotation movements (either passive or active) of a limb at the point of limitation. As muscular relaxation is obtained, the limb is moved slowly into the new range. When tension is observed, more rhythmic rotation movements are necessary. RRo is a PNF technique producing inhibition.

Slow Stroking (SS): applied to paravertebral spinal region causes generalized inhibition and a calming effect. SS is applied by alternating, firm strokes (using a flat hand) downward on paravertebral muscles for 3 to 5 minutes while the patient is lying prone (or sitting and resting forward on a table top). Indications for SS: increased SNS activity; increased arousal. Precaution for SS: patients with large amounts of body hair can be less responsive to the calming effect and may become irritated. SS is a sensory stimulation technique producing inhibition.

Slow vestibular stimulation (SVS): slow repetitive rolling or rocking movements applied through passive or active-assisted techniques. Examples of SVS include sitting and rocking; rolling side lying; using a rocking chair; using the therapy ball, a bolster, equilibrium board, or a swing; riding a wheelchair. Indications for SVS: patients with hypertonia or being hyperactive; high arousal; combative stage TBI. SVS can be combined with deep breathing exercises, imagery relaxation techniques, and quiet environment. SVS is a vestibular stimulation technique producing inhibition.

continues

Table 4-43   (continued)

Vestibular Stimulation (VS) of head and body: using fast spinning in a chair; spinning in a hammock; prone on a scooter board; using equilibrium board, wobble boards, or therapy ball. Indications for VS: hypotonia; children with hyperactivity; coordination problems; akinesia and bradykinesia (in PD). VS is a vestibular stimulation technique producing inhibition.

Locomotion Training

Table 4-44   Locomotion Training Sequence[1]

Activities to prepare for locomotion using instruction and training: (1) Bridging (focus on lower trunk, hip and pelvis, and LEs); (2) Quadruped (focus on the trunk, proximal and intermediate UEs, and proximal LEs); (3) Sitting (focus on upper trunk, pelvis, and proximal and intermediate UEs); (4) Sit to stand; (5) Kneeling/half kneeling (focus on trunk, pelvis, proximal and distal LEs, and reciprocal control of LEs); (6) Modified plantigrade (focus on trunk, UEs, and proximal, intermediate, and distal control of LEs); (7) Standing (focus on trunk and LEs).

Activities at the parallel bars using instruction and training: (1) Moving from sitting to standing and back; (2) Standing balance training; (3) Stepping, sidestepping, and cross-stepping; (4) Training in an appropriate gait pattern; (5) Using the appropriate gait pattern to ambulate forward and to turn; (6) Training to transfer with the assistive device from sitting to standing and back; (7) Standing and weight shifting balance training with assistive device; (8) Gait training with the appropriate assistive device forward and turning.

Indoor locomotion activities using instruction and training: (1) Walking forward and backward; (2) Resisted progression; (3) Sidestepping and cross-stepping; (4) Braiding; (5) Stair climbing; (6) Falling techniques for patients who ambulate independently with assistive devices for long term.

Outdoor locomotion activities using instruction and training: (1) Opening doors and passing through thresholds that go outdoors; (2) Climbing curbs; (3) Negotiating ramps, stairs, and sloped surfaces; (4) Walking on even and uneven surfaces; (5) Walking and crossing at stoplights; (6) Entering and exiting buildings in the community; (7) Entering and exiting vehicles; (8) Using elevators and revolving doors.

Constraint-Induced Movement Therapy as a Form of Functional Training

Table 4-45   CIMT as a Form of Functional Training

Constraint-induced movement[5] therapy (CIMT) forces the use of the affected extremity by restraining the unaffected extremity. For example, for a patient having hemiplegia of the right (involved) upper extremity, the therapist constrains the patient's left (uninvolved) upper extremity in a sling. Then the patient uses his or her right (involved) upper extremity repetitively and intensively for 2 weeks.

CIMT is becoming more and more successful in the United States. It was developed by Dr. Edward Taub[6] (a professor of psychology) at the University of Alabama in Birmingham. Dr. Taub calls CIMT "learned non-use." Dr. Taub's idea of "learned non-use" includes three principles[6, 7,8] of constraining the unaffected limb, forced use of the affected limb, and massed practice. In order to start CIMT, a patient (client) needs to be able to extend his or her wrist and move his or her arm and fingers. In addition, patients (clients) need to demonstrate basic head and trunk stability during upright positioning.

Research showed[6,7 8,9] that CIMT helps patients (clients) by improving functional use of their affected extremity much more than the regular therapy. The results[6] of a 2003 study proved that plastic changes occurred in the motor cortex of patients with TBI who received CIMT intensively (7 hours daily) for 2 weeks. Other studies[7,8,9] showed that CIMT can produce a use-dependent cortical reorganization of the brain in patients (clients) who had CNS injury-related paresis of the upper limb (including chronic hemiparesis from stroke). In other studies,[7,8 9] CIMT was found to help the use of affected (hemiparetic) upper extremity of children with cerebral palsy. The studies[8,9] suggested that CIMT leads to recruitment of a large number of neurons adjacent to those originally involved in the control of the stroke-affected limb. The research conclusion supports the effectiveness of CIMT in a clinical setting by providing a neurophysiological basis[6,7] for the therapy-induced effects on the brain's neural network.

CIMT is a form of "functional training" or "task oriented training" therapy. CIMT can be applied to patients (clients) after CVA, TBI, and CP. Tasks significant for daily function such as standing, walking, grasping, and releasing are emphasized. Motor learning strategies are used to enhance function.

Physical therapy goals using functional training based on CIMT may consider: training patient early to avoid learned nonuse; consider patient's history, health status, age, and experience when designing stimulating and interesting activities; involving patient in goal setting and decision making; structure the practice using task-related training; structure the patient's practice as context specific; maintain

continues

Table 4-45   (continued)

focus on the therapist's role as training coach (minimizing hands on therapy); monitor recovery closely; document progress using valid and reliable functional outcome measures; be cautious about timetables and predictions (because the recovery may be longer).

Neurologic Intervention Patterns

Table 4-46   Therapeutic Exercises[10]

Strength, power, and endurance training for head, neck, limb, pelvic floor, trunk, and ventilatory muscles (such as active assistive, active, and resistive exercises, including concentric, dynamic, isotonic, eccentric, isokinetics, isometric, and plyometric; aquatic programs; standardized, programmatic, complementary exercise approaches task-specific performance training).

Flexibility exercises (such as muscle lengthening; range of motion; stretching).

Relaxation exercises (such as breathing strategies; movement strategies; relaxation techniques; standardized, programmatic, complementary exercise approaches).

Balance, coordination, and agility training (such as developmental activities training; motor function training and retraining such as motor control and motor learning; neuromuscular education and reeducation; perceptual training; posture awareness training; standardized, programmatic, complementary exercise approaches task-specific performance training; sensory training or retraining; task specific performance training; vestibular training).

Body mechanics and postural stabilization (such as body mechanics training; posture awareness training; postural control training; postural stabilization activities).

Gait and locomotion training (such as developmental activities training; gait training; implement and device training; perceptual training; standardized, programmatic, complementary exercise approaches for wheelchair training).

Neuromotor development training (such as developmental activities training; motor training; movement pattern training; neuromuscular education or reeducation).

Table 4-47   Functional Training in Self-Care and Home Management Including ADL and IADL[10]

ADL training (such as: bathing; bed mobility and transfer training; developmental activities; dressing; eating; grooming; toileting).

Devices and equipment use and training (such as: assistive and adaptive device and equipment training during ADL and IADL; orthotic, protective, or supportive device or equipment training during ADL and IADL; prosthetic device or equipment training during ADL and IADL).

Functional training programs (such as: simulated environments and tasks; task adaptation; travel training).

IADL training (such as: caring for dependents; home maintenance; household chores; shopping; structured play for infants and children; yard work).

Injury prevention or reduction (such as: injury prevention education during self-care and home management; injury prevention or reduction with use of devices and equipment; safety awareness training during self-care and home management).

Table 4-48   Prescription, Application, and as Appropriate, Fabrication of Devices and Equipment (Assistive, Adaptive, Orthotic, Protective, Supportive, and Prosthetic)[10]

---

1. Adaptive devices (such as: environmental controls; hospital beds; raised toilet seats; seating systems).
2. Assistive devices (such as: canes; crutches; long-handled reachers; walkers; power devices; static and dynamic splints; wheelchairs).
3. Orthotic devices (such as: braces; casts; splints; shoe inserts).
4. Protective devices (such as: braces; cushions; helmets; protective taping).
5. Supportive devices (such as: compression garments; corsets; elastic wraps; neck collars; serial casts; slings; supplemental oxygen; supportive taping).

Table 4-49   Functional Training in Work (Job/School/Play), Community, and Leisure Integration or Reintegration Including IADL, Work Hardening, and Work Conditioning[10]

---

1. Devices and equipment use and training (such as: assistive and adaptive device and equipment training during IADL; orthotic, protective, or supportive device or equipment training during IADL; prosthetic device or equipment training during IADL).
2. Functional training programs (such as: simulated environments and tasks; task adaptation; task training; travel training).
3. IADL training (such as: community service training involving instruments; school and play activities training including tools and instruments; work training with tools).
4. Injury prevention or reduction (such as: injury prevention education during work at job, school, or play; community and leisure integration or reintegration; injury prevention or reduction with use of devices and equipment; safety awareness training during work at job, school, or play; community and leisure integration and reintegration).
5. Leisure and play activities and training.

Neurologic Intervention Patterns   **311**

Table 4-50   Manual Therapy Techniques (Excludes Joint Mobilization)[10]

1. Manual traction
2. PROM
3. Massage (such as: connective tissue massage; therapeutic massage).
4. Soft tissue mobilization.

Table 4-51   Physical Agents and Mechanical Modalities[10]

1. Physical agents (such as cryotherapy—cold pack, ice massage, vapocoolant spray; hydrotherapy—pools, whirlpool tanks; sound agents—phonophoresis and ultrasound; thermotherapy—dry heat, hot packs; athermal agents—pulsed electromagnetic fields).
2. Mechanical modalities (such as compression therapies—taping, contact casting, compression garments, total contact casting, and vasopneumatic compression devices; gravity-assisted compression devices—standing frame and tilt table).

Table 4-52   Electrotherapeutic Modalities[10]

1. Biofeedback
2. Electrical muscle stimulation (such as EMS, FES, NMES, TENS, HVPC).
3. Electrotherapeutic delivery of medications (such as iontophoresis).

Table 4-53   Patient/Client Related Instruction[10]

Instruction, education, and training of patients/clients and caregivers regarding current condition (pathology; pathophysiology—disease, disorder, or condition; impairments, functional limitations, or disabilities); enhancement of performance; health, wellness, and fitness; plan of care; risk factors (for pathology; pathophysiology—disease, disorder, or condition; impairments, functional limitations, or disabilities); transitions across settings; transitions to new roles.

Table 4-54   Airway Clearance Techniques[10]

1. Breathing strategies (such as active cycle of breathing or forced expiratory techniques; assisted cough/huff techniques; autogenic drainage; paced breathing; pursed lip breathing; techniques to maximize ventilation: maximum inspiratory hold; staircase breathing; manual hyperinflation).

2. Positioning (such as positioning to alter work of breathing; positioning to maximize ventilation and perfusion; pulmonary postural drainage).
3. Manual and mechanical techniques (such as assistive devices; chest percussion, vibration, and shaking; chest wall manipulation; suctioning; ventilatory aids).

Intervention Patterns for Cerebral Vascular Accident

Table 4-55   CVA Intervention Patterns

Interventions to improve sensory function: (1) encourage patient to use the affected extremity; (2) use sensory stimulation techniques (such as stroking, approximation, superficial, and deep pressure) for functional training; (3) use feedback and encouragement with stimulation techniques; (4) use stimulation techniques encouraging patient's extremities to cross the midline (reaching, PNF); (5) provide visual, tactile, or proprioceptive stimuli on the affected side (maximizes patient's attention to affected side); (6) do not use intense stimulation to produce withdrawal effects; use pressure splints for deep pressure and joint sensation sensory stimulations; (7) use patient and patient's family education for protection of affected extremity (to prevent trauma to affected side).

Interventions to improve flexibility and joint integrity: (1) use daily PROM and AROM exercises in all motions (PT can also apply joint mobilization) to prevent contractures; (2) use positioning (with resting splints); (3) place the affected scapula in protraction and upward rotation to prevent impingement with overhead activities (do not use overhead pulleys); (4) patient education for self ROM (using the affected UE to horizontally abd/add the unaffected UE to 90°; sitting and leaning forward toward the floor with bilateral UEs); (5) weight shifting activities forward in modified plantigrade to stretch affected plantarflexors; (6) patient positioning in supine at edge of mat with affected hip in abduction and extension, knee flexion, and foot placed flat on the floor (or stool) to break scissoring synergy pattern.

Interventions to improve muscular strength: (1) strengthening exercises starting with gravity eliminated powder boards or aquatics (for very weak patients) and continuing with free weights, elastic bands, and isokinetics; (2) functional activities and resistive exercises such as step-ups and stair climbing with ankle weights; (3) use exercise precaution (Valsalva) with HTN and patients with cardiopulmonary dysfunctions; (4) use eccentric exercises to decrease cardiovascular stress; use exercises in sitting upright position for HTN; (5) use safety precautions for patients taking medications (see safety precautions in Part 1); (6) decrease risk of injury for older adults with CVA immobilized for long periods of time by starting with con-

continues

Table 4-55   (continued)

centric low intensity exercises (instead of eccentric and high intensity), allowing enough rest periods, and monitoring for fatigue and DOMS.

Interventions to decrease spasticity: (1) positioning (see positioning techniques below); (2) use rhythmic rotation and prolonged stretch; (3) use slow rocking movements (rocking the patient's body over the elongated limb); (4) use weight-bearing positioning in kneeling and quadruped; (5) use rotational upper trunk movements in PNF diagonal patterns; (6) ask patient to perform side sitting on the affected side to stretch spastic flexor muscles; (7) use reciprocal inhibition to reduce tone in the agonist muscles; (8) use ice wraps or ice packs to decrease neural firing rates; (9) use relaxation techniques; (10) use air splints for affected upper extremity with patient in quadruped position and elbow extended.

Interventions to improve postural control and functional mobility: (1) rolling[1] (focus on rolling toward the unaffected side to challenge the affected side; use the hands' prayer position to assist the movement); (2) supine to sit and back (focus on rising from the affected side); (3) sitting (focus on achieving a symmetrical posture of spine and pelvis and feet flat; provide verbal and tactile cues to help symmetry; use UEs in front or at sides for support in early sitting; use gentle bouncing on a therapy ball to promote pelvic and trunk alignment; focus on lateral weight shifts to affected side to challenge patient; scooting in sitting helps with putting pants on; coming to end of seat to place feet back under the body helps with transitional movements); (4) bridging (to develop trunk and hip extensor control for bedpan, pressure relief, scooting, and sit to stand transfers; include weight shifts and placing hips to the side while bridging; in beginning stabilize foot to achieve affected LE hook-lying position; use more difficult task such as the patient to placing unaffected foot on a ball while bridging); (5) sit to stand and sitting down transfers (ask patient to use momentum to shift body forward; have patient's feet well back to allow ankle DF and assist with forward rotation; have patient's hands in prayer position or place hands clasp together on therapy ball while patient is moving forward; in the beginning elevate the patient's seat to decrease hip/knee extension, later lower the seat; practice small range movements such partial squats with patient against a wall); (6) standing modified plantigrade (early standing posture to develop postural and extremity control assisting quads in extension); (7) standing (first using high table or wall support for stabilization, then weight shifting in all positions, and finally reaching in all directions and stepping); (8) Transfers (to both sides focusing toward affected side; use different surfaces and heights).

Interventions to improve upper-extremity function: (1) extended arm weightbearing[1] with hand placed on a support surface (promotes stabilization and decreases flexion synergy); (2) approximation (for stimulation of shoulder and scapula stabilizers and elbow extensors); (3) quadruped position (offers maximal challenge); (4) reaching (to improve scapular protraction, upward rotation, and elbow, wrist, and finger extension; beginning reaching starts in side lying; advanced reaching includes independently lifting and reaching forward and standing and reaching to pick an object from a shelf); (5) grasp and manipulation (begins with voluntary gross grasp and release; voluntary release is more difficult than grasp; patient needs positioning, stretching, and inhibitory techniques to decrease flexion and increase extension; use task training such as reaching for an object off a shelf; practice advanced wrist and finger extension activities such as using utensils to eat, writing, drinking from a cup, or picking up coins).

Interventions to improve lower-extremity function: (1) to activate hip extensors[1] and abductors, dorsiflexors, and knee extensors (use PNF LE D1 extension; use supine PNF LE D1 flexion; sitting, crossing and uncrossing the affected LE; standing; step ups; bridging to promote hip extension with knee flexion; lower trunk rotation in side lying, kneeling, or standing to decrease retraction and elevation for pelvic control; pelvic shifts while sitting on a therapy ball; hip abduction in hook lying, supine, side lying, modified plantigrade, and standing); (2) to break up knee hyper-extension in standing (use foot slides in supine hook lying and in sitting; use partial squats).

Interventions to improve balance: (1) weight shifts first in sitting, then in standing; symmetrical weightbearing in sitting and standing; (2) shifting toward the affected side in sitting and standing; (3) weightbearing on the affected hip in sitting and on the affected foot in standing with prohibited unaffected LE movement or weight-bearing; (4) decrease base of support (in sitting; LE uncrossed to crossed; in standing from wide to narrow and tandem; standing on one LE); (5) change sup-port surfaces (sitting on mat to therapy ball; standing on floor to dense foam); (6) use sensory inputs (feet on firm surface or foam); (7) use UE position and support; (8) use UE movements; (9) use LE movements; (10) use trunk movements; (11) use destabilizing functional activities; (12) perform dual task training; (13) change envi-ronments (open and closed); (14) use postural strategies (ankle, hip, medial lateral hip); (15) use stepping strategies.

Interventions to improve locomotion: (1) gait training (progress patient from parallel bars and use of assistive devices to no assistive devices; may use an overhead harness and partial body weight support; maintain the natural rhythm of walking and speed; encourage patient to take even steps using verbal cues and/or foot markers placed on the floor; patient to progress from smaller steps to longer steps, increased distance and faster speeds; patient to walk in different environ-ments); (2) analysis of gait abnormalities; (3) practice of functional locomotion

continues

Table 4-55   (continued)

skills (walking forward, backward, sideward; sidestepping, braiding, step up, step down, lateral step up; stair climbing, step over step; walking on ramps, curbs, uneven terrain, over and around obstacles; crossing the street; stepping on and off elevator and escalator); (4) dual task activities (carrying a tray wile walking; walking and talking; bouncing a ball while walking; holding a ball while walking); (5) use treadmill, cycle ergometer, and isokinetic training; (6) use of orthotics to improve safety (use temporarily the dorsiflexor assist for early stages; use posterior leaf spring AFO that controls for foot drop; use solid ankle AFO for maximum stabilization; AFO set in 5° DF limits knee hyperextension; AFO set in 5 PF° stabilizes knee during midstance).

Interventions to improve motor learning: (1) patient learns the skill in the cognitive stage (therapist gives simple, clear, verbal instructions trying not to overload patient; patient practices the learned skill or learned component parts of the skill; correct performance is reinforced; interventions should be provided for errors; patient active participation is important; patient practice skills on unaffected side first, then on affected side; patient can use mental practice; patient examines his or her performance; if patient cannot examine himself or herself accurately, therapist helps patient in proper decision making); (2) feedback (intrinsic occurring naturally as part of movement response or extrinsic provided by the therapist; visual inputs such as patient looking at the movement are important in early interventions; proprioception stimulations such as manual contacts, tapping, stretching, antigravity postures or vibration are important in later learning to enhance the learned skill; therapist to limit immediate feedback and increased sensory stimulations in later training; pain and fatigue should always be avoided); (3) practice (patient needs constant practice and repetition for motor learning and recovery; in the beginning, in the hospital, patient needs adequate rest periods due to decreased endurance; later patient needs variable practice using random practice order to improve performance and for better retention; learning environment is important with a closed environment with reduced distractions in the beginning and an open environment with interferences toward the end; patient motivation needs to be considered by making therapy session positive experience and having patient and family involved in goal setting.

Table 4-56   Strategies for Right CVA

Use verbal cues; do not use demonstration or gestures; give frequent feedback; focus on slowing down and controlling movements; focus on patient's safety; avoid environmental and spatial clutter; do not overestimate patient's ability to learn.

Table 4-57   Strategies for Left CVA

Develop an appropriate communication base using words, gestures, and pantomime; assess patient's level of understanding; give frequent feedback and support; do not underestimate patient's ability to learn.

Table 4-58   Intervention Strategies for Flaccid, Spastic, and Relative Recovery Stages

In the flaccid stage, the PTA must concentrate on the following interventions: bed mobility turning from supine to side lying and sitting and back; pressure splints to provide sensory input and stabilization of affected extremity and decrease edema; use arm slings to prevent shoulder subluxation and improve shoulder function; use arm board or lap tray to provide support for the upper extremity; preparation for sitting up; preparation for standing up (focus on LEs control); trunk balance; stimulation and facilitation techniques to increase tone and voluntary movements.

In the spasticity stage, the PTA must concentrate on the following interventions: rehabilitation of patient in the sitting and standing positions as much as possible; some treatments started in the flaccid stage in supine position will continue in sitting and standing positions; inhibition techniques to decrease spasticity; weight-bearing on the involved extremity; sitting; standing; progression to treatment in prone lying and kneeling; gait training with assistive device; working for independent control of affected extremity; facilitation techniques for voluntary movement; placing.

In the relative recovery stage, the PTA must concentrate on treatments to improve patient's gait, balance, and coordination; dissociation of mass patterns of movement; ADLs.

Table 4-59 CVA Positioning Techniques

Position the patient with CVA in supine: trunk in midline with head and neck in neutral and symmetrical; a small pillow or towel under the scapula to assist with scapular protraction; affected upper limb positioned (on a pillow) in external rotation and abduction with elbow extended, wrist neutral, fingers extended; hip forward (pelvis protracted) and in neutral (in regard to rotation) with a small towel under knee to prevent hyperextension; foot and ankle in neutral (if there is PF, use a splint); do not use anything against the soles of the feet.

Position the patient with CVA side lying on the unaffected side: head/neck in neutral and symmetrical; trunk straight in midline; a small pillow can be placed under the affected rib cage to elongate the affected side; affected scapula protracted and affected shoulder placed well forward on a supporting pillow; elbow extended, wrist neutral, fingers extended; thumb abducted; affected hip forward, pelvis protracted; affected knee flexed and supported on a pillow.

Position the patient with CVA side lying on the affected side: head/neck in neutral and symmetrical; trunk straight in midline; affected upper scapula protracted; affected shoulder well forward with elbow extended; forearm supinated; wrist neutral; fingers extended; thumb abducted; affected hip in extension; affected knee flexed (another position may be hip and knee in slight flexion with protraction of pelvis).

Position the patient with CVA sitting in the wheelchair (chair): head and neck in neutral and symmetrical; spine in extension and aligned in midline; equal weightbearing on both buttocks; affected shoulder protracted and forward with elbow supported on a lapboard (or a trough); wrist neutral with finger extended and thumb abducted; both lower extremities are flexed to 90° and in neutral in regard to rotation.

Intervention Patterns for Parkinson's Disease

Table 4-60 PD Intervention Patterns

Interventions to improve motor learning:[1] (1) use structured instruction (use task-specific learning; use structured activities; use simple tasks; use many repetitions of one activity until learning is achieved; do not overload the patient with new tasks until the initial task is learned); (2) use visual cues (use brightly colored floor markings during gait training; improve stride length and velocity; decrease shuffling gait); (3) use rhythmic auditory stimulation (use music or a metronome to increase gait cadence; use music for marching in place).

Interventions to improve relaxation: (1) use slow rhythmic rotational movements of extremities and trunk (use PNF diagonal patterns to incorporate rotation; use gentle trunk rocking to reduce rigidity; use hook lying, lower trunk rotation, rolling in side lying; use rhythmic initiation; use diaphragmatic breathing during PNF diagonal patterns such as PNF D2 flexion and PNF D2 Extension).

Interventions to improve flexibility: (1) use PROM and AROM exercises; (2) use PNF diagonal patterns (use PNF D2 for bilateral UEs flexion to improve trunk extension and decrease thoracic kyphosis; use PNF D1 LE extension to decrease LE flexed and adducted positions); (3) use PNF hold relax or contract relax; (4) use light and gentle stretching (of hip and knee flexors, ankle plantarflexors, and elbow flexors); (5) use prone daily positioning to prevent contracture (early in the disease); (6) use weights to stretch hip and knee flexion contractures (later in the disease).

Interventions to increase muscular strengthening: (1) use aquatic exercises (walking pool program; supervised aerobic pool program); (2) use aerobic training exercise program (individualized; established by the PT); (3) during strength training, focus on antigravity muscles; (4) use a HEP of daily exercises with moderate duration and intensity (standing corner wall stretches are effective for kyphotic and forward head posture; overhead flexion and abduction with a cane; modified plantigrade exercises holding lightly at the kitchen countertop; use group exercises to increase patient's motivation; patient should not overdo activities and become fatigued); (5) use functional training exercises (use rhythmic initiation for strengthening exercises; use segmental rotation of upper and lower trunk during bed mobility activities; use PNF D1 UEs and LEs flexion patterns for movement initiation; use anterior and posterior pelvic tilts on a therapy ball to improve pelvic mobility; use weight shifting; use PNF D2 flexion and D2 extension of UE to increase upper trunk extension; strengthen hip and knee extensors using modified wall squats; use modified plantigrade with upper limbs extended on a wall; use lateral side stepping; practice quadruped creeping to teach patient how to get up from falling; practice half kneeling and kneeling as transitional activities).

Interventions to improve gait: (1) use gait training techniques to increase speed, broaden base of support, lengthen stride, improve stepping, facilitate heel to toe pattern, improve trunk rotation and arm swing; (2) decrease kyphotic and forward head posture during gait (use gait training with an overhead harness instead of assistive device; walking on a motorized treadmill using an overhead harness); (3) use visual (such as floor markings) and auditory cues (to walk faster, take larger steps, or swing arms); (4) use marching in place with music techniques (to improve step height and increase speed); (5) highlight lower trunk rotation during gait (using braiding technique of side stepping with alternate crossed stepping); (6) use different gait training surfaces and techniques (from tile flooring to carpet and outside grass; from eyes open to eyes closed; from closed environment to open environments; from straight flooring to curbs, ramps, and stairs); (7) reduce freezing episodes during gait (by encouraging rotational movements or stepping over obstacles).

continues

Neurologic Intervention Patterns **319**

Table 4-60 (continued)

Interventions to improve balance: (1) use dynamic stability training (weight shifting, reaching, trunk rotation combined with reaching, sitting on a therapy ball); (2) use balance challenging techniques (such as arms to side, arms folded across chest, feet together, feet apart, arms overhead, single leg raises, stepping, marching in place, functional reach; change the support surface by adding foam or asking patient to close his or her eyes; as a safety precaution do not use manual displacement at all since can cause increase rigidity); (3) use standing exercises (such as toe offs, heel rises, chair rises, modified wall squats, single limb stance with side kicks, marching in place; as a safety precaution allow patient to maintain light touch support during standing exercises).

Interventions to improve cardiopulmonary function: (1) use diaphragmatic breathing exercises; (2) use deep breathing training to increase vital capacity; (3) use UEs exercises (wrist cuff weights, ergometer, PNF UE bilateral D2 flexion and extension); (4) use LE resistance exercises (ergometer and/or daily walking program; aquatic therapy); (5) use the PT's individualized aerobic exercise program (based on ACSM guidelines for frequency, intensity, duration, and progression).

Interventions to promote patient, family, and caregiver education: use one on one instruction, group sessions, printed materials, and/or computer or video presentations; use a supportive and positive attitude; recommend support groups.

Intervention Patterns for Multiple Sclerosis

Table 4-61 MS Intervention Patterns

Interventions to increase muscular strength: (1) use the PT's individualized exercise program for each patient (PT considers the frequency, intensity, type, and time duration of exercise); (2) avoid patient's exercise fatigue; (3) have patient perform exercises in the morning; (4) use moderate exercise intensity; (5) use resistance exercises (free weights, elastic bands, and weight and isokinetic machines); (6) use circuit training (different stations alternating upper and lower extremities exercises); (7) use adequate rest periods between exercises; (8) use slow progression of exercises; (9) avoid patient's overwork; (10) have patient exercise in a cool environment (prevent overheating; use cooling suits or vests; use aquatic exercises); (11) do not use free weights with patients having proprioception, incoordination, or tremors; (12) use written instructions or diagrams with patients having cognitive or memory deficits; (13) include functional strengthening activities (closed chain exercises and balance training); (14) use group exercises to improve patient's motivation.

Interventions to increase flexibility: (1) use stretching and ROM exercises (stretch pectoralis and latissimus dorsi for forward posture deficits; stretch hip flexors, adductors, hamstrings, and heel cords for patients confined to a wheelchair; stretch hip and knee extensors and plantarflexors for patients confined to bed).

Interventions to improve cardiopulmonary function:[1] (1) use the PT's individualized aerobic exercise program (PT needs to test the patient prior to exercise; be cautious with medications' effects and patient's fatigue); (2) for stable MS the individualized aerobic exercise program is recommended three times per week, 10 minutes sessions, at 50% to 75% or 50% to 65% peak VO_2 (recommended exercises are cycling, walking, swimming, water aerobics, or circuit training; patient education is important for understanding, self-monitoring, safety, and modifications of exercise program).

Interventions to improve sensory deficits: (1) instruct patient to use adequate lighting all of the time to compensate for visual deficits (use bright light at night; reduce clutter); (2) give the patient an eye patch for one eye for double-vision deficit (eye patch to be used when driving, watching television, or reading; eye patch should not be used all the time); (3) instruct patient in skin care, protection, and pressure relief for superficial sensations deficits to prevent decubitus ulcers (patient to keep skin clean and dry; to inspect the skin daily; to wear comfortable clothes that are soft and not tight; to do push ups in the chair every 15 minutes; to be repositioned in bed every 2 hours; to use pressure relieving devices such as special mattresses, cushions, cuffs, or boots; to avoid activities that can traumatize skin during transfers; to avoid skin contact with hot water or hot objects; to be aware of and seek immediate medical attention for skin blisters or open sores).

Interventions to decrease spasticity: (1) use cold packs, ice packs, or cool wraps (caution with patients with intact sensations that may develop ANS responses such as increased heart and respiratory rate and nausea); (2) use ROM exercises early in the disease process; (3) use stretching exercises (intermittent static stretching for 30 to 60 seconds for 5 to 10 repetitions; use serial casts or air splints; use stretching as a HEP for patient/caregiver; teach patient/caregiver proper stretching techniques; prevent ballistic stretching; emphasize stretching quadriceps, adductors, and plantarflexors, and hamstrings and hip flexors for patients in wheelchair); (4) reduce extensor tone (use lower trunk rotation in side lying or hook lying; patient hook lying, with a therapy ball under lower legs, and PTA gently rocking the ball back and forth; patient moving from quadruped to side sitting position); (5) reduce hypertonicity using inhibitory techniques; (6) use positioning schedule for patient confined to bed or wheelchair.

Interventions to decrease pain: (1) instruct patient in daily stretching exercises to decrease pain; (2) use massage and ultrasound to relieve pain; (3) use postural retraining exercises and orthotic and adaptive devices to decrease pain; (4) use a

continues

Table 4-61   (continued)

soft collar to limit neck flexion for Lhermitte's sign pain; (5) use aquatic therapy (cooler water) for pain from dysesthesia; (6) have patient wear stockings and gloves (neutral warmth technique) for chronic pain relief (be careful that patient is not hot).

Interventions to decrease fatigue: (1) instruct patient to avoid heat caused by strenuous activities or environmentally; (2) use energy conservation (modification of tasks or the environment; using crutches, walkers or orthotics; breaking down difficult activities into small parts); (3) use activity pacing (an activity can be interspaced throughout the day with periodic rest periods; patient needs to set priorities and limit activities to the most important and enjoyable ones); (4) PTA to work with rehab team to help patient.

Interventions to increase balance and coordination (especially for patients with ataxia): (1) increase postural stability (use joint approximation for shoulders, hips, head and spine; use rhythmic stabilization technique); (2) promote dynamic postural control (use weight shifting, reaching, and stepping activities; use aquatic therapy in 85°F water); (3) promote functional activities (use bridging, sit to stand and scooting activities; use real life functional tasks such as reaching, turning, or bending while sitting or standing; practice transfers from sit to stand and back); (4) use challenging balance activities (change balance surfaces; decrease base of support; eyes open and eyes closed; use platform training); (5) stabilize movements (use light weight cuffs for ankles or wrists to reduce tremors of limbs and trunk in ambulation; use weighted canes or walkers in ambulation; use a soft collar for head and neck tremors; caution not to fatigue the patient); (6) use Frenkel's exercises.

Interventions to improve ambulation: (1) use stretching and strengthening exercises (stretch iliopsoas and hamstrings regularly especially if sitting in wheelchair; strengthen mostly hip flexors, ankle dorsiflexors, quadriceps, and hip abductors); (2) use aquatic exercises (can reduce tone and fatigue and control ataxia); (3) use the motorized treadmill (and an overhead harness); (4) use orthotic devices as necessary (AFO for foot drop and knee hyperextension control; can use Rocker shoes for ankle mobility); (5) use assistive devices as necessary (walker or crutches to help with fatigue, strength, sensory deficits, and balance); (6) use wheeled mobility devices for later in the disease (use three- or four-wheeled scooters; manual or power wheelchair for postural support and fatigue; prevent sacral sitting with kyphosis; use gel-cushioned seating, footrests, lap belt, heel loops); (7) teach transfers and wheelchair mobility (use transfer board or hydraulic lift).

Interventions to improve functionality: (1) use functional mobility training (bed mobility, transfers, gait training); (2) work with OT/COTA in ADLs; (3) use adaptive equipment training (raised seats, transfer board, wrist rests for writing or typing, long-handled shoe horns, button hooks, Velcro closures, socks aids; voice amplification for speech, computer assisted communication system for speech).

Interventions to improve speech and swallowing: (1) use diaphragmatic breathing; (2) use coughing techniques; (3) use upright positioning with slight forward head position and chin parallel to table (to avoid aspiration and help with swallowing); (4) use oral motor exercises to improve function of the mouth (for lip closure, tongue movements, and jaw control).

Interventions to improve cognitive function: (1) use memory book (to log daily events and reminders); (2) structure the environment (labeling the furniture for immediate use); (3) give written directions for functional tasks or HEP (such as transfers, positioning, ambulation, self-stretching and strengthening); (4) assist caregiver/family to help with directions and cueing.

Intervention Patterns for Traumatic Brain Injury

Table 4-62   TBI Intervention Patterns

RLA, levels 1, 2, and 3: (1) prevent contracture development[1] (use positioning: position head in neutral, rolls placed behind neck and parallel to head for support and to prevent lateral flexion and rotation; position trunk with normal alignment and rolls behind shoulders and hips to prevent rotation; position upper extremity with cone or towel in hand to prevent finger flexion; position lower extremity with hips and knees in slightly flexed position and a roll between legs to prevent adduction or IR; turn the patient every 2 hours; position the patient in wheelchair/chair: use reclining wheelchair or tilt in space wheelchair; position head and pelvis in wheelchair/chair; prevent foot drop by using boots; use gentle PROM); (2) decrease abnormal tone (use PROM and positioning by maintaining the head and neck in neutral position; discourage primitive posturing that increases tone; keep the entire body in proper alignment; use serial casting for plantarflexion contracture); (3) maintain skin integrity, prevent decubiti development through frequent position changes (turning every 2 hours); (4) maintain respiratory status, prevent complications through postural drainage, percussion, vibration, suctioning to keep airway clear; (5) use sensory stimulation to improve arousal and elicit movements (stimulate auditory, olfactory, visual, tactile, gustatory, kinesthetic, and vestibular sys-

continues

Table 4-62   (continued)

tems; after stimulation monitor patient for changes in BP, HR, respiration; watch for diaphoresis; document patient's motor responses such as grimacing, head turning, vocalization, or changes in posture); (6) teach family about the recovery stages, performing ROM exercises, positioning, and sensory stimulation (work with a social worker (SW) to provide support and guidance); (7) promote early return of functional mobility skills through upright positioning for improved arousal and proper body alignment (support patient's neck and head in upright posture; may use a tilt table to allow weightbearing through lower extremities).

RLA level 4: (1) provide consistency through use of team-determined behavioral modification techniques (all team members should be consistent especially when addressing inappropriate behaviors); (2) use the same therapist for treatments; (3) use a daily routine; (4) use calm, comforting, and focus behavior; (5) provide structure and orientation; (6) do not expect carryover (patient learns functional tasks; use charts or graphs to progress the patient with new skills); (7) expect patient to be self-centered and do not attempt to change the patient's attitude; (8) provide safe and functional choices for therapy (allow patient to have control over treatment but in a safe way such as asking whether he or she wants to walk or to play with the ball; either choice would be helpful allowing patient to have some control without making wrong choices); (9) provide closed supervision in a closed environment to maintain patient's safety; (10) teach the family about the patient's aggressive behaviors (to understand and accept them as temporary and short-term behaviors; teach family consistency).

RLA levels 5 and 6: (1) continue interventions from level 4 and focus in maximizing patient's motor abilities (watch for mental and physical fatigue signs such as irritability and decreased performance); (2) use specific and clear feedback in plain words (do not overwhelm the patient with feedback); (3) provide verbal and physical assistance; (4) allow rest periods; (5) teach compensatory techniques such as dressing with one hand if hemiparesis is present in one upper extremity; (6) involve the patient in task specific training; (7) break down complex tasks into component parts; (8) provide structure and prevent overstimulation (provide a daily schedule; use memory logs; work with patient in a closed, reduced stimulus environment); (9) restore movement and functional mobility by using developmental sequence postures; (10) use relaxation techniques; (11) teach and emphasize safety with patient and patient's family; (12) teach family how to assist patient with functional mobility (such as bed mobility, transfers, gait training, wheelchair mobility), PROM, and strengthening exercises.

RLA levels 7 and 8: (1) physical therapy general goals are geared toward increasing patient's independence through weaning from structure and using open environments (instead of closed); (2) patient should be involved in decision-making; (3) patient needs assistance with behavioral, cognitive, and emotional reintegration (through honest feedback and preparation for community reentry). Other patient's needs are: (4) promotion of independence in functional tasks through mobility skills, and ADLs (using real-life environments); (5) improvement of postural control, symmetry, and balance; (6) encouragement of an active lifestyle (and how to increase cardiovascular endurance); (7) provision of emotional support, and encouraging socialization, behavioral control, and motivation; (8) patient and family education for patient compensation for impairments or disabilities (family acquainted with the community resources for TBI).

Intervention Patterns for Spinal Cord Injury

Table 4-63   SCI Intervention Patterns

Improve respiratory capacity by using: (1) deep breathing exercises, glossopharyn-geal breathing, and strengthening exercises to respiratory muscles (especially diaphragm by using manual contacts below the xiphoid process or weights); (2) assist coughing (manual contacts over epigastric region by pushing quickly inward and upward while patient is trying to cough); (3) use respiratory hygiene with postural drainage, percussion, vibration, suctioning; (4) use abdominal support (abdominal corset to support abdominal contents and assist the diaphragm to rest; it decreases possibility of orthostatic hypotension); (5) stretch pectoral muscles.

Maintain ROM, prevent contracture: (1) use PROM (daily; watch for contraindicated trunk and hip motion in paraplegia such as SLR more than 60° and hip flexion more than 90° and head/neck motion in tetraplegia); (2) use positioning (increase patient's tolerance to prone positioning; position ankles at 90° angle); (3) use splinting (mostly for wrists, hands, and fingers in the early interventions and ankles and hips later); (4) use selective stretching to preserve function (for example keeping tight long finger flexors for tenodesis grasp or tight lower trunk for stability).

Maintain skin integrity, free of decubiti and other injury: (1) use positioning program (prone positioning; gradual upright positioning when patient is medically stabilized using abdominal corset and elastic stockings and monitoring vital signs); (2) use pressure-relieving devices (using cushions, gel cushion, ankle boots); (3) perform patient education for pressure relief, and pressure relief activities (push ups) and daily skin inspection (using a long-handled or adapted mirror); (4) provide prompt treatment of pressure sores.

continues

Table 4-63   (continued)

Improve strength of all remaining innervated muscles: (1) use selective strengthening during acute phase to reduce stress on spinal segments; (2) use resistive exercises (manually, or with cuff weights in straight planes or PNF patterns); (3) strengthen anterior deltoid, shoulder extensors, biceps, and lower trapezius with tetraplegia and all upper-extremity muscles with paraplegia (emphasize shoulder depressors, triceps, and latissimus dorsi for transfers and gait training).

Reorient patient to vertical position: (1) use tilt table, and wheelchair; (2) use abdominal binder, elastic lower-extremity wraps to decrease venous pooling; (3) check for signs and symptoms of orthostatic hypotension (such as lightheadedness, syncope, mental or visual blurring, sense of weakness).

Promote early return of functional mobility skills and ADLs: (1) emphasize independent rolling (using the head, neck, upper extremity and momentum; avoid adaptive devices such as bed rails or trapezes; from supine to prone use flexion of head and neck with rotation; from prone to supine use extension of head and neck with rotation; use bilateral upper-extremities rocking from supine to prone; cross the patient's ankles with upper limb in direction of roll; use PNF D1 flexion and D2 extension patterns in early rolling); (2) use bed mobility activities (such as prone on elbows for head and neck control, prone on hands with paraplegia, supine on elbows and pull ups with tetraplegia; strengthen biceps and shoulder flexors for wheelchair training); (3) train patient to assume sitting (for ADLs, transfers, self ROM, and wheelchair training; for tetraplegia is required 100° SLR to assume long sitting position and avoid posterior tilt and sacral sitting; teach to sit from supine on elbows or prone on elbows' positions); (4) train patient in quadruped positioning (lead up activity for ambulation; can assume quadruped from prone on elbows by first moving backward on elbows and then, when the hips are positioned over the knees, putting weight on each hand by extending the elbows; can assume quadruped from long sitting by rotating the trunk, putting weight on each hand by extending the elbows, and using momentum and strength in the upper extremities and trunk to move in quadruped); (5) train patient in kneeling position (to increase functionality in trunk and pelvis and promote upright control; is important for ambulation with crutches and KAFOs; can assume kneeling position from quadruped by moving the hands backward until the pelvis drops toward the heels while the therapist gives patient mat crutches to start practicing); (6) train patient in transfers (when patient has good sitting balance; start with mat transfers using first a sliding board then without sliding board; advance to other surfaces transfers; patient needs to use momentum and muscle substitution depending on functional levels to transfer; patient to train and practice first, components of transfers, before performing the entire transfer); (7) teach wheelchair mobility (in a customized wheelchair; the wheelchair prescription will be different for each patient depending on level of injury; special wheelchair considerations are needed: seat depth 1 to 2 inches back from popliteal space, floor to seat height measurement considering the seat cushion, back height to allow functionality, fitted seat width and depth, heel loops on footrest, and removable armrests and detachable swing way leg rests); (8) train patient to use orthotic devices in ambulation (such as KAFOs, reciprocal gait orthosis—RGO, and AFOs); (9) train patient in ambulation (using forearm crutches for paraplegia; using 4-point, 2-point, swing to, or swing through gait patterns); (10) train patient in locomotor techniques (where equipment is available).

Intervention Patterns for Guillain-Barré Syndrome

Table 4-64   Guillain-Barré Syndrome Intervention Patterns

Acute phase interventions (in the ascending phase): (1) monitor respiratory system (use pulse oximetry for oxygen saturation level in the arterial blood—normally higher than 96%; use pulmonary physical therapy by facilitating coughing and airway clearance); (2) prevent indirect impairments (use PROM exercises, positioning, specialty bed, gentle passive stretching, and skin care); (3) prevent injury to denervated muscles (use positioning and splinting and do not overuse the denervated muscles; do not overstretch; provide light exercises using the water buoyancy in the Hubbard tank).

Subacute phase interventions (in the descending phase): (1) provide muscle reeducation (start with active assistive and active ROM exercises in straight planes and PNF patterns; continue with low to moderate intensities resistive exercises; avoid overuse and fatigue with exercises; allow necessary resting periods between repetitions); (2) provide functional training (gradual return to ADLs and locomotion; teach energy conservation and activity pacing; avoid overuse and fatigue with activities); (3) provide cardiovascular fitness and general aerobic conditioning; (4) provide patient and patient's family education and support.

Intervention Patterns for Amyotrophic Lateral Sclerosis

Table 4-65   ALS Intervention Patterns

Early-stage interventions: (1) patient education to continue with normal activities as long as possible (promote patient's health and wellness; teach alternative means to accomplish functional activities as the disease progresses; teach patient to avoid overworking weakened denervated muscles; teach energy conservation and activity pacing; teach patient to monitor fatigue; teach patient and patient's family to use equipment and community resources as the disease progresses); (2) use preventative treatments (AROM, AAROM, stretching, strengthening, and endurance exercises).

Middle-stage interventions: (1) continue interventions from the early stage; (2) maintain patient's respiratory status (use postural drainage and pectoral muscles stretching); (3) maintain patient's functional activities (avoid overuse of denervated muscles, modify tasks and activities, and monitor patient's fatigue; teach patient wheelchair mobility; make environmental modifications for patient's home or work such as installing grab bars in the bathroom or wheelchair ramps); (4) consider the rate of disease progression, the area involved, the extent of the disease, patient's acceptance and motivation, and available psychosocial resources.

Late-stage interventions: (1) prevent indirect impairments (use PROM exercises, positioning, pressure relieving devices such as pressure distributing mattress and gel cushions, hospital specialty bed, skin care, and pulmonary physical therapy if needed); (2) relieve pain, muscular spasms and/or spasticity (use modalities such as massage; use stretching and PROM; use positioning; provide family or caregiver education about using a daily PROM program to prevent adhesions especially for the shoulder, transfer training, positioning, turning in bed, and skin care; use mechanical lift if necessary); (3) address patient's cervical muscular weakness and pain (use orthotic cervical collar—can be soft for mild to moderate weakness or rigid for moderate to severe weakness; use recliner chair; use tilt in space or reclining wheelchair); (4) address patient's respiratory muscle weakness (use patient and caregiver education about energy conservation and activity pacing techniques, signs of aspiration, how to avoid choking, and manual assisted coughing techniques; use breathing exercises and positioning); (5) address patient's functional activities (use adaptive equipment to help patient with ADLs, including eating or feeding utensils; use orthotic devices especially for ankles and knees to assist with ambulation; use wheeled walker or forearm crutches to assist with ambulation).

Review of Nervous System Anatomy and Physiology

Parts of the Brain and Functions

See Figures 4-2–4-4.

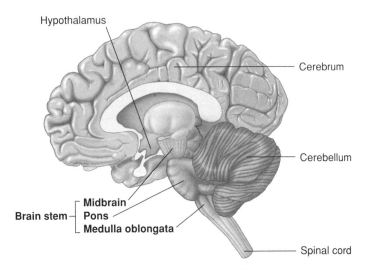

Hypothalamus

Cerebrum

Cerebellum

Midbrain
Brain stem — Pons
Medulla oblongata

Spinal cord

Figure 4-2 Brain stem. From Anatomy and Physiology: Understanding the Human Body by Robert K. Clark, page 196, Figure 12.9 "The brainstem consists of the medulla oblongata, pons, and midbrain."

Table 4-66   Brain Stem, Diencephalon, Cerebrum, and Cerebellum and Their Functions

Brain Stem, Diencephalon Cerebrum, and Cerebellum	Functions
Brainstem consists of (1) midbrain; (2) pons; (3) medulla oblongata	(1) Contains ascending and descending tracts and specific cranial nerve nuclei; important for motor control; (2) contains nuclei for regulation of respiration and for cranial nerves V, VI, and VII; (3) regulates respiratory, cardiac, and vasomotor centers; contains nuclei for cranial nerves VIII through XII.

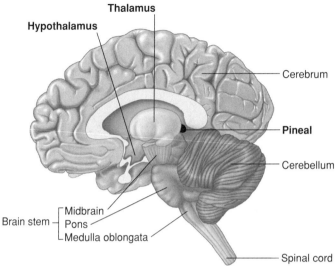

Thalamus

Hypothalamus

Cerebrum

Pineal

Cerebellum

Brain stem ⎡ Midbrain
         ⎢ Pons
         ⎣ Medulla oblongata

Spinal cord

Figure 4-3   Diacephalon. From Anatomy and Physiology: Understanding the Human Body by Robert K. Clark, page 197, Figure 12.10 "The thalamus, hypothalamus, and epithalamus represented here by the pineal gland are included in the diencephalon."

Diencephalon consists of (1) thalamus and (2) hypothalamus.	(1) Relays information to specific cortical sensory areas; (2) controls body temperature, emotions, aggression, eating, drinking, sleep/wake cycles, sexual behaviors, and regulation of the autonomic nervous system.
Cerebrum (1) cerebral hemispheres, (2) basal ganglia.	(1) See functions of each lobe in Table 4-67; (2) forms an associated motor system called the extrapyramidal system; important in formation of motor plans and adjustment of movements.
Cerebellum (1) archicerebellum, (2) paleocerebellum, and (3) neocerebellum.	(1) Equilibrium and regulation of muscle tone; (2) maintenance of posture and control of voluntary movement; (3) smooth coordination of voluntary movements.

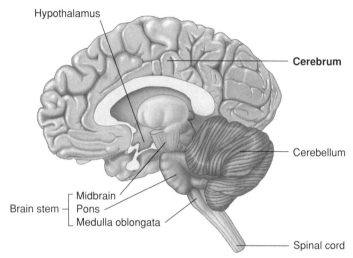

Figure 4-4 Cerebrum. From Anatomy and Physiology: Understanding the Human Body by Robert K. Clark, page 199, Figure 12.12 "The cerebrum."

Cerebral Hemispheres and Functions

See Figures 4-5 and 4-6.

Table 4-67   Lobes and Their Functions

Lobes	Functions
Frontal: (1) precentral gyrus, (2) prefrontal cortex, (3) Broca's area.	(1) Primary motor cortex for voluntary muscle activation of the contralateral side of the body; (2) controls emotions, abstract thinking, and judgments; (3) controls the motor (expressive) aspect of speech for the left hemisphere.
Parietal: postcentral gyrus.	Primary sensory cortex; integrates sensations from the contralateral side of the body for pain and temperature, touch, proprioception, and combined sensations; important for short-term memory.

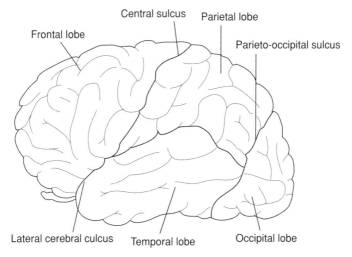

Central sulcus   Parietal lobe

Frontal lobe

Parieto-occipital sulcus

Lateral cerebral culcus   Temporal lobe   Occipital lobe

Figure 4-5   Lobes of the Cerebrum. From Anatomy and Physiology: Understanding the Human Body by Robert K. Clark, page 201, Figure 12.16 "The lobes of the cerebrum."

Occipital: (1) primary visual cortex, (2) associative visual cortex.	(1) Receives and processes visual stimuli; (2) gives meaning to visual information by processing visual stimuli.
Temporal: (1) primary auditory cortex, (2) associative auditory cortex, (3) Wernicke's area.	(1) Receives and processes auditory stimuli; important for long-term memory; (2) processes auditory stimuli; (3) controls the comprehension (receptive) aspect of speech.
Limbic: the oldest part of the brain.	Functions: instincts, emotions, preservation of individual, feeding, aggression, and endocrine sexual responses.

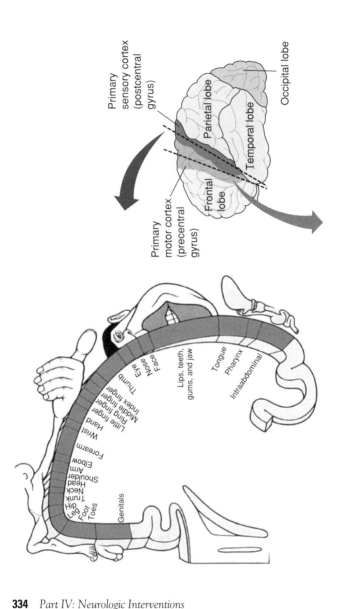

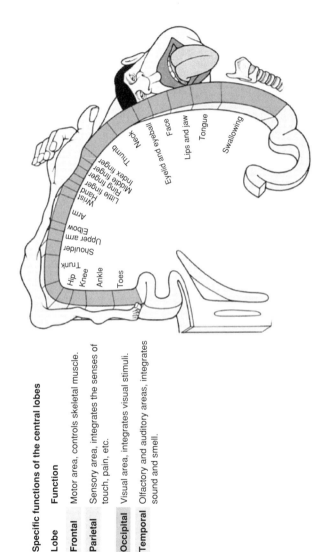

Specific functions of the central lobes

Lobe	Function
Frontal	Motor area, controls skeletal muscle.
Parietal	Sensory area, integrates the senses of touch, pain, etc.
Occipital	Visual area, integrates visual stimuli.
Temporal	Olfactory and auditory areas, integrates sound and smell.

Figure 4-6 Specific Functions of the Central Lobes. From Anatomy and Physiology: Understanding the Human Body by Robert K. Clark, page 203, Figure 12.19 "Specific functions of the central lobes."

Spinal Cord

See Figure 4-7a,b and Figures 4-8 and 4-9.

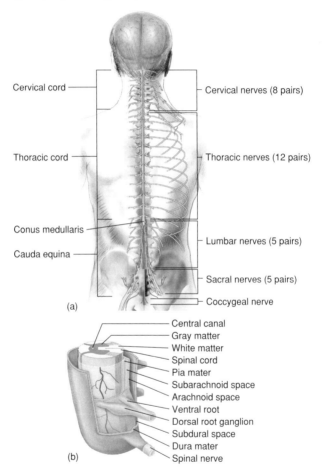

Figure 4-7 Spinal Cord and Its Protective Structures. From Anatomy and Physiology: Understanding the Human Body by Robert K. Clark, page 214, Figure 12.25 a, b "The spinal cord and its protective structures."

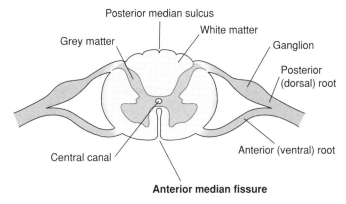

Posterior median sulcus

White matter

Grey matter

Ganglion

Posterior
(dorsal) root

Central canal

Anterior (ventral) root

Anterior median fissure

Figure 4-8 Spinal Nerve Roots. From Anatomy and Physiology: Understanding the Human Body by Robert K. Clark, page 215, Figure 12.27 "A transverse section of the spinal cord showing spinal nerve roots."

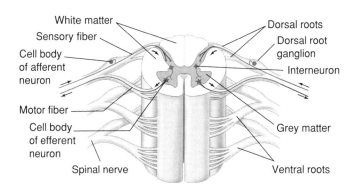

White matter

Sensory fiber

Cell body
of afferent
neuron

Dorsal roots

Dorsal root
ganglion

Interneuron

Motor fiber

Cell body
of efferent
neuron

Grey matter

Spinal nerve

Ventral roots

Figure 4-9 Spinal Cord and Dorsal Root Ganglia. From Human Biology: Fifth Edition by Daniel D. Chiras, page 181, Figure 10-8 "The Spinal Cord and Dorsal Root Ganglia."

Review of Nervous System Anatomy and Physiology **337**

NEUROLOGIC
INTERVENTIONS

Table 4-68   Spinal Cord (SC)

SC is a cylindrical mass of nerve tissue; situated in the vertebral canal; protected by bone, and surrounded by meninges.

SC is a continuation of medulla oblongata; starts at foramen magnum in the skull; ends at conus medullaris (L1–L2).

SC contains gray matter (cell bodies and unmyelinated axons) and white matter (myelinated ascending and descending tracts).

The gray matter is situated in the center of the cord (in shape of letter H) and is made of cell bodies and dendrites of neurons. The white matter is arranged in tracts around the gray matter.

The gray matter contains two anterior (ventral) horns and two posterior (dorsal) horns. Anterior horns contain efferent (motor) neurons. Posterior horns contain afferent (sensory) neurons.

SC is divided into 31 segments with 31 pairs of spinal nerves (SNs): 8 cervical, 12 thoracic, 5 lumbar, 5 sacral, and 1 coccygeal. Each SN has an anterior and a posterior root. The anterior root has motor fibers and posterior root has sensory fibers. There is no posterior root for C1. In cervical spine, nerve roots exit above corresponding vertebral body (C8 exits below C7 and above T1). In thoracic/lumbar spine, nerve roots exit below corresponding vertebral body.

SC gives rise to C4–T1 nerve roots (supply UEs) and L1–S5 nerve roots (supply LEs).

SC is a pathway for motor impulses from the brain and sensory impulses to the brain.

SC mediates stretch reflexes and the defecation and urination reflexes.

Ascending (Sensory) Tracts

Table 4-69   Sensory or Afferent Tracts

Dorsal columns convey sensations of proprioception, kinesthesia, vibration, stereognosis, barognosis, graphesthesia, two-point discrimination, and tactile localization.

Spinothalamic tracts convey sensations of pain and temperature and crude touch.

Spinocerebellar tracts convey sensations of proprioception (from muscle spindles and GTO), and touch and pressure receptors.

Spinoreticular tracts convey sensations of deep and chronic pain.

Descending (Motor) Tracts

Table 4-70 Motor or Efferent Tracts

Corticospinal (or pyramidal) tracts function: voluntary motor control.
Vestibulospinal tracts function: control of muscle tone, antigravity muscles, and postural reflexes.
Rubrospinal tract function: assists in motor function.
Reticulospinal system function: modifies transmission of sensation of pain.
Tectospinal tract function: assists in head turning in response to visual stimuli.

Autonomic Nervous System

Table 4-71 Sympathetic Nervous System (SNS)

Thoracolumbar division of ANS: prepares the body to cope with stressful situations (fight or flight); has afferent and efferent nerve fibers.

SNS effects: increased HR and BP; constriction of peripheral blood vessels; dilation of the pupil; dilation of the bronchioles; slowing of peristalsis; secretion of epinephrine and norepinephrine by adrenal medulla.

Table 4-72 Parasympathetic Nervous System (PNS)

Craniosacral division of ANS: conserves and restores homeostasis; has afferent and efferent nerve fibers.

PNS effects: decreased HR and BP; dilation of peripheral blood vessels; constriction of the pupil; constriction of the bronchioles; increasing of peristalsis and glandular activity.

Brain Meninges and Ventricles

See Figures 4-10 and 4-11.

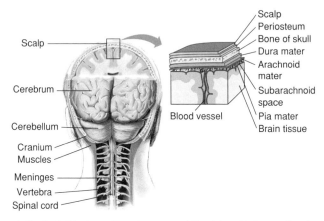

Figure 4-10 Brain Meninges. From Anatomy and Physiology: Understanding the Human Body by Robert K. Clark, page 190, Figure 12.5 " In addition to the bone, the central nervous system is protected by meninges."

Table 4-73   Brain Meninges and Ventricles

Meninges	Ventriles Filled with Ceregrospinal Fluid (CSF)
Dura Mater: outside, tough, and fibrous membrane.	Lateral ventricles: large and irregularly shaped; communicate with third ventricle.
Arachnoid: middle, delicate, and vascular membrane.	Third ventricle: located posterior and deep; communicates with fourth ventricle.
Subarachnoid space: contains CSF and major arteries.	Fourth ventricle: located in pons and medulla; communicates with subarachnoid space.
Pia Mater: inside, thin, and vascular membrane covering the brain surface.	

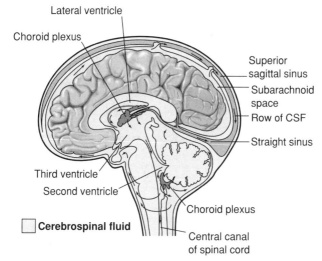

Lateral ventricle

Choroid plexus

Superior sagittal sinus

Subarachnoid space

Row of CSF

Straight sinus

Third ventricle

Second ventricle

Choroid plexus

Cerebrospinal fluid

Central canal of spinal cord

Figure 4-11   Brain Ventricles. From Anatomy and Physiology: Understanding the Human Body by Robert K. Clark, page 191, Figure 12.6 "The location and flow of cerebrospinal fluid."

The Role of Cerebrospinal Fluid (CSF)

Table 4-74   Role of CSF

CSF protects the brain and helps in the exchange of nutrients and waste products. It is produced in the choroid plexus in ventricles. CSF normal pressure = 70–180 mm/H_2O. Total CSF volume = 125–150 cc.

Brain Blood Supply

Table 4-75   Brain Blood Supply

Carotid system: supplies the frontal, parietal, and parts of temporal lobe.	Carotid system originates from the aortic arch that becomes right and left common carotid arteries (divide and form internal and external carotid arteries). Internal carotid artery enters the cranium and forms anterior and middle cerebral arteries.
Vertebrobasilar system: supplies the brain stem, cerebellum, temporal, occipital lobes, and part of thalamus.	Vertebrobasilar system originates from the subclavian artery and vertebral artery (that unite and form the basilar artery). Basilar artery forms right and left posterior cerebral arteries.
Circle of Willis: connects the carotid and vertebrobasilar systems.	Circle of Willis consists of anterior and posterior communicating arteries.

Muscle Sensory Receptors and Functions

Table 4-76   Sensory Receptors and Functions

Sensory Receptors	Functions
Muscle spindles: situated in the belly of the muscle and parallel to the muscle fibers.	Monitor changes in muscle length and the velocity of these changes; monitor position, movement sense, and motor learning.
Golgi tendon organ: situated at the musculotendinous insertion of the muscle.	Monitors tension within the muscle; provides a protective mechanism to the muscle.

References

1. O'Sullivan, SB, Schmitz, TJ. *Physical Rehabilitation*, 5th ed. Philadelphia: F.A. Davis Company; 2007.
2. Rothstein, JM, Roy, SH, Wolf, SL, Scalzitti, DA. *The Rehabilitation Specialist's Handbook*, 3rd ed. Philadelphia: F.A. Davis Company; 2005.
3. Hart-Hughes, S. *Balance Assessment Handbook: A Component of the Falls Toolkit.* Available at http://www.va.gov/NCPS/. Accessed November 2006.
4. American Spinal Injury Association. *Standard Neurological Classification of Spinal Cord Injury.* Available at: http://www.asia-spinalinjury.org/publications/index.html. Accessed January 2007.
5. American Heart Association. *Constraint-Induced Movement Therapy.* Available at: http://www.strokeassociation.org. Accessed November 2006.
6. Taub, E, et al., Improved motor recovery after stroke and massive cortical reorganization following constraint-induced movement therapy. *Phys Med Rehabil Clin North Am* 2003;14(1 Suppl):S77–S91.
7. Yun-Hee, K, et al., Plastic changes of motor network after constraint-induced movement therapy. *Yonsei Med J* 2004;45:241–246.
8. Taub, E, et al., Constraint-induced movement therapy: A new approach to treatment in physical rehabilitation. *Rehabil Psychol* 1998;43:152-170.
9. Liepert, J, et al., Motor cortex plasticity during constraint-induced movement therapy in stroke patients. *Neurosci Lett* 1998;250:5–8.
10. The American Physical Therapy Association. *Guide to Physical Therapist Practice*, 2nd ed. Alexandria, VA: APTA; 2001; Revised 2003.

NEUROLOGIC
INTERVENTIONS

Part V

Cardiopulmonary Interventions

Section 5-3: Patient Safety During Cardiopulmonary Interventions
Basic Cardiac Life Support for Adults
Effects of Medications in Cardiac Rehab
Common Bronchodilators Used in Pulmonary Rehab
Signs/Symptoms to Discontinue Cardiac Interventions
Signs and Symptoms to Change or Discontinue Interventions in
    Pulmonary Rehab
Postural Drainage Possible Complications and Safety Interventions
    during Pulmonary Rehab
Oxygen Safety
Cardiac Safety Rehab Guidelines After Medical Cardiac Procedures
Orthostatic Hypotension in Cardiopulmonary Rehab

Section 5-4: Types of Cardiopulmonary Interventions
Target Heart Rate
Patient Education: Rating of Perceived Exertion
Metabolic Equivalents and Activities
Patient Education Topics for Cardiac Disease
Phases of Cardiac Rehabilitation After Myocardial Infarction (MI)
Prevention Interventions for Coronary Artery Disease (CAD)
Pulmonary Interventions: Terms Related to Postural Drainage
Postural Drainage Positions: Indications, Contraindications, and
    Precautions
Percussion and Shaking Techniques: Indications, Precautions, and
    Contraindications
Other Interventions for Pulmonary Rehab
Examples of Pulmonary Exercises

Section 5-5: Cardiopulmonary Intervention Patterns
APTA's Guide to Physical Therapist Practice—APTA's
    Cardiopulmonary Intervention Patterns
Coronary Artery Disease Intervention Patterns
Congestive Heart Failure Intervention Patterns
Chronic Obstructive Pulmonary Diseases (COPDs) Intervention
    Patterns

Cardiopulmonary Data
Collection

Vital Signs and Normatives[1]

Table 5-1 Procedures for Taking Blood Pressure at the Brachial Artery

1. Cuff width and length need to be appropriate for the size of the patient; cuff width needs to be 20% wider than the diameter of the arm.
2. Cuff is placed 1 to 2 inches above the antecubital fossa and inflated until no radial pulse can be palpated.
3. During cuff deflation, brachial artery is auscultated over the antecubital fossa with a stethoscope.
4. Korotkoff's sounds begin: systolic blood pressure (SBP)—the first clear tapping sound that is heard; tapping sounds increase in intensity.
5. The tapping sounds are replaced by a muffled, soft blowing sound.
6. Diastolic blood pressure (DBP)—disappearance of the muffled, soft blowing sound.

Table 5-2 Blood Pressure Normatives—Adult[1]

Category	Systolic BP	Diastolic BP
Normal BP	120 mmHg or less	80 mmHg or less
Prehypertension	120–140 mmHg	80–90 mmHg
Stage I hypertension (HTN)	140–159 mmHg	90–99 mmHg
Stage II hypertension	160–179 mmHg	100–109 mmHg
Stage III hypertension	More than 180 mmHg	More than 110 mmHg

Table 5-3 Blood Pressure Normatives Infant/Child/Adolescent[1]

Normal BP infant = 80/50 mmHg
Normal BP child = 100/55 mmHg
Normal BP adolescent = 115/70 mmHg

CARDIOPULMONARY
INTERVENTIONS

Table 5-4   Location of Pulses for Monitoring Heart Rate

Brachial: over the medial portion of antecubital fossa for an adult; inside of the upper arm for an infant; it is the most common area to check for a pulse on an infant when performing CPR.

Carotid: on either side (only on one side) of the neck between the trachea and the sternocleidomastoid muscle; it is the most common side to check for a pulse on an adult or a child when performing CPR.

Femoral: in the inguinal area (inguinal triangle) at the crease between the abdomen and the thigh.

Pedal: area over the dorsal, medial aspect of the foot.

Popliteal: in the back of the knee at the popliteal space; patient needs to bend the knee slightly.

Temporal: in the area superior and lateral to the eye.

Table 5-5   Heart Rate Normatives Adult/Infant/Child/Adolescent[1]

Normal heart rate (HR) Adult = 70 bpm (range = 60–100)

Abnormal HR adult = bradycardia = less than 60 bpm; tachycardia = more than 100 bpm

Normal HR infant = 120 bpm (range = 70–170)

Normal HR child = 125 bpm (range = 75–140)

Normal HR adolescent = 85 bpm (range = 50–100)

Table 5-6   Temperature and Respiratory Rate of Adult/Infant/Child/Adolescent

Temperature Adult/Infant/Child/Adolescent	Respiratory Rate (RR) Adult/Infant/Child/Adolescent
Normal temperature adult = 98.6°F	Normal RR adult = 12–18 breaths/min
Normal temperature infant = 98.2°F	Normal RR infant = 30–50 breaths/min
Normal temperature child = 98.6°F	Normal RR child = 20–40 breaths/min
Normal temperature adolescent = 98.6°F	Normal RR adolescent = 15–22 breaths/min

Abnormal Breathing Patterns

Table 5-7   Abnormal Breathing Patterns[2]

Tachypnea (rapid shallow breathing) may be observed in restrictive lung disease, pleuritic chest pain, or elevated diaphragm (because of atelectasis, pleurisy, or rib fracture).

Bradypnea (slow breathing) may be observed secondary to increased intracranial pressure, diabetic coma, or drug-induced respiratory depression.

Hyperpnea (rapid deep breathing) may be observed after exercise (a certain degree is normal), anxiety (may get hyperventilation), metabolic acidosis, comatose patients, myocardial infarction, hypoxia, or hypoglycemia. Kussmaul's breathing = deep gasping breathing associated with severe diabetic ketoacidosis. In general, Kussmaul's breathing is also a sign of impending death.

Cheyne-Stokes breathing (hyperpnea for 10 to 60 seconds, followed by apnea or no breathing) may be observed in congestive heart failure, drug-induced respiratory depression, uremia, or brain damage (both sides of cerebral hemispheres or diencephalon). It also may be observed in coma or basal ganglia disease. It indicates a grave prognosis in adults but may be a normal finding in children.

Obstructive breathing (prolonged expiration and air trapping in the chest; breathing becomes shallow) may be observed in obstructive lung diseases.

Ataxic breathing or Biot's breathing (several short breaths followed by long irregular periods of apnea) may be observed in cases of increased intracranial pressure (as in brain injury).

Sighing breathing (a deep inspiration followed by a slow audible expiration)—sighs in large number may be observed in dyspnea and dizziness. Occasional sighs are normal.

CARDIOPULMONARY INTERVENTIONS

Blood Values and Normatives

Table 5-8   Blood Values and Normatives[2]

Normal calcium serum level: 8.5–10.5 mg/dL (slightly higher in children). Is an electrolyte. Calcium blood levels are regulated by the parathyroid hormone. Blood without calcium will not clot. Calcium deficiency produces hypocalcemia (symptoms: muscular twitching, spasms, convulsions).

Normal creatinine level: 0.6–1.5 mg/dL. It is a source of energy for muscular contraction. It is excreted daily by kidneys. Increased creatinine values are found in renal disease.

continues

Table 5-8 (continued)

Fasting glucose level: 70–110 mg/dL. Higher levels (more than 126 mg/dL) cause hyperglycemia (in diabetes mellitus). Lower levels cause hypoglycemia (patient can have confusion, anxiety, and neurological problems).

Normal hematocrit level: men = 40% to 54 %; females = 37% to 47%; children in general (depends on age) = 35% to 49%; newborns = 49% to 54%. Hematocrit is the volume of erythrocytes (mature red blood cells) packed by centrifugation in a given volume of blood.

Normal hemoglobin level: men = 14 to 18 g/100 ml; females = 12 to 16 g/100 ml. Hemoglobin is an iron-containing pigment of red blood cells that carries oxygen from lungs to body's tissues.

Normal iron level: 50–150 μg/dL (higher in males). Iron is essential in oxygen transport in blood; is used to make hemoglobin.

Normal lipids level: equal or less than 200 mg/dL; LDL equal or less than 130 mg/dL; HDL equal or more than 35 mg/dL. Normal triglycerides level = 40–150 mg/dL.

Oxygen saturation (arterial): adult and child = 95% to 98%.

PCO_2 (partial pressure of carbon dioxide) normatives: adult and child = 35–45 mmHg; infant = 35–55 mmHg. PCO_2 measures carbon dioxide concentration in arterial blood gas; levels vary in asthma, chronic obstructive lung disease, CHF, ketoacidosis, and others.

pH (potential of hydrogen) normatives: adults = 7.35–7.45; children = 7.39–7.41; infants = 7.26–7.41. Potential of hydrogen (pH) measures acidity or alkalinity in blood.

PaO_2 (partial pressure of oxygen while breathing room air) normatives: adult and child = 75–100 mmHg; infant = 75–80 mmHg. PaO_2 measures oxygen concentration in arterial blood.

Normal potassium level: 3.5–5.0 mEq/L. Potassium is an electrolyte. Potassium deficiency causes hypokalemia (symptoms: muscle weakness, dizziness, thirst, confusion, arrhythmias, and changes in the EKG). Potassium excess causes hyperkalemia (symptoms: impaired electrical conduction of heart; ventricular fibrillations).

Normal sodium level: 135–145 mEq/L. Sodium is an electrolyte. Sodium deficiency causes hyponatremia (that can originate because CHF, renal failure, cirrhosis, dehydration, side effects of drugs; symptoms: weakness, confusion, anorexia). Sodium excess causes hypernatremia (that can originate because dehydration and fluid deficits in the blood; symptoms: thirst, orthostatic hypotension, dizziness, altered mental status, neuromuscular dysfunctions).

Normal uric acid level: 3.0–7.0 mg/dL. Uric acid is a crystalline acid as end product of purine metabolism. Increased eliminations of uric acid can be found in gout and leukemia; decreased elimination can be found in renal failure and lead poisoning.

Heart and Lung Sounds

Table 5-9   Heart and Lung Sounds[3]

S_1—the normal heart sound (called also "lub") that occurs when the bicuspid (mitral) and tricuspid valves close; beginning of systole. S_1 can be auscultated over the left lower sternal border (called the apex of the heart).

S_2—the normal heart sound (called also "dub") that occurs when the aortic and pulmonary valves close; end of systole (the period between S_1 and S_2); beginning of diastole (the period between S_2 and the next S_1). S_2 can be auscultated over the left upper sternal border (called the base of the heart).

S_3—the abnormal heart sound that can be heard only with a stethoscope; it is called a ventricular gallop; occurs after S_2 and is associated with left ventricular failure. S_3 can be found in congestive heart failure (CHF).

S_4—the abnormal heart sound that can be heard only with a stethoscope; it is called an atrial gallop. S_4 occurs before S_1 and is associated with hypertension, myocardial infarction, coronary artery disease (CAD), or aortic stenosis.

Pericardial friction rub—the abnormal heart sound that can be heard only with a stethoscope; it is heard as high pitch and rough and creaking or squeaking sound. Pericardial friction rub is associated with inflammation of the pericardial sac with or without excessive fluid (called pericardial disease). Pericardial disease or pericarditis can result from myocardial infarction, trauma, or infection (bacterial, viral, fungal, or tuberculosis).

Murmur—the abnormal heart sound that can be heard without the stethoscope for murmur grades of 1, 2, 3, and 4; it can be heard only with a stethoscope for murmur grades of 5 and 6. Heart murmurs can be rumbling, soft, blowing, loud, or booming and can be heard during systole, diastole, or both. Diastolic murmur is a turbulence between S_2 and S_1; systolic murmur is a turbulence between S_1 and S_2. Murmurs do not necessarily indicate heart disease; many heart diseases do not necessarily produce murmurs. Murmurs can be heard in a stenotic valve (valve that has an impaired opening) or in a regurgitant valve (valve that has an impaired closing).

Vesicular breath sounds—the normal breath sounds heard over the lungs that are low pitched. Vesicular breath sounds are produced by air passing in and out of the airways. Bronchial and tracheal breath sounds—the normal breath sounds heard

continues

CARDIOPULMONARY INTERVENTIONS

Table 5-9 (continued)

over the bronchi and trachea; are higher pitched and louder than vesicular sounds; are produced by air passing over the walls of bronchi and trachea.

Wheezes—the abnormal lung sounds that can be heard with a stethoscope during expiration; are whistling, musical sounds caused by narrowing of the lumen of the airways. Wheezes are the result of asthma, bronchitis, mitral stenosis, emphysema, airway obstruction (caused by foreign bodies), pulmonary infections, pulmonary edema, or other chronic obstructive pulmonary diseases (COPDs).

Crackles—the abnormal lung sounds that can be heard with a stethoscope; are rustling or bubbling sounds also called rales. Crackles are the result of atelectasis (collapsed lungs). Crackles can also be caused by air passing over airway secretions or opening of collapsed airways.

Friction—the abnormal lung sounds that can be heard with a stethoscope; are produced by rubbing together of roughened pleural surfaces; are similar to crackles but more superficial.

Stridor – the abnormal high pitched (harsh) sound occurring during inspiration that can be heard without a stethoscope. It is a sign of upper airway obstruction indicating a life-threatening condition (such as epiglottitis). When not hearing stridor in patients having difficulty breathing, it should never be interpreted as an unobstructed upper airway.

Sputum Analysis

Table 5-10 Sputum Analysis

Sputum should be analyzed and documented for quantity, viscosity, color, odor, frequency, time of day, and ease of expectoration.

Types of sputum are: (1) fetid (foul smelling; signifies anaerobic infection; occurs with bronchiectasis, lung abscess, or cystic fibrosis)[4]; (2) mucoid (white or clear; present with chronic cough due to acute or chronic bronchitis and cystic fibrosis; not necessarily associated with bronchopulmonary infection); (3) frothy (white or white with a shade of pink; foamy; thin frothy sputum can be associated with pulmonary edema); (4) hemoptysis (blood or bloody sputum expectoration; can be a small amount or massive hemorrhage; present in a variety of pathologies); (5) purulent (pus; yellow or greenish sputum; sometimes thick and copious sputum; common in acute and chronic infection); (6) mucopurulent (mix of mucoid sputum and pus; yellow to green color; common in infection); (7) tenacious (thick and very sticky sputum); (8) rusty (rusty color sputum; common in pneumococcal pneumonia).

Cardiopulmonary Signs and Symptoms

Table 5-11 Cardiopulmonary Signs and Symptoms

Cyanosis—blue, gray, or dark purple discoloration of the skin, lips, nails, and tongue caused by deoxygenated or reduced hemoglobin in the blood; oximetry of the arterial blood saturation may be 85% or less. Cyanosis of the mucous membrane such as the mouth indicates hypoxemia and respiratory failure. Cyanosis of retinae indicates congenital heart disease or cardiac failure. Peripheral cyanosis of the digits (of fingers and toes) indicates chronic hypoxia; it may indicate respiratory obstruction, reduced pulmonary function, or inadequate ventilation. For African-American patients (clients), cyanosis can be seen by close inspection of lips, tongue, conjunctiva (of the eyelids), palms of the hands, and the soles of the feet. One method of testing is pressing the palms. Slow blood return indicates cyanosis. Another sign is ashen gray lips and tongue.

Clubbing—enlarged terminal phalanx of the finger; excessive growth of the soft tissues of the ends of the fingers (giving a beak appearance from the side and a sausage appearance from above). Clubbing indicates chronic obstructive pulmonary disease (COPD), lung fibrosis, lung carcinoma, and other pulmonary illnesses.

Diaphoresis—profuse sweating and cold clammy skin. Diaphoresis indicates inadequate cardiovascular response or excessive effort.

Pulse palpation: (1) normal or regular pulse—a pulse when the force and frequency are the same; it is documented as 3+; (2) bounding pulse—an abnormal pulse that reaches a high intensity and then disappears quickly; it is also called a collapsing pulse; it is documented as 4+; (3) thready pulse—an abnormal pulse characterized as fine, scarcely perceptible; it is documented 1+; (4) weak or slow pulse—an abnormal pulse characterized by a rate of less than 60 beats per minute; it is documented 2+.

Pitting edema—edema of the extremities characterized by maintenance of the skin depression after moderate pressure was applied; bilaterally it may indicate congestive heart failure (CHF).

Electrocardiogram (EKG or ECG)

Table 5-12   Electrocardiogram (EKG or ECG)

Electrocardiogram (EKG or ECG): records the electrical activity of the heart; determines different waves patterns in cardiac rhythm; evaluates the abnormal heart rhythms. EKG is used with the exercise tolerance test (ETT), also called the graded exercise test, to record patient's/client's electrical activity of the heart during graded increases in the rate of exercise.

See Figure 5-1.

Table 5-13   Electrocardiogram (EKG) Waves

P wave[4]: first wave caused by atrial depolarization; a normal P wave is upright, rounded, and 1 to 3 mm tall. Abnormally shaped P waves can be: flutter (F) waves; fibrillation (f) waves (small with irregular deflections on the baseline); premature (P) waves (have a different PR interval in a rhythm group and look different than regular P waves).

QRS complex[4]: ventricular depolarization. Irregularities in the ventricular conduction can be flutter and fibrillation (develop with ventricular tachycardia). Premature ventricular contractions (PVCs) are wide, bizarre QRS complexes.

ST segment: beginning of ventricular repolarization; can identify ischemia, injury or infarction. Abnormal ST segment can be: depressed ST segment that means ischemia or a nontransmural myocardial injury (part of the tissue of a portion of the cardiac wall is injured); elevated ST segment that means transmural myocardial injury (such as an infarction, in which the tissue in the entire thickness of a portion of the cardiac wall dies).

T wave: completion of ventricular repolarization.

Regular sinus rhythm: each QRS complex is preceded by a P wave; QRS complexes are equally spaced.

Cardiac Cycle

Table 5-14   Cardiac Cycle

Atrial systole: contraction of the heart muscles (myocardium) involving the right and left atria (that contract at the same time). There is an electrical systole (that stimulates the myocardium of the chambers of the heart to contract), and mechanical

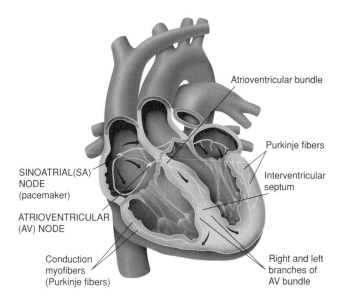

CARDIOPULMONARY
INTERVENTIONS

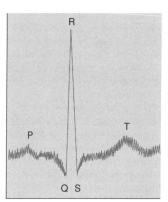

Figure 5-1   Conduction system of the heart and normal EKG. From Anatomy and
              Physiology: Understanding the Human Body by Robert K. Clark, page
              296, Figure 16.9 "The impulse generation and conduction system of
              your heart."

Table 5-14   (continued)

systole (that is contraction of the heart). As the atria contract, the blood pressure
in each atrium increases forcing additional blood into the ventricles. The additional flow of blood is called the atrial kick. If normal electrical conduction of the
heart is absent (such as in atrial fibrillation, atrial flutter, or complete heart block),
the atrial kick is absent. Electrical systole of the atria begins with the onset of the
P wave on the EKG.

Ventricular systole: contraction of the myocardium involving the right and left ventricles. At the beginning of ventricular systole, both, bicuspid (mitral) and tricuspid
valves (known together as the atrioventricular valves) close. When these valves
close the S_1 takes place. At the end of the ventricular systole, the aortic and pulmonic valves close. When these valves close the S_2 takes place. As the left ventricle empties, its pressure falls below the pressure in the aorta, and the aortic valve
closes. Also, as the pressure in the right ventricle falls below the pressure in the
pulmonary artery, the pulmonic valve closes. Ventricular systole occurs between
S_1 and S_2. In an EKG, the electrical systole of the ventricles begins at the beginning of the QRS complex.

Cardiac diastole (complete cardiac diastole): period of time when the heart relaxes
after the contraction (in preparation for refilling with blood). Diastole is the filling
stage of the heart. It has two phases: the ventricular diastole (when the ventricles
are relaxing), and atrial diastole (when the atria are relaxing). During ventricular
diastole, the pressure in the ventricles (right and left) drops (from the peak that it
reached in the systole). When the pressure drops in the left ventricle (below the
pressure in the left atrium), the bicuspid (mitral) valve opens, and the left ventricle
fills with blood (that was accumulating in the left atrium). Also, when the pressure
drops in the right ventricle (below the pressure in the right atrium), the tricuspid
valve opens, and the right ventricle fills with blood (that was accumulating in the
right atrium). Diastole occurs between S_2 and S_1.

During the cardiac cycle, the rhythmic sequence of contractions is coordinated by
the sinoatrial (SA) and atrioventricular (AV) nodes. SA node is also called the cardiac pacemaker of the heart (and is located in the upper wall of the right atrium).
SA node is responsible for the electrical stimulation (action potential) that initiates
atrial contraction. Then, the electrical wave reaches the AV node (situated in the
lower right atrium) and through the Bundles of His and Purkinje fibers leads to
contraction of the ventricles.

Cardiac Terminology and Normatives

Table 5-15 Cardiac Terminology and Normatives

Cardiac output (CO): amount of blood/minute that leaves the right or left ventricles; it is expressed in L/min. CO normative = 4–6 L/min; it is influenced by the heart rate and the stroke volume; it is calculated by multiplying the stroke volume by the heart rate.

Stroke volume (SV): amount of blood that is ejected by the left ventricle with each heartbeat (myocardial contraction). SV is influenced by contractility (ability of ventricle to contract), preload (amount of blood in the ventricle at the end of diastole), and the afterload (the left ventricle force to overcome aortic pressure and open the aortic valve during systole). SV is also influenced by the patient's age and gender, and the amount of exercise performed by the patient. SV average normative = 60–80 ml.

Ejection fraction (EF): percentage of blood emptied from the ventricle during systole. EF of the left ventricle averages (in healthy hearts) = 60% to 70%. After myocardial infarction EF can be reduced. EF is used as an index of contractility.

Cardiac index (CI): it is similar and more accurate than CO; takes into consideration the relationship between CO and the body surface area (BSA); it can be expressed as CI = CO/BSA.CI normative (average adult at rest) = 3.0 L/min/m^2

Pulmonary Terminology and Normatives

Table 5-16 Pulmonary Terminology and Normatives[3]

Ventilation: movement of air into and out of the lungs; physiologically, it is the amount of air inhaled per day; can be estimated by spirometry

Tidal volume (TV): volume of air inhaled (inspired) and exhaled (expired) in a normal, quiet breath; can be 500 ml for a child and an adult; can be 20 ml for an infant

Inspiratory reserve volume (IRV): maximal amount of air that can be forcefully inhaled after a normal inspiration

Expiratory reserve volume (ERV): maximal amount of air that can be forcefully expelled from the lungs after a normal expiration

Residual volume (RV): volume of air remaining in the lungs after a maximal, full expiration; RV is necessary for continuous gas exchange

Inspiratory capacity (IC): volume of air that can be inspired after a resting exhalation (expiration); calculated as the formula: IC = IRV + TV

continues

Table 5-16 (continued)

Vital capacity (VC): volume of air that can be exhaled from the lungs after a maximal inspiration; calculated as the formula: VC = IRV + TV + ERV. VC is important to evaluate the ability of the lung to exchange O_2 and CO_2; normal VC is more than 80% of predicted; mild VC is between 66% and 80% of predicted; moderate VC is between 50% and 65% of predicted; severe VC is less than 50% of predicted

Functional residual capacity (FRC): amount of air remaining in the lungs after a normal expiration (exhalation); calculated as the formula: FRC = ERV + RV

Total lung capacity (TLC): volume of air in the lungs after a maximal inspiration (inhalation); calculated as the formula: TLC = IRV + TV + ERV + RV; normal TLC is more than 80% of predicted; mild TLC is between 66% and 80% of predicted; moderate TLC is between 50% and 65% of predicted; severe TLC is less than 50% of predicted

Forced expiratory volume (FEV): amount of air expired after a full inspiration (inhalation); when testing FEV, the expiration is performed quickly as possible and the volume is measured at 0.5 second, at 1 second, at 2 seconds, and at 3 seconds; normal FEV is more than 80% of predicted; mild FEV is between 66% and 80% of predicted; moderate FEV is between 50% and 65% of predicted; severe FEV is less than 50% of predicted

Respiration: act of breathing (inhaling and exhaling); diffusion of gas across the alveolar and capillary membranes; normal respiratory exchange of oxygen and carbon dioxide in the lungs

Arterial oxygenation: ability of arterial blood to carry oxygen; normal adult and child arterial blood oxygen saturation is between 95% and 98%

Alveolar ventilation: ability to remove carbon dioxide from the pulmonary circulation and maintain the normal potential of hydrogen = pH (measures the concentration of free floating hydrogen ions within the body; it is a solution that is not acid or alkaline; normal body's blood plasma pH is between 7.35 and 7.45)

Contraindications to Exercise Tolerance Tests

Table 5-17   Contraindications to Exercise Tolerance Test (ETT)

Absolute Contraindications to ETT	Relative Contraindications to ETT
Recent complicated MI; any acute cardiac event or injury	More than 200 mmHg resting systolic BP or more than 115 mmHg resting diastolic BP
Unstable angina; uncontrolled ventricular arrhythmia	Electrolyte imbalances (such as hypokalemia or hypomagnesemia)
Uncontrolled atrial arrhythmia; third-degree AV heart block (without pacemaker)	Frequent and complex ventricular ectopy; ventricular aneurysm
Aortic aneurysm (known or suspected); myocarditis (or pericarditis)	Uncontrolled diabetes or other metabolic disease
Thrombophlebitis; pulmonary embolus	Moderate valvular disease
Acute infections; psychosis	Neuromuscular, musculoskeletal, or rheumatoid disorders that can be exacerbated by exercise
Acute CHF; severe aortic stenosis	Advanced or complicated pregnancy

Termination Criteria to Exercise Tolerance Test

Table 5-18   ETT Termination Criteria

Fall in arterial blood gas for oxygen (PaO_2) of more than 20 mmHg or PaO_2 being less than 55 mmHg

Rise in arterial blood gas for oxygen (PaO_2) of more than 10 mmHg or an increase in PaO_2 more than 65 mmHg

Maximal shortness of breath (dyspnea); symptoms of fatigue; total fatigue

Cardiac ischemia or cardiac arrhythmia

Increase in diastolic BP of more than 20 mmHg; increase in systolic BP of more than 250 mmHg; decrease in BP with increased exercises

Leg pain; pallor; cold sweat (diaphoresis); ataxia; signs of insufficient cardiac output

Patient/client delayed (several hours) responses to ETT: insomnia; prolonged fatigue; sudden weight gain caused by fluid retention

Medical Cardiac Tests and Procedures: Left Heart Cardiac Catheterization, Echocardiogram, Coronary Artery Bypass Graft Surgery, Percutaneous Transluminal Coronary Angioplasty

Table 5-19   Medical Cardiac Tests and Procedures

Left heart cardiac catheterization: percutaneous intravascular insertion of a catheter into any chamber of the heart or great vessels for diagnosis, assessment of abnormalities, interventions, and evaluation of the effects of pathology on the heart and great vessels. During left heart cardiac catheterization, the following diagnostic cardiac tests can be performed: assessment of coronary artery anatomy and its normality, estimation of the cardiac ejection fraction (of left ventricle function), assessment of the cardiac valves, measurements of the intracardiac pressures, and biopsies of the endocardium. In regard to estimation of the cardiac ejection fraction, the normal fraction is 60% to 70% of the volume of blood left in the left ventricle at the end of the diastole that has been ejected into the aorta during the systole. A lower cardiac ejection fraction indicates an impaired left ventricle. During cardiac catheterization, the patient may also receive a coronary angiogram to record the size, shape, and location of the heart and blood vessels. The angiogram can be of the aorta (to diagnose aneurysm or tumors) and/or of the heart (to determine the size and shape of the chambers and the valves).

Echocardiogram: noninvasive procedure using ultrasound waves to evaluate cardiac structures (such as the heart's valves, chambers, walls, and abnormal intracardiac masses or blood clots). Echocardiogram: (1) can be dobutamine stress echocardiogram (dobutamine is given to patient to increase the heart's workload and evaluate the adequacy of blood flow; (2) can diagnose prior myocardial infarction); (3) can be multidimensional visualization echocardiogram (using computer technology to visualize three-dimensional cardiac structures); (4) can be stress echocardiogram (identifies segments of the heart when the patient is performing a treadmill test or is taking a vasodilator medication); (5) can be transesophageal echocardiogram (invasive echocardiogram into the esophagus; detects cardiac sources of emboli, valves' malfunctions, endocarditis, or congenital heart disease).

Coronary Artery Bypass Graft Surgery (CABG): surgical procedure to treat severe coronary artery disease by using a shunt (or a graft from a donor artery or vein) to install an alternate route for the blood flow and to bypass an obstruction (blockage) in one or more of the coronary arteries. The graft can be taken from the radial artery of the nondominant hand or from the saphenous vein. In the CABG surgery, the graft is attached and sutured above (into the aorta) and below into the obstructed artery (beyond the occlusion) so that blood flows around it and to the area of the heart below the obstruction. The graft improves the blood flow and the heart's function, relieves angina pectoris symptoms, and prevents a myocardial infarction. CABG surgery techniques are continually improving with less sternal cutting involved or no sternal cutting at all. After CABG surgery, typically, the patient will be postoperatively monitored in the intensive care coronary unit (ICCU) with breathing/suctioning tube (and ventilator), vascular catheters (including pulmonary artery pressure monitor, arterial catheter for BP monitoring, and IV tubes), heart monitor, chest drainage tubes, bladder catheter, and nasogastric tube.

Percutaneous Transluminal Coronary Angioplasty (PTCA): also called balloon angioplasty or angioplasty. PTCA is a nonsurgical method of treating localized coronary artery narrowing. During PTCA, under x-ray guidance, a special double lumen catheter with a deflated balloon on the tip is inserted transcutaneously in an artery (in the femoral or radial artery). X-ray guides the catheter up into the involved (narrowed by plaque) coronary artery of the heart. Then the balloon is inflated and deflated several times to open the narrow artery by compressing the plaque deposits against the wall of the artery. In some cases during a PTCA, stents are placed permanently inside the opened artery to hold it open. Stents are made of tiny mesh-like tubes of stainless steel that are inserted in the involved artery (that was just opened) using the catheter with a deflated balloon on the tip. The balloon is inflated, expanding the stent and pressing it against the artery wall. The stent is coated with a special medication to prevent endothelial cell proliferation (as a result of endothelial cell trauma and having a foreign object placed into the artery). At the end of the PTCA, the balloon is deflated and the catheter and balloon removed. The stent remains permanently expanded and in place to help keep the narrowed portion of the artery open.

Artificial cardiac pacemaker: device used to trigger mechanical contractions of the heart by emitting periodic electrical discharges. Pacemakers are used for bradycardia, A-V conduction block (may be post MI), other types of A-V block (bifascicular or trifascicular second degree), recurrent syncope (due to carotid sinus abnormalities), sinus node dysfunction, certain arrhythmias, and certain types of CHF (class III CHF).

Automatic Implantable Cardioverter Defibrillator (AICD): surgically implanted defibrillator for patients at high risk for sudden cardiac arrhythmia (that can be life threatening).

Impairments of
Cardiopulmonary Conditions

Coronary Artery Disease Impairments

Table 5-20   CAD Impairments

CAD: narrowing of the coronary arteries due to atherosclerosis; it is more common in men than women. In the CAD, blockages within the coronary arteries limit the flow of oxygenated blood to the myocardium causing infarction or ischemia of the heart muscle.

Angina pectoris (classic CAD symptom) impairment: pain, burning, or pressure in the chest. Chest pain or discomfort is caused by ischemia that is a temporary condition (secondary to an imbalance of myocardial oxygen supply and demand). Angina can start with exertion, emotion, exposure to cold air, or eating of a large meal. Angina can also be precipitated by exertion and can progress to a full myocardial infarction (MI) if symptoms are not treated. Levels of angina: light pain (1+) to most severe (4+); on a 1 to 10 pain scale, patients may rate the pain as 10. Classical presentation of angina includes the Levine sign, when the patient is clenching his or her fist over the sternum; however, angina symptoms can also present with radiating pain down the left arm, pain going up into the chin or the jaw, and pain between the shoulder blades. Angina can be confirmed by a 12-lead EKG showing ischemia with an ST depressed segment and an inverted (flipped) T wave.

Angina is classified in stable angina and unstable angina. Stable angina has less intensity (pain 5/10 that improves to 0/10 with rest and administration of oxygen and nitroglycerin). Unstable angina (also called preinfarction angina) does not improve (as the stable angina) and requires immediate (emergency) medical intervention. In general, any angina symptoms require medical interventions.

Other CAD impairments: (1) cough, (2) dyspnea, (3) orthopnea (labored breathing while lying flat; is relieved by sitting up; is the classic symptom of left ventricular heart failure), (4) weakness, (5) weight gain and venous stasis (due to peripheral edema), (6) anorexia, (7) nausea, (8) increased pulmonary arterial pressure, (9) hypertension, (10) sweating, (11) lightheadedness, (12) possible hypotension (depending on the cardiac disease).

Myocardial infarction (loss of living heart muscle as a result of coronary occlusion) occurs when the atherosclerotic plaque in a coronary artery ruptures, forming a thrombus that obstructs the injured blood vessel. Most MIs heal initially without incident, but complications can occur. EKG identifies MI with a (pathologic) Q wave (that is the transmural MI with full thickness of the ventricular wall) or a non-Q wave (that is the nontransmural MI involving the endocardium). Newer MI classification indicates that a non-Q wave EKG (absent Q wave) may also be a transmural MI.

continues

Table 5-20   (continued)

Typically, after an hour from the transmural MI, the EKG will show ST elevated. After a few hours from the transmural MI, the EKG will show a pathologic Q wave. A nontransmural MI will show on the EKG an ST depression (without a Q wave).

Congestive Heart Failure Impairments

Table 5-21   CHF Impairments

CHF is a result of CAD. CHF is the inability of the heart to circulate blood effectively to meet the body's metabolic demands; can affect left ventricle, right ventricle, or both.

CHF impairments: (1) dyspnea, (2) orthopnea, (3) dyspnea with exertion, (4) muscular fatigue, (5) tachycardia, (6) cyanosis, (7) productive cough, (8) pulmonary edema (increased hydrostatic pressure in the pulmonary veins and interstitial space of the lung), (9) peripheral edema (with bilateral pitting edema), (10) fluid weight gain, (11) presence of an abnormal S_3 heart sound, (12) renal dysfunction, (13) heart murmurs (from mitral regurgitation of enlarged left ventricle), (14) obstructive sleep apnea.

Chronic Obstructive Pulmonary Diseases (COPDs) Impairments

Table 5-22   COPDs Impairments

COPDs: most common chronic respiratory disorders affecting normal expiratory volumes; cause narrowing obstruction or destruction of the bronchi/bronchioles and alveolar (bronchial) tissue. The main COPD is emphysema (characterized by airflow limitation that is not fully reversible). COPD causes: tobacco smoking (most common); exposure to environmental dust, smoke, or particular pollution; deficiency of α1 antitrypsin (inadequate protection against destructive enzyme activity in the lungs).

Classification of COPD: 0 = at risk for COPD (may have chronic impairments such as cough and sputum production); I = mild COPD (FEV in 1 second is equal or more than 80% of the predicted; may have or not have chronic impairments such as cough and sputum production); II = moderate COPD (FEV in 1 second is less than 80% of the predicted; may have or not have chronic impairments such as cough and sputum production); III = severe COPD (FEV in 1 second is less than 50% of the predicted; may have or not have chronic impairments such as cough and sputum production); IV = very severe COPD (FEV in 1 second is less than 30% of the predicted; has chronic respiratory failure).

Emphysema impairments: (1) chronic cough, (2) expectoration (of pink thin sputum), (3) exertional dyspnea, (4) enlarged thorax (due to loss of elastic recoil of the lungs), (5) increase in the anterior–posterior diameter of the chest, (6) dorsal kyphosis, (7) barrel chest appearance, (8) distant breath and heart sounds, (9) expiratory wheezing, (10) crackles, (11) mild to moderate weight loss, (12) decreased exercise tolerance, (13) repeated respiratory infections. In advanced stages, there is (14) hypertrophy of accessory muscles, (15) cyanosis, (16) digital clubbing, and (17) breathing using only pursed-lip breathing.

Other specific pulmonary impairments of emphysema are: (1) decreased vital capacity, (2) increased residual volume and functional residual capacity, (3) decreased FEV, (4) hypoxemia (decreased oxygen concentration in the arterial blood—PaO_2), (5) hypercapnia (increased in partial pressure of carbon dioxide in the blood—$PaCO_2$—to levels of 45 or 50 mmHg).

Asthma: is a type of COPD characterized by increased sensitivity to irritants such as cold air, chemicals, exercise, infection, or stress; manifests as spasms in the bronchi resulting in narrowing of the airways producing mucus and secretions in bronchial area. Asthma impairments are: (1) cough, (2) dyspnea, (3) wheezing during expiration, (4) crackles, (5) anxiety, (6) tachycardia, (7) tachypnea, (8) cyanosis, and (9) increased use of accessory muscles.

Chronic bronchitis is a type of COPD characterized by chronic cough and sputum production mostly from cigarette smoking. Chronic bronchitis impairments are: (1) crackles, (2) wheezing, (3) increased respiratory infections, (4) hypoxemia, (5) variable $PaCO_2$ to levels, (6) edema from right sided heart failure, and (7) decreased expiratory rates.

Cystic fibrosis is a type of COPD. It is also a genetic pulmonary disease transmitted by an autosomal recessive trait and a malfunction of the exocrine glands resulting in increased secretions in the lung. Cystic fibrosis affects other organs. Cystic fibrosis impairments are: (1) thick secretions (lead to obstructions), (2) frequent respiratory infections, (3) weight loss (despite caloric intake), (4) skin tastes salty, (5) chronic cough, (6) viscous secretions, (7) cyanosis, (8) dyspnea, (9) tachypnea, (10) decreased expiratory flow (decreased forced expiratory volume in 1 second), (11) increased residual volume, (12) hyperinflation of lungs, (13) poor endurance, (14) gastrointestinal dysfunction (or diabetes).

Bronchiectasis is a type of COPD characterized by chronic dilation of a bronchus or bronchi caused by the damaging effects of a long standing infection usually in

continues

Impairments of Cardiopulmonary Conditions **367**

Table 5-22   (continued)

patient's childhood. Bronchiectasis impairments are: (1) dyspnea, (2) copious thick secretions, (3) productive cough, (4) crackles, (5) digital clubbing, (6) hemoptysis (expectoration of blood), (7) recurrent secondary infections, and (8) decreased breath sounds.

Chronic Restrictive Lung Diseases Impairments

Table 5-23   CRLDs Impairments

CRLDs: grouping of disorders with different etiologies resulting in difficulty expanding the lungs and reduced lung volume. Causes: pleural disease, trauma, surgery, infections, radiation therapy, inorganic dust, oxygen toxicity, asbestos exposure, inhalation of noxious gases, pulmonary edema (effusion of serous fluid into the alveoli and interstitial tissue of the lungs), pulmonary embolism, pulmonary fibrosis, hyaline membrane disease, normal aging. Types of CRLDs: (1) idiopathic pulmonary fibrosis (the most common CRLD characterized by formation of scar tissue in the parenchyma of the lungs following inflammation of the alveoli), (2) asbestosis (results from inhalation of asbestos particles), (3) oxygen toxicity, (4) radiation pneumonitis.

CRLDs general impairments: (1) dyspnea, (2) nonproductive cough, (3) early fatigue, (4) rapid shallow breathing, (5) limited chest expansion, (6) decreased ability to take a deep breath, (7) use of accessory muscles for ventilation, (8) cyanosis, (9) crackles, (10) weight loss, (11) postural deviations (kyphosis) for breathing difficulties, (12) decreased chest mobility, (13) hypoxemia, (14) hypocapnia, and (15) reductions in vital capacity (VC), forced residual capacity (FRC), and total lung capacity (TLC). Hypercapnia is the terminal stage of the idiopathic pulmonary fibrosis.

CRLDs can also be caused by alterations in the neuromuscular apparatus characterized by decreased muscular strength and inability to expand the rib cage. It may occur with multiple sclerosis (MS), muscular dystrophy (MD), Parkinson's disease (PD), spinal cord injury (SCI), or cerebral vascular accident (CVA). CRLDs impairments with the above conditions are: (1) dyspnea; (2) hypoxemia; (3) crackles; (4) digital clubbing; (5) cyanosis; (6) decreased breath sounds; (7) reduced cough effectiveness; (8) reduced lung volumes; (9) atelectasis (collapsed lungs). CRLDs can also be caused by pulmonary restrictions as a result of pulmonary or cardiac surgery (secondary to lung abscesses, lung abnormalities, tuberculosis, tumors, CAD, arrhythmias, aneurysm, congenital heart abnormalities, or cardiac valve disorders).

In addition, CRLDs can be caused by trauma to the chest area resulting in rib fractures and puncture of the lungs (causing pneumothorax—air in the pleural space, hemothorax—blood in the pleural space or lung contusions). Impairments: shallow breathing, pain with deep inspiration or cough, crepitation, dyspnea, absent or decreased breath sounds, cyanosis, cough with hemoptysis.

Patient Safety During Cardiopulmonary Interventions

Basic Cardiac Life Support for Adults

Table 5-24   CPR Performed by One Rescuer[5]

* The rescuer is a professional (PT, PTA, Nurse, MD, EMT, etc.)

Assessment: Determine unresponsiveness (tap or gently shake patient or client and shout). If unresponsive, activate the EMS system.

Airway: Position patient (or client) and open the airway by the head tilt-chin lift or jaw-thrust maneuver.

Breathing: Assess breathing to identify absent or inadequate breathing.

• If patient is unresponsive with normal breathing and spinal injury is not suspected, place patient (client) in a recovery position, maintaining an open airway. If an adult patient (client) is unresponsive and not breathing, provide two initial breaths.

• If you are unable to give initial breaths, reposition the head and reattempt ventilation. If you are still unsuccessful in making the chest rise with each ventilation after an attempt and reattempt, follow the unresponsive foreign body airway occlusion (FBAO) sequence.

• Be sure that the patient's (client's) chest rises with each rescue breath you provide. After you deliver the effective breaths, assess for signs of circulation.

Circulation: Check for signs of circulation; look for normal breathing, coughing, or movement and feel for a carotid pulse (take no more than 10 seconds to do this). If there are no signs of circulation, begin chest compressions: 15 chest compressions at rate of approximately 100 per minute, depressing chest 1.5 to 2.0 in (4 to 5 cm) with each. Then open the airway and deliver two breaths; begin 15 more compressions at 100 per minute.

Reassessment: After four complete cycles of 15 compressions and two ventilations, re-evaluate patient (client), checking for signs of circulation. If there are no signs of circulation, resume CPR, beginning with chest compressions.

• If signs of circulation are present, check for breathing. If breathing is present, place patient (client) in a recovery position and monitor breathing and circulation. If breathing is absent but signs of circulation are present, provide rescue breathing at 10 to 12 times per minute and monitor for signs of circulation every few minutes.

• If there are no signs of circulation, continue compressions and ventilations at a ratio of 15:2. Stop and check for signs of circulation and spontaneous breathing every few minutes. Do not interrupt CPR except in special circumstances.

CARDIOPULMONARY INTERVENTIONS

Table 5-25 CPR Performed by Two Rescuers[5]

*Having two professional rescuers give CPR is less fatiguing; the performance may be extended over longer time periods.

In two-rescuer CPR, one person is positioned at the patient's (client's) side and performs chest compressions while the other remains at the patient's (client's) head, maintains an open airway, monitors the carotid pulse, and provides rescue breathing. Compression rate is 100 per minute. The compression–ventilation ratio is 15:2 with a pause for ventilation of 2 seconds after each compression until airway is secured.

To determine whether victim has resumed spontaneous breathing and circulation, chest compressions must be stopped for 10 seconds at approximately the end of the first minute of CPR and every few minutes thereafter.

Warning: Prolonged CPR is frequently associated with increases of serum PSA; therefore, PSA cannot be used for diagnosis of adenocarcinoma of prostate during the first weeks after CPR.

Table 5-26 Foreign Body Airway Occlusion (FBAO)[5] Sequence

Finger sweep and tongue-jaw lift should be used only in unresponsive/unconscious patient (client) with complete FBAO sequence. Finger sweep and tongue-jaw lift: with patient (client) face up, open patient's (client's) mouth by grasping both the tongue and lower jaw between the thumb and fingers and lifting the mandible (tongue-jaw lift). This maneuver alone may be sufficient to relieve an obstruction. Insert index finger of other hand deeply into patient's (client's) throat to base of tongue. Use a hooking action to dislodge the foreign body and maneuver it into the mouth. It is sometimes necessary to use the index finger to push the foreign body against the opposite side of the throat to dislodge and remove it.

Table 5-27 Heimlich Maneuver (for Removal of a Foreign Body Blocking the Air Passage)[4]

Maneuver for victim who is standing: Clasped hands placed just below middle of rib cage. The rescuer forms a fist with one hand and places it below the sternum. The rescuer then grasps the wrist of the hand forming the fist. The hands are then rapidly brought inward and upward.

Maneuver for victim who is supine: Hands placed just below rib cage at distal end of sternum. As in the standing position, the rescuer then grasps the wrist of the hand forming the fist. The hands are then rapidly brought distal to proximal.

Effects of Medications in Cardiac Rehab

Table 5-28   Effects of Medications in Cardiac Rehab[3]

Angiotensin-Converting Enzyme (ACE) inhibitors: group of drugs that treat HTN, CHF, and other diseases; suppress the rennin–angiotensin–aldosterone system. Examples of ACE inhibitors are Captopril, Lotensin, Prinivil, Zestril, Minoxidil, and Univasc. ACE inhibitors: (1) have no effect on HR; (2) decrease BP at rest and with exercise; (3) have no effect in exercise capacity; (4) increases or have no effect in exercise capacity in patients with CHF.

Beta blockers: group of drugs that treat angina pectoris, HTN, dysrhythmias; stimulate SNS; contain epinephrine and norepinephrine. Examples are Acebutolol, Atenolol, Metoprolol, Propranolol, Nadolol, Penbutolol, Timolol. Beta blockers: (1) decrease HR and BP at rest and with exercise; (2) increase exercise capacity in patients with angina; (3) decrease exercise capacity or have no effect in exercise capacity in patients without angina.

Calcium channel blockers: group of drugs that treat angina pectoris, HTN, vascular spasm, CHF, supraventricular tachycardia, intracranial bleeding; slow the influx of calcium into smooth muscles and decrease arterial resistance and oxygen demand. Examples are Felodipine, Nicardipine, Diltiazem, Verapamil. Some calcium channel blockers such as Felodipine or Nicardipine: increase HR at rest and with exercise. Other calcium channel blockers such as Diltiazem or Verapamil: decrease HR at rest and with exercise. All calcium channel blockers: (1) decrease BP at rest and with exercises; (2) increase exercise capacity in patients with angina; (3) have no effect in exercise capacity in patients without angina.

Digitalis: drug that treats CHF, atrial fibrillations, atrial flutter, supraventricular tachycardia. Digitalis is an antiarrhythmic and cardiotonic drug; increases the force of myocardial contraction and affects the AV and SA nodes. Examples of digitalis are Digoxin or Lanoxin. Digitalis: (1) decreases HR in patients with CHF and atrial fibrillations; (2) has no effect on BP; (3) increases exercise capacity in patients with CHF and atrial fibrillations.

Diuretics: group of drugs that treat HTN, CHF, edema; increase urine secretion. Examples are Furosemide, Isosorbide, Bendroflumethiazide, Metolazone. Diuretics: (1) have no effect on HR; (2) have no effect on BP at rest or with exercise; (3) have no effect on exercise capacity except for patients with CHF.

Nicotine: drug used as an aide to stop smoking (in conjunction with a smoking cessation program). Examples are Nicorette Gum or Habitrol. Nicotine: (1) increases HR and BP at rest and with exercise; (2) has no effect on exercise capacity; (3) decreases exercise capacity (or has no effect) in patients with angina.

continues

Patient Safety During Cardiopulmonary Interventions   **373**

Table 5-28 (continued)

Nitrates: group of drugs that treat angina pectoris, HTN, CHF; they are arteriovenous dilators. Examples are Amyl Nitrate, Isotrate, Novo Sorbide, Sorbitrate, Isordil. Nitroglycerin (NTG) is also a type of nitrate used as an arterial and venous dilator. NTG treats angina pectoris, CHF, and acute pulmonary edema. NTG is available as intravenous infusion in critical care, as ointment (applied to the chest), as transdermal patches, and as oral drug (either tablet dissolving under tongue or a spray of the mouth). NTG is contraindicated for men using Sildenafil for erectile dysfunction (can cause a fatal heart attack). Nitrates: (1) increase HR at rest; (2) increases HR or have no effect with exercise; (3) decrease BP at rest; (4) decrease BP or have no effect with exercise; (5) increases exercise capacity in patients with angina; (6) have no effects in exercise capacity in patients without angina or patients with CHF.

Vasodilators (non-nitrates): group of drugs that treat mostly severe to moderate HTN and CHF; dilate blood vessels by relaxing smooth muscles; depress heart conduction and irritability. Examples are Hydralazine; Minoxidil, Nifedipine. Vasodilators: (1) increase HR or have no effect at rest or with exercise; (2) decrease BP at rest or with exercise; (3) have no effect on exercise capacity; (4) increase or have no effect on exercise capacity with CHF.

Common Bronchodilators Used in Pulmonary Rehab

Table 5-29   Common Bronchodilators and Their Side Effects[3]

β_2 agonists (such as Albuterol, Terbutaline, or Isoproterenol) are taken orally or by inhalation; are used for intermittent attacks of wheezing and exercises induced asthma. Side effects are palpitations, tachycardia, and nervousness.

Methylxanthines (such as Theophylline or Dyphylline) are taken orally or intravenously; are used for asthma and COPD. Side effects are palpitations, tachycardia, vomiting, nausea, and seizures.

Anticholinergics (such as Ipratropium bromide) are taken by inhalation; are used for COPD, and acute asthma (are combined with β_2 agonist medication). Side effects are dry mouth, nausea, and cough.

Signs/Symptoms to Discontinue Cardiac Interventions

Table 5-30   Signs/Symptoms to Discontinue Cardiac Interventions[1]

Temperature of more than 100°F
Systolic BP of more than 240 mmHg
Diastolic BP of more than 110 mmHg
Fall in systolic BP of more than 20 mmHg.
Rise in heart rate (HR) of more than 20 bpm
Resting HR of more than 130 bpm and/or less than 40 bpm
Chest pain, palpitations, and/or irregular pulse
Oxygen saturation of less than 90%
Blood glucose of more than 250 mg/dL
Cyanotic and/or diaphoretic
Dizziness and/or syncope
Bilateral leg/foot edema

Signs and Symptoms to Change or Discontinue Interventions in Pulmonary Rehab

Table 5-31   Signs and Symptoms to Change/Discontinue Interventions in Pulmonary Rehab

Increased cyanosis
Severe dyspnea
Decreased oxygen saturation levels
Moderate to severe blood streaked sputum
Severe fatigue
Severe pain
Deep vein thrombosis (DVT)
Pneumothorax
Pulmonary embolism
Severe pulmonary edema
Cardiac arrhythmia
Congestive heart failure
Severe hypertension
Severe pleural effusion

continues

CARDIOPULMONARY INTERVENTIONS

Table 5-31   (continued)

Intervention over an area of fracture or tumor

Unstable angina or recent myocardial infarction

Intervention involving direct pressure on the xiphoid process

Uncontrolled coughing

Forced expiration should not be used during pursed lip breathing

Avoid prolonged expiration and hyperventilation

PTA needs to immediately report to PT any change in patient's condition during interventions or any new contraindication and precaution to intervention. When any
patient's life-threatening condition occurs, the PTA needs to provide CPR, call
EMS, reposition the patient, and report to PT or nursing personnel.

Postural Drainage Possible Complications and Safety Interventions During Pulmonary Rehab

Table 5-32   PD Possible Complications and Safety Interventions

1. Hypoxemia—decreased oxygen concentration of the arterial blood. Safety interventions for hypoxemia: need to call the physical therapist and the nursing staff (if
   in hospital or SNF); need to call the physical therapist and EMS (for home health
   care); patient needs higher oxygen concentrations during procedure if potential
   for or observed hypoxemia exists. If patient becomes hypoxemic during treatment,
   patient needs to have administered 100% oxygen, stop pulmonary therapy immediately, return patient to original resting position, and consult physical therapist (and
   nursing staff/EMS—depending where the interventions were rendered). Ensure
   adequate ventilation until help arrives. Hypoxemia during postural drainage may
   be avoided in unilateral lung disease by placing the involved lung in the uppermost
   position with patient on his or her side.

2. Increased intracranial pressure—increased pressure of the cerebrospinal fluid in
   the head. Normal intracranial pressure is between 0 and 10 mmHg. Pressure
   higher than 20 mmHg can cause risk of compression or herniation of the brain or
   brain stem. Safety interventions for increased intracranial pressure: stop pulmonary therapy, return patient to original resting position, and consult physical
   therapist (or nursing staff/EMS—depending where the interventions were rendered).

3. Acute hypotension—decreased blood pressure below the normal. Safety interventions for acute hypotension: stop pulmonary therapy, return patient to original
   resting position, monitor patient, and consult physical therapist.

4. Pulmonary hemorrhage—hemorrhage from the lung, with bright red and frothy blood that is typically coughed up. Safety interventions for pulmonary hemorrhage: stop pulmonary therapy, return patient to original resting position, and call physical therapist, nursing staff/EMS—depending where the interventions were rendered. Administer oxygen and maintain an airway until nursing or EMS respond.

5. Pain or injury to muscles, ribs, or spine. Safety interventions for pain or injury: stop pulmonary therapy that appears directly associated with pain or injury, be careful in moving patient, and consult physical therapist.

6. Vomiting and aspiration (vomit material aspirated into the nose, throat, or lungs). Safety interventions for vomiting and aspiration: stop pulmonary therapy, administer oxygen, maintain airway, return patient to previous resting position, and contact physical therapist, and nursing staff/EMS immediately—depending where the interventions were rendered. Patient needs to have the airway cleaned using suctioning.

7. Bronchospasm—abnormal narrowing and partial obstruction of the lumen of the bronchi (caused by spasm of the peribronchial smooth muscle). Patient experiences coughing and wheezing. Safety interventions for bronchospasm: stop pulmonary therapy, return patient to previous resting position, administer or increase oxygen delivery while contacting physical therapist. The patient may need the physician-ordered bronchodilators.

8. Dysrhythmia—irregular heart rate (disordered or disrupt heart rhythm). Safety interventions for dysrhythmia: stop pulmonary therapy, return patient to previous resting position, administer or increase oxygen delivery while contacting physical therapist and nursing staff/EMS immediately—depending where the interventions were rendered.

Oxygen Safety

Table 5-33 Oxygen Safety in Home Health Pulmonary Rehab

Long-term home oxygen is available from three different delivery systems: electrically driven oxygen concentrators, liquid systems, and compressed gas. Inside the home, liquid and compressed gas systems use large tanks to store oxygen. Small, portable tanks of compressed oxygen also may be needed for brief periods (such as a few hours) outside the home. Each system has advantages and disadvantages. Oxygen is typically administered with continuous flow through a two-pronged nasal tube (cannula), even though this system is highly wasteful of

continues

Table 5-33   (continued)

oxygen (delivering only up to 40% oxygen concentrations). To improve efficiency and increase the patient's (client's) mobility, several devices, including reservoir cannulas, Ambu bags, demand-type systems, and transtracheal catheters (cannula placed directly into the trachea), can be used. Usually, a respiratory therapist or a physician instructs the patient about the proper oxygen use.

When the patient (client) is using oxygen therapy at home, it is important to stabilize the tank (possibly using a stand) and store it in an area that is out of the way so it will not fall. The tank should be closed tightly when not in use. Because oxygen can cause an explosion, it is also important to be careful to keep the tank away from any flammable source, such as matches, heaters, or hair dryers. No one in the house should smoke when oxygen is in use.

Cardiac Safety Rehab Guidelines After Medical Cardiac Procedures

Table 5-34   Safety Guidelines Post Medical Cardiac Procedures

Guidelines after Percutaneous Transluminal Coronary Angioplasty (PTCA): physical therapy interventions immediately after PTCA may consist of transfers, ambulation, and ADLs at comfortable low intensity. Aerobic training may start 2 to 3 weeks after PTCA (to allow a decrease in the inflammatory response). The exercise prescription for aerobic training should be based on the post-PTCA ETT (not pre-PTCA ETT).

Guidelines after Coronary Artery Bypass Graft (CABG) surgery: physical therapy interventions immediately after CABG surgery may consist of: (1) transfers and early ambulation; (2) upper extremity flexibility exercises (as per the surgeon's choice; some doctors limit upper extremity flexibility exercises in first 4 or 6 weeks postoperative); (3) postural training; (4) functional training; (5) pain management for areas of incision (using PNF UE diagonal patterns, and ROM exercises with 10 repetitions for one to two times per day); (6) patient education after CABG surgery to avoid lifting, pushing, and pulling objects until sternum is healed. After CABG surgery, patients may have postoperative fatigue and need to increase ambulation gradually. At 6 weeks after CABG surgery, cardiac rehab can begin with aerobic training after a maximal ETT.

Guidelines after Automatic Implantable Cardioverter Defibrillator (AICD) or pacemaker implant: physical therapy interventions need to check with the doctor when to start upper extremity aerobic exercises. Also, the PT/PTA should consider patient's heart rate settings and limit activities (such as functional training or ambulation) at the programmed heart rate. Interventions should avoid intensities that accidentally may activate the device. Initially, upper extremity aerobic exercises should be avoided not to accidentally dislodge the device. In addition, patients with AICD or pacemakers should receive education about keeping away from electromagnetic signals (such as antitheft devices) that may discharge or cause pacemakers to slow down or speed up.

Orthostatic Hypotension in Cardiopulmonary Rehab

Table 5-35   Orthostatic Hypotension[1]

Orthostatic hypotension occurs when a person assumes an upright position when getting up from bed (or chair). During orthostatic hypotension, the patient's blood pressure suddenly drops more than 20 mmHg when changing positions from lying to sitting or standing. At the same time, a patient with orthostatic hypotension may have a blood pressure of 100 mmHg (or less) in standing. During orthostatic hypotension, patient's symptoms are lightheadedness, dizziness, and loss of balance. Patients at risk for orthostatic hypotension are: patients who were in bed rest for long periods of time; patients who took vasodilators or antihypertensive medications; patients who became dehydrated; patients who have peripheral vascular disease (PVD) or muscular atrophy. Suggested interventions for orthostatic hypotension include: (1) using a slow, stepwise progression from supine to sit; (2) elevating the head of the bed gradually; (3) supporting patient's feet while patient is sitting at the edge of the bed; (4) patient education for deep breathing and ankle pumps while patient is sitting at edge of the bed; (5) using support stocking; (6) using a tilt table.

Types of Cardiopulmonary Interventions

Target Heart Rate

Table 5-36   Target Heart Rate (THR)

THR needs to be determined by PT. In cardiopulmonary rehab, THR can also be determined during an ETT (also called a graded exercise test).

During exercises, the patient must be monitored not to exceed the determined THR.

Formula for THR is: (1) First, calculate patient's maximal heart rate (HR_{max}). Patient's HR_{max} is calculated by subtracting patient's age from 220 (220 − patient's age). For example, for a patient who is 60 years old, the HR_{max} is 220 − 60 = 160. (2) Second, calculate the patient's THR. A patient having a cardiac pathology needs to exercise starting between 50% and 75% of the HR_{max}. As in the previous example, the THR for a patient who is 60 year old having cardiac disease would be 160 (50% − 75%) = 80 bpm − 120 bpm. This patient should start exercises that do not exceed a THR of 80 bpm (which is 50% of the HR_{max}). Then, the patient can start to gradually build up his or her exercise program to a THR of 120 bpm (which is 75% of the HR_{max}).

When using the THR formula, the therapist must take into consideration patient's medications (such as beta blockers that may decrease the HR_{max}).

Patient Education: Rating of Perceived Exertion

Table 5-37   Patient Education About the RPE Scales

Physical activity for patients who have cardiopulmonary dysfunctions needs to be monitored carefully. A rapid assessment done by the patient (client) himself is very important especially for patients (clients) who experience dyspnea. The assessments tools that are commonly used to teach the patient (client) to monitor physical activity intensity are: (1) Borg Rating of Perceived Exertion (RPE) scale[6] (a 15-point scale that starts at 6 as "very light" and ends up at 20 with 19 being very, very hard); (2) Modified Borg scale (a 10-point scale scientifically tested in a research study in California[7]).

Research studies[7,8] evaluating these RPE scales showed that the Borg scale had a high correlation with a person's actual heart rate during physical activity and provided a fairly good estimate of the actual heart rate during activity. Other studies[6] found that the Borg RPE scale correlated with many physiological variables such as heart rate, lactate concentration, percentage of VO_{2max}, VO_2, ventilation, and respiratory rates; however, inconsistencies existed showing that some variables affected the validity of the RPE score as a measure of exercise intensity. For

continues

Table 5-37   (continued)

example, although the RPE correlated with the heart rate in some studies, research that used sedentary patients as subjects, found that there were weaker correlations (between RPE and the heart rate) in studies that used trained subjects. Studies[7,8] also found that there were variations between the scale and the exercise protocols or the subjects' gender. Male RPE scores showed weaker correlations than female RPE scores.

Because the 15-point RPE Borg scale is used the most in the clinical facilities, the patient should be introduced to this scale before starting the exercise or activity. The following is an example of *patient education information* about the 15-point RPE Borg scale:

1. While doing exercises or physical activity, we want you to rate your perception of exertion. This feeling should reflect how heavy and strenuous the exercise feels to you, combining all sensations and feelings of physical stress, effort, and fatigue.

2. Try to appraise your feeling of exertion as honestly as possible without thinking about what the actual physical load is. Your own feeling of effort and exertion is important, not how it compares to other people's feelings.

3. Number six (#6) on the RPE scale corresponds to "no exertion at all" such as lying in bed or sitting in a chair relaxed.

4. Number nine (#9) on the RPE scale corresponds to "very light" exercises. For a healthy person, it is like walking slowly at his or her own pace for a few minutes.

5. Number thirteen (#13) on the RPE scale is "somewhat hard" exercise, but it still feels okay to continue.

6. Number seventeen (#17) on the RPE scale is "very hard." It means that the exercise is very strenuous. A healthy person can still go on, but the person needs to push himself or herself. The exercise or activity feels very heavy and the person is very tired.

7. Number nineteen (#19) on the RPE scale is an extremely strenuous exercise level. For most people, this is the most strenuous exercise they have ever experienced.

Metabolic Equivalents and Activities

Table 5-38   Metabolic Equivalents (METs) Overview

METs—metabolic equivalents estimate the metabolic cost of physical activity by evaluating the basic oxygen requirements at rest. One MET = approximately 3.5 ml of O_2/kg/min. Clinically, every activity can be expressed in METs comparing the activity METs with the METs at rest.

Table 5-39 METs and Activities[3]

1 – 2 METs: walking at 1 mph (on a level surface); active exercises to the upper or lower extremities (can be in supine or standing); driving a car; desk work; light housework; electric calculating machine operation; washing clothes; polishing furniture; feeding self; needlework; sewing; standing; motorcycling; playing cards

2 – 3 METs: walking at 2 mph (on a level surface); biking at 5 mph (on a level surface); active exercises in standing; light exercises on a mat; playing billiards; bowling; shuffleboard; driving a powerboat; golfing with power cart; canoeing; horseback riding at a walk; light wood working; riding lawn mower; auto repair; radio and television repair; bartending; janitorial work

3 – 4 METs: biking at 6 mph; walking at 3 mph; walking stairs slowly; playing volleyball with another five people (noncompetitive); golfing and pulling the bag cart; sailing in a small boat; horseback riding (trotting); playing badminton (socially, doubles); vacuuming; pushing light power mower; cleaning windows; mopping floors; laying bricks; plastering; using a wheelbarrow (with 100-pound load); welding (with moderate load); machine assembly

4 – 5 METs: biking at 8 mph; walking at 3.5 mph (on a level surface); active exercises to the upper or lower extremities (can be in supine or standing); playing table tennis; golfing and carrying the golf clubs; dancing foxtrot; playing badminton (single); playing tennis (doubles); ballet; raking leaves; scrubbing floors; washing the car; painting; performing masonry work; performing paperhanging work; performing light carpentry work

5 – 6 METs: biking at 10 mph; walking at 4 mph; performing step aerobics to tolerance; canoeing at 4 mph; horseback ridding (posting to trotting); stream fishing; ice or roller skating at 9 mph; digging a garden; shoveling light earth

6 – 7 METs: walking at 5 mph; biking at 11 mph; playing tennis (singles); swimming (20 yards/min); playing competitive badminton; skiing (light) down the hill; water skiing; folk and square dancing; shoveling light snow; shoveling 10 times/min (4.5 kg or 10 pounds); splitting wood; hand lawn mowing

7 – 8 METs: jogging at 5 mph; biking at 12 mph; playing basketball; skiing (vigorous) downhill; mountain climbing; canoeing at 5 mph; playing ice hockey; playing touch football; playing paddle ball; sawing hardwood; carrying 36 kg or 80 pounds; digging ditches

8 – 9 METs: running at 5.5 mph; bicycling at 13 mph; swimming (at 30 yards/min); skipping rope; playing squash (socially); playing handball (socially); playing basketball (vigorous); ski touring at 4 mph; shoveling 10 times/minute (5.5 kg or 14 pounds)

10 METs and more: running at 6 mph (for 10 METs); running at 9 mph (for 15 METs); running at 10 mph (for 17 METs); playing competitive handball; playing competitive squash; swimming (greater than 40 yards/min); ski touring of more than 5 mph; shoveling 10 times/min (7.5 kg, or 16 pounds)

Patient Education Topics for Cardiac Disease

Table 5-40   Patient Education Topics Offered by the Entire Medical Team

Medications: action of medications; effects of medications considering quality of life and survival; general side effects and what to do about it; dosage; lower cost availability and financial assistance; patient's disclosure of herbal remedies and supplements.

Dietary recommendations: patient's regular dietary habits; instructions how to reduce fat intake (for most of the heart diseases); instructions how to monitor salt and fluid intake (for CHF); restrictions on alcohol consumption.

Activity guidelines: education about the planned exercises, activities at home (including sex, sexual difficulties, and coping strategies), leisure activities, and work activities.

Patient self monitoring during activities: education about monitoring HR if patient is able to feel the pulse; monitoring activities or exercises using the Borg RPE scale; awareness of signs and symptoms suggesting exercise intolerance (such as light-headedness, dyspnea, mental confusion, inability to carry a brief conversation while performing activities or exercises). Patients having CHF may use the Borg dyspnea scale (uses numbers that correspond to patient's current perceived respiratory effort, such as 10 = completely out of breath; 5 = somewhat breathless; 1 = breathing easily) or the Borg RPE scale.

Patient's recognition of symptoms and patient's response: written information about patient's action when symptoms occur (such as calling the physician or going to hospital); recognizing weight gain (2 pounds or over in 1 to 2 days for CHF); expected symptoms; explanation of the medical treatment plan by the physician; clarification of patient's responsibilities; importance of smoking cessation; role of the family members (or other caregivers) in the medical treatment plan.

Lifestyle topics: resumption of sexual activity (it depends on the patient being comfortable to bring up the issue; patient and patient's partner need to be encouraged to bring up the issue). In general, when patients are able and comfortable to climb stairs or walking outdoors, they may be ready for sexual activity. Patient needs to know that in regard to the amount of energy used, sexual activity is different than other physical activities, and needs planning, pacing, and warm up.

Psychosocial and social topics: patient may have emotional depression. Studies showed emotional depression post CABG surgery (especially for women as compared with men). Patient needs encouragement to seek guidance and counseling

Phases of Cardiac Rehabilitation After Myocardial Infarction

Table 5-41   Interventions for Cardiac Rehab Phases

Cardiac rehab post-MI uses team approach. The multidisciplinary team includes MD/DO, Nurse, PT, PTA, OT, COTA, exercise physiologist, nutritionist, and social worker. Cardiac rehab includes three phases: phase I—inpatient phase; phase II—outpatient phase; phase III—community-based phase

Phase I/inpatient phase[3] uses different inpatient cardiac rehab programs based on increasing MET levels. General interventions in phase I include: (1) patient and patient family education for life changes, risk factor modifications, family support, self-monitoring of vital signs (precautions: HR not to rise with activity more than 20 bpm above the resting HR), recognizing adverse symptoms with activity (teaching Borg RPE Scale), and HEP (walking on a level surface at 1 mph); (2) bed mobility skills (ankle pumps to decrease possibility of DVT; transfers with assistance to decrease possibility of pneumonia); (3) activities starting at 1 MET and continuing gradually to 2 METs (some hospitals may progress patient's activities to 4 – 5 METs depending on the patient's individual response and medical history).

Phase II/outpatient phase is based on the results of ETT (at 4 to 6 weeks post-MI); uses an exercise prescription of 70% to 85% of maximum heart rate; uses a more conservative exercise prescription for a negative ETT (positive for ischemia). General interventions include: (1) patient education (continuing from phase I) for self-monitoring of vital signs, lifestyle changes, regulation of diet, performing independent ADLs, and an HEP (to include up to 5 METs); (2) activities at 5 METs (treadmill walking at 3.5 mph on a level surface; active exercises to the upper or lower extremities in supine or standing; stationary bicycling; golfing using a power cart; vacuuming; mild resistance exercises); (3) resistance exercises (starting at approximately 5 weeks post-MI) must teach the patient to exercise first large muscle groups before small; patient to focus on the Borg RPE scale at 11 to 13 (light to somewhat hard); patient to use slow, controlled movements; patient to stop exercises if becoming uncomfortable.

Phase III/community-based or voluntary program: long-term physical fitness and cardiopulmonary function; patient self-monitoring of vital signs during exercise; patient to be aware of his or her target rate; MET activity to be set considering patient's individual activities at work and play.

CARDIOPULMONARY INTERVENTIONS

Prevention Interventions for Coronary Artery Disease

Table 5-42   Prevention Interventions for CAD[3]

Dietary guidelines (provided by nutritionist or dietician): (1) patient needs to adopt a low-fat diet (decrease saturated fats and avoid trans fatty acids), to decrease salt intake, and have adequate fiber, minerals, and vitamins in the diet; (2) patient may require a sensible diet plan designed by a nutritionist in order to lose weight.

Exercise guidelines (provided by PT/PTA): (1) patient needs to gradually increase the endurance activity (such as increasing walking as the aerobic exercise to 40 to 45 minutes per session); (2) patients over age 40 with two or more risk factors for heart disease need an ETT before starting an aerobic program or a strengthening exercise program; (3) the ETT can identify latent ischemia; (4) exercise program (prescription) for patients over age 40 with 2 or more risk factors and a normal ETT can start at 70% to 80% of the HR_{max} for 30 to 40 minutes, 3 to 4 times per week with 5 to 10 minutes of warm up and cool down.

Community-based smoking cessation programs (or medically supervised smoking cessation programs) can be recommended for patients who smoke to assist them to stop smoking.

Stress management programs of different types; can be recommended and adapted to the patient's individual needs.

Use of medications: patient to control risk factors such as hypertension, diabetes mellitus, hypercholesterolemia, anxiety or depression with medications; medications to be used in a proper and consistent mode.

Control of hypertension: patient to control hypertension using a multifactorial approach that involves, in addition to medications, lifestyle modifications (including weight reduction), dietary reduction of sodium intake, and increased physical activity.

Pulmonary Interventions: Terms Related to Postural Drainage

Table 5-43   Postural Drainage Terms

Turning—turning is the rotation of the body around the longitudinal axis to promote unilateral or bilateral lung expansion and improve arterial oxygenation. Regular turning can be to either side or the prone position, with the bed at any degree of inclination (as indicated and tolerated). Patients may turn themselves or they may be turned by the caregiver or by a special bed or device.

Postural drainage—postural drainage is the drainage of secretions, by the effect of gravity, from one or more lung segments to the central airways (where they can be removed by cough or mechanical aspiration). Each position consists of placing the target lung segment(s) superior to the carina tracheae (the ridge at the lower end of the trachea separating the openings of the two primary bronchi). Positions should generally be held for 3 to 15 minutes (longer in special situations). Standard positions are modified as the patient's condition and tolerance warrant.

Percussion is a massage technique for mobilizing secretions from the lungs by striking the chest wall. It is also referred to as cupping, clapping, and tapotement. The purpose of percussion is to intermittently apply kinetic energy to the chest wall and lung. This is accomplished by rhythmically striking the thorax with cupped hand or mechanical device directly over the lung segment(s) being drained. No convincing evidence demonstrates the superiority of one method over the other. Vibration is another massage technique that involves the application of a fine tremulous action (manually performed) by pressing in the direction that the ribs and soft tissue of the chest move during expiration (over the draining area).

Postural Drainage Positions: Indications, Contraindications, and Precautions

Table 5-44 Postural Drainage: Indications, Contraindications, and Precautions

Postural drainage uses gravity to assist the removal of secretions from specific lobes of the lung, bronchi, or lung cavities. Postural drainage positions increase anteroposterior lung expansion and height allowing effective breathing. Indications for postural drainage positions: aspiration; increased pulmonary secretions; atelectasis (lung collapse) due to excess mucus. To perform postural drainage: the patient should be positioned that the involved segmental bronchus is uppermost.

Contraindications for all postural drainage positions: (1) intracranial pressure (ICP) > 20 mmHg; (2) head and neck injury until stabilized; (3) active hemorrhage with hemodynamic (circulating blood forces) instability; (4) recent spinal surgery (such as laminectomy); (5) acute spinal injury or active hemoptysis (expectoration of blood from larynx, trachea, bronchi, or lungs); (6) emphysema (COPD); (7) bronchopleural fistula (an abnormal opening between the pleural space and an airway in the lung); (8) pulmonary edema associated with congestive heart failure; (9) large pleural effusions (fluid in the pleural cavity); (10) pulmonary embolism (obstruction of pulmonary artery or one of its branches); (11) aged, confused, or anxious patients who do not tolerate position changes; (12) rib fracture, with or

continues

Table 5-54 (continued)

without flail chest (in flail chest, the affected rib segment is not attached on either end, and moves in and out during breathing); (13) surgical wound or healing tissue.

Contraindications for Trendelenburg position (patient's head is low and body and legs are on an elevated and inclined plane): (1) intracranial pressure (ICP) > 20 mmHg; (2) patients in whom increased intracranial pressure is to be avoided (such as after neurosurgery, aneurysms, or eye surgery); (3) uncontrolled hypertension; (4) distended abdomen; (5) esophageal surgery; (6) recent gross hemoptysis related to recent lung carcinoma treated surgically or with radiation therapy; (7) uncontrolled airway at risk for aspiration (tube feeding or recent meal). Precautions for the Trendelenburg position: (1) pulmonary edema, (2) shortness of breath, (3) congestive heart failure, (4) medication-controlled hypertension, (5) hiatal hernia, (6) obesity, and (7) nausea. Contraindications for reverse Trendelenburg position (patient's head is elevated and body and legs are low): hypotension or vasodilators medications.

Precautions for the side-lying positions: (1) arthritis, (2) recent rib fracture, (3) shoulder tendonitis/bursitis, (4) patient's discomfort, and/or (5) axillofemoral bypass graft.

Table 5-45   Bronchial Drainage Positions and Percussion[4]

Upper lobes—apical segments: the patient can be positioned on a bed or a drainage table (that is flat). Patient leans back on pillow at 30° angle against the therapist. Therapist clasps with markedly cupped hand over area between clavicle and top of scapula on each side.

Upper lobes—posterior segments: the patient can be positioned on a bed or a drainage table (that is flat). Patient leans over folder pillow at 30° angle. The therapist stands behind and clasps over upper back on both sides.

Right middle lobe (on a foot of table or bed elevated 16 inches): the patient lies head down on left side and rotates one-fourth turn backward. A pillow may be placed behind from shoulder to hip. Patient's knees should be flexed. Therapist clasps over right nipple area. In females with breast development or tenderness, use cupped hand with heel of hand under armpit and fingers extending forward beneath the breast.

Left upper lobe—lingular segments (foot of table or bed elevated 16 inches): the patient lies head down on right side and rotates one-fourth turn backward. A pillow may be placed behind from shoulder to hip. Patient's knees should be flexed. Therapist clasps with moderately cupped hand over left nipple area. In females with breast development or tenderness, use cupped hand with heel of hand under armpit and fingers extending forward beneath the breast.

Lower lobes—lateral basal segments (foot of table or bed elevated 20 inches): the patient lies on abdomen, head down, and then rotates one-fourth turn upward. Patient's upper leg is flexed over a pillow for support. The therapist clasps over uppermost portion of lower ribs. For left lateral basal segment, the patient should lie slightly on his or her right side in the same position, whereas for the right lateral basal segment, the patient should lie slightly on his or her left side in the same position.

Lower lobes—posterior basal segments (foot of table or bed elevated 20 inches): the patient lies on abdomen. Head is down, and pillow is under hips. The therapist clasps over lower ribs close to spine on each side.

Upper lobes—anterior segments (bed or drainage table that is flat): the patient lies on back with pillow under the knees. Therapist clasps between clavicle and nipple on each side.

Lower lobes—anterior basal segments (foot of table or bed elevated 20 inches): the patient lies on his or her side, with head down, and a pillow under the knees. The therapist clasps with slightly cupped hand over lower ribs. To drain the right anterior basal segment, the patient should lie on his or her left side in the same position, whereas for the left anterior basal segment, the patient should lie on his or her right side on the same position.

Lower lobes—superior segments (bed or table that is flat): the patient lies on abdomen with two pillows under the hips. The therapist clasps over middle back at tip of scapula on either side of the spine.

Percussion and Shaking Techniques: Indications, Precautions, and Contraindications

Table 5-46   Percussion and Shaking Techniques: Indications, Precautions, and Contraindications

Percussion is a tapotement massage technique used in pulmonary physical therapy to strike the chest wall with cupped hands to mobilize lung secretions. Indications for percussion: (1) aspiration; (2) increased pulmonary secretions; (3) atelectasis (lung collapse) caused by excess mucus. Percussion can be applied in combination with postural drainage positions for specific lung segments. Precautions when applying percussion and/or shaking: (1) fractured ribs, (2) degenerative bone disease, (3) hemoptysis (expectoration of blood), (4) coagulation disorders, (5) increased partial thromboplastin time (PTT—blood coagulation) to more than 38 seconds (normal = 25 to 38 seconds), and (6) platelet count below 50,000.

continues

Table 5-46   (continued)

Contraindications for percussion (in addition to postural drainage contraindications): (1) subcutaneous emphysema; (2) recent epidural spinal infusion or spinal anesthesia; (3) recent skin grafts, or flaps, on the thorax; (4) burns, open wounds, and skin infections of the thorax; (5) recently placed transvenous (temporary pacemaker inserted transvenously into right ventricular apex) pacemaker or subcutaneous pacemaker (particularly if mechanical devices are to be used); (6) suspected pulmonary tuberculosis; (7) lung contusion; (8) bronchospasm; (9) osteomyelitis (inflammation of bone and marrow) of the ribs; osteoporosis; (10) coagulopathy (blood clotting defect); (11) complaint of chest-wall pain.

Shaking is a vibration massage technique used in pulmonary physical therapy to mobilize lung secretions. Indications for shaking: (1) aspiration; (2) increased pulmonary secretions; (3) atelectasis (lung collapse) caused by excess mucus. PTA may use five to seven shaking techniques for a specific lung segment in combination with postural drainage positions. Less than five techniques are ineffective and more than ten (with inhalations) can cause hyperventilation. Precautions and contraindications are the same as for percussion.

Other Interventions for Pulmonary Rehab

Table 5-47   Breathing Techniques, Activity Pacing, Coughing, and Aerobic Training

*For relaxation exercises, see Part III.

Breathing exercises are taught in a quiet environment, with the patient in a relaxed and comfortable position (free of restrictive clothing). At the beginning of the exercises, the patient should be sitting in a semireclined position with the head and the trunk elevated at approximately 45°, allowing the abdominal musculature to relax. The patient's knees and hips are flexed and supported with a pillow.

Precautions during breathing exercises: (1) do not allow the patient to perform forced expiration (because it can cause bronchospasm); expiration should be passive, relaxed, or controlled; (2) do not allow the patient to start inspiration using the accessory muscles and the upper chest; upper chest should be quiet during breathing; (3) do not allow the patient to take a very prolonged expiration (because it causes the patient to gasp with the next inspiration and becomes an irregular breathing pattern); (4) allow the patient to perform deep breathing for only three or four inspirations and expirations at a time (to avoid possibility of hyperventilation).

Glossopharyngeal breathing is a breathing technique for patients who have weakness in the muscles of inspiration (diaphragm and accessory muscles). The patient is taking several "gulps" of air. Then the patient closes his/her mouth forcing the air into the lungs.

Pursed-lip breathing is an expiratory breathing technique for patients who have dyspnea caused by mostly COPD. It may prevent premature closing of intrapulmonary airways. First patient inhales through the nose for several seconds with the mouth closed. Then the patient exhales through puckered lips (such as whistling or kissing) to slow the expiratory flow. This creates slight back pressure allowing better gas exchange. During pursed-lip breathing, there should not be expiratory flow through the nose.

Diaphragmatic breathing is a breathing technique retraining the patient to use the diaphragm while relaxing abdominal muscles during inspiration (such as having the abdomen rising while the chest wall remains stationary). Patient inhales slowly that the abdomen swells out, and the lower part and the upper part of the chest expand and slightly lift. Then the patient holds the breath momentarily and releases the expiratory flow slowly (exhaling) as the abdomen is drawn in, the diaphragm is lifted, and the chest relaxes. Diaphragmatic breathing is used for COPD and CRLD. Diaphragmatic breathing is also a relaxation technique. The therapist may use a biofeedback machine to help use of diaphragm and inhibit use of accessory muscles.

Diaphragmatic breathing is performed as the following: (1) The patient is relaxed in a semireclined position, and the procedure is explained to the patient. (2) The therapist places his or her hand gently over the subcostal angle of the patient's thorax. (3) The therapist applies gentle pressure throughout the exhalation phase of breathing. Toward the end of the exhalation, the therapist increases to firm pressure. The patient is asked to inhale against the resistance of the therapist's hand. (4) As the therapist feels the diaphragm moving, the hand resistance is released allowing the patient a full inhalation. (5) Patient is taught the technique first in a semireclined sitting position (also called semi-Fowler position) and then in sitting, standing, walking, and stair climbing positions.

Segmental breathing is a breathing technique to help the hypoventilated segments of the lungs in patients with pleuritic pain, splinting (from surgery or trauma), and segmental atelectasis. Before segmental breathing, the patient needs clear airways (of mucous) by using secretion removal techniques. Patient inhales against the resistance of the therapist's hand (placed at the thorax over the area of hypoventilation). As the therapist feels the local expansion of the thorax, the hand resistance is slowly released to allow full inhalation.

Activity pacing is teaching the patient how to perform an activity (such as ADLS, ambulation, stair climbing, and other tasks) within his or her breathing capacity

continues

Table 5-47   (continued)

limits. The patient needs to break an activity in several small components. Then the patient performs each component with rest periods between them, eliminating dyspnea and fatigue. While performing each small component of the activity, the patient may use pursed-lip breathing technique. For example, to climb one flight of stairs, the patient inhales at rest and then on exhalation using pursed-lip breathing ascends one or two steps. Then the patient stops to rest until full recovery. The patient repeats the process until the whole flight is ascended without dyspnea and fatigue.

Coughing is the easiest way to clear the airway. Assisted cough takes place with the patient in sitting (against a wall), and PTA placing both hands below the patient's subcostal angle (against the patient's abdomen between the navel and the rib cage). As patient inhales deeply and attempts to cough, the PTA's hands push inward and upward assisting the exhalation of air. Huffing is similar to coughing (patient to take a deep breath and immediately to forcibly expel the air saying: "ha, ha, ha").

Mucous (phlegm) expulsion through coughing may need to be sent to the laboratory for analysis. In pneumonia, the mucous is viscid, tenacious, and sticky. Its appearance is rusty and containing blood. In bronchitis is mucoid, streaked with blood, and greenish yellow (from pus).

Suctioning is removal of secretions from the larger airways. How to perform: (1) use aseptic technique; (2) provide supplemental oxygen; (3) insert suction catheter without applying suction, as fully as possible (be gentle); (4) apply suction while withdrawing the catheter; (5) re-expand lung with mechanical ventilator or manual inflation by resuscitator bag attached to tracheal tube. Warning: Suctioning procedure should be done by an experienced PT (check your state practice act). Tracheal suctioning can be used only with patients who have an artificial airway in place. Avoid hypoxemia, cardiac dysrhythmias, mechanical trauma, bacterial contamination of tracheobronchial tree, and increase in intracranial pressure.

Bagging: provides artificial ventilation; restores oxygen; re-expands the lungs after suctioning. How to perform: (1) attach manual resuscitator bag to oxygen source; (2) connect manual resuscitator bag to tracheal tube; (3) squeeze bag rhythmically to deliver volume of air to patient; (4) patient exhales passively. Bagging is used before and after suctioning for patients who are not mechanically ventilated.

Turning, passive positioning, using splints, PROM, AROM, sitting, standing, ambulation: are used with every patient in cardiopulmonary acute care (ICU/CCU); are dependent on patient's diagnosis and tolerance. The therapist should be careful with intravascular lines and tubes. In addition, the therapist should watch the patient for orthostatic hypotension, dyspnea, and changes in vital signs.

Aerobic training is part of cardiopulmonary rehab post acute care. It includes warm up, aerobic exercise, and cool down. Stretching exercises during exhalation (to prevent Valsalva) are recommended before aerobic training. The warm up period (5 to 15 minutes) consists of the same exercise as the aerobic but performed at a lower intensity and using controlled breathing. The aerobic exercise (20 to 60 minutes) should maintain the calculated THR of the exercise prescription. The patient can be monitored using a rating of perceived shortness of breath, heart rate values, respiratory rate, and oximetry (oxygen saturation measurement). The cool down (5 to 15 minutes) consists of low level aerobic activities that slowly return the cardiopulmonary system to pre-exercise levels.

Examples of Pulmonary Exercises

Table 5-48   Examples of Pulmonary Exercises

Lateral chest mobilization exercises (during inspiration and expiration): mobilizes the lateral rib cage. To perform mobilization to the lateral side of the chest: (1) during inspiration, the patient (sitting) is bending away from the tight side of the chest (to lengthen hypomobile structures and expand the chest); (2) during expiration, the patient (sitting) is pushing a fisted hand onto the lateral aspect of the chest while bending toward the tight side. (3) to progress these exercises, ask the patient to raise his or her arm on the tight side over the head and side-bend away from the tight side (increasing the stretch on the hypomobile structures).

Upper chest mobilization exercises: stretch the pectoralis muscles. To perform upper chest mobilization for pectoralis stretch: (1) patient position during the exercise is sitting in a chair with hands clasped behind the head; (2) during inspiration, the patient is abducting the arms horizontally; (3) during expiration, the patient is bringing the elbows together while is bending forward.

Upper chest mobilization exercises: for upper chest expansion and stretching the shoulders. To perform upper chest mobilization for chest expansion and shoulders stretch: (1) patient position during the exercise is sitting in a chair; (2) during inspiration, the patient is reaching with both arms overhead (at 180^0 bilateral shoulder flexion and slight abduction); (3) during expiration, the patient is bending forward at the hips while reaching forward with both arms toward the floor.

Cardiopulmonary Intervention Patterns

APTA's Guide to Physical Therapist Practice—APTA's Cardiopulmonary Intervention Patterns

Table 5-49   Therapeutic Exercises[9]

1. Strength, power, and endurance training for head, neck, limb, pelvic floor, trunk, and ventilatory muscles (such as active assistive, active, and resistive exercises, including concentric, dynamic, isotonic, isometric, and plyometric; aquatic programs; standardized, programmatic, complementary exercise approaches task-specific performance training).
2. Flexibility exercises (such as muscle lengthening, range of motion, stretching).
3. Relaxation exercises (such as breathing strategies; movement strategies; relaxation techniques; standardized, programmatic, complementary exercise approaches).
4. Aerobic capacity and endurance conditioning and reconditioning (such as aquatic programs, gait and locomotor training, increased workload over time, task-specific performance training, walking and wheelchair propulsion programs).
5. Body mechanics and postural stabilization (such as body mechanics training, posture awareness training, postural control training, postural stabilization activities).
6. Gait and locomotion training (such as developmental activities training; gait training; implement and device training; perceptual training; standardized, programmatic, complementary exercise approaches wheelchair training).
7. Neuromotor development training (such as developmental activities training, motor training, movement pattern training, neuromuscular education or reeducation).
8. Balance, coordination, and agility training (such as developmental activities training; motor function such as motor control and motor learning training and retraining; neuromuscular education and reeducation; standardized, programmatic, complementary exercise approaches.

Table 5-50   Functional Training in Self-Care and Home Management, Including ADL and IADL[9]

1. ADL training (such as bathing, bed mobility and transfer training, developmental activities, dressing, eating, grooming, toileting)
2. Devices and equipment use and training (such as assistive and adaptive device and equipment training during ADL and IADL; orthotic, protective, or supportive device or equipment training during ADL and IADL; prosthetic device or equipment training during ADL and IADL)

continues

Table 5-50 (continued)

3. Functional training programs (such as simulated environments and tasks)
4. IADL training (such as caring for dependents, home maintenance, household chores, shopping, structured play for infants and children, yard work)
5. Injury prevention or reduction (such as safety awareness training during self-care and home management, injury prevention or reduction with use of assistive devices and equipment)

Table 5-51 Prescription, Application, and as Appropriate, Fabrication of Devices and Equipment (Assistive, Adaptive, Orthotic, Protective, Supportive, and Prosthetic)[9]

1. Adaptive devices (such as seating systems)
2. Assistive devices (such as canes, crutches, long-handled reachers, walkers, power devices, static and dynamic splints, wheelchairs)
3. Orthotic devices (such as braces, casts, splints, shoe inserts)
4. Protective devices (such as braces, cushions)
5. Supportive devices (such as compression garments, corsets, elastic wraps, neck collars, supplemental oxygen, mechanical ventilators)

Table 5-52 Functional Training in Work (Job/School/Play), Community, and Leisure Integration or Reintegration Including IADL, Work Hardening, and Work Conditioning[9]

1. Devices and equipment use and training (such as assistive and adaptive device and equipment training during IADL; orthotic, protective, or supportive device or equipment training during IADL; prosthetic device or equipment training during IADL)
2. Functional training programs (such as simulated environments and tasks, task adaptation, task training, work conditioning, work hardening)
3. IADL training (such as community service training involving instruments, school and play activities training including tools and instruments, work training with tools)
4. Injury prevention or reduction (such as injury prevention education during work at job, school, or play, community, and leisure integration or reintegration; injury prevention or reduction with use of devices and equipment; safety awareness training during work at job, school, or play, community, and leisure integration and reintegration)
5. Leisure and play activities and training

Table 5-53   Manual Therapy Techniques (Excludes Joint Mobilization)[9]

1. Manual lymphatic drainage
2. PROM
3. Massage (such as connective tissue massage, therapeutic massage)
4. Soft tissue mobilization

Table 5-54   Electrotherapeutic Modalities[9]

Electrical muscle stimulation (such as EMS, TENS).

Table 5-55   Patient/Client Related Instruction[9]

Instruction, education, and training of patients/clients and caregivers regarding: risk factors for pathology and pathophysiology (disease, disorder, or condition) impairments, functional limitations, or disabilities; enhancement of performance; health, wellness, and fitness programs; plan for intervention; current condition—pathology and pathophysiology (diseases, disorder, or condition), impairments, functional limitations and disabilities; plan of care; transitions across settings; transitions to new roles

Table 5-56   Airway Clearance Techniques[9]

Breathing strategies (such as: active cycle of breathing or forced expiratory techniques; assisted cough/huff techniques; autogenic drainage; paced breathing; pursed lip breathing; techniques to maximize ventilation: maximum inspiratory hold, staircase breathing, manual hyperinflation)

Positioning (such as positioning to alter work of breathing, positioning to maximize ventilation and perfusion, and pulmonary postural drainage)

Manual and mechanical techniques (such as assistive devices; chest percussion, vibration, and shaking; chest wall manipulation; suctioning; ventilatory aids)

Coronary Artery Disease Intervention Patterns

Table 5-57 Basic Physical Therapy Goals for CAD Interventions (Included in the APTA's Guide to Physical Therapist Practice)[9]

To improve physiological response to increased oxygen requirements; to decrease symptoms associated with increased oxygen requirements

To increase power, strength, endurance, and aerobic capacity

To increase capability of performing ADLs, IADLs, home management, and community and work integration/reintegration

To improve ability to recognize a recurrence and seek immediate interventions; to decrease the risk of recurrence

To acquire behaviors that promote wellness, healthy habits, and prevention

To increase patient/client, family, and caregiver decision-making ability in regard to patient (client) health and use of health care resources

Table 5-58 Exercise Guidelines for CAD

The aerobic exercise prescriptions should be based on FITT equation: F = frequency, I = intensity, T = time (duration), T = type (mode).

In regard to the frequency, aerobic exercise training is recommended three to five times per week for 12 or more weeks.

In regard to the time, aerobic exercise training session can be 20 to 40 minutes of aerobic exercise, 5 to 10 minutes of warm up, and 5 to 10 minutes of cool down. Patients (clients) who are deconditioned may need rest periods of 5 minutes between exercises.

The aerobic exercise intensity may start at approximately 70% to 85% of the HR_{max}. Patients (clients) who are deconditioned may need to start at a lower intensity of 50% to 60% of the HR_{max}. However, the safest method of calculating the exercise intensity for patients/clients having CAD is using the medically supervised ETT. During ETT, EKG monitoring can detect exercise-induced ischemia.

Exercise intensity can also be based on exercise prescription or patient (client) report of rating of perceived exertion (Borg RPE scale). As per the RPE Borg scale, patients (clients) need to limit their exertion between "fairly light" (11) to "somewhat hard" (13).

During exercises, patient (client) should not experience fatigue as a result of exercises. If fatigue occurs, the exercises intensity or frequency should be decreased. Patients (clients) should be aware that: symptoms of fatigue and overexertion may occur during the exercises (activities), or may occur later in the day or the following day.

The type (mode) of exercise or activity can be treadmill, bicycle, stair climber, rower, reclining bicycle, stepper, cross-country ski stimulator, and arm ergometer. Patients (clients) have a large variety of equipment to choose from. It is important to allow patients (clients) to choose the equipment that they enjoy the most.

The exercise or activity should be progressively increasing in a logical fashion of increasing energy costs (such as METs) with appropriate BP and HR monitoring.

The contraindications to aerobic exercise training are: (1) unstable angina, (2) symptomatic heart failure, (3) uncontrolled arrhythmia, (4) moderate to severe aortic stenosis, (5) uncontrolled diabetes, (6) acute systemic illness or fever, (7) uncontrolled tachycardia, (8) resting systolic BP of equal or more than 200 mmHg, (9) resting diastolic BP of equal or more than 110 mmHg, (10) thrombophlebitis.

As a safety precaution, patients (clients) need to know to stop the exercise (activity) immediately with any ischemia symptom.

If ischemia occurs when the patient is in the outpatient facility, the PTA should stop the activity, have the patient lie down, take the patient's BP and HR, and call the PT. From the results of the BP and HR, the PT will determine patient's ischemic threshold (maximum volume of oxygen when the patient experienced ischemia). In outpatient facility, patients (clients) may use nitroglycerin (NTG) medication to reduce ischemia. NTG is taken sublingually or using a spray. The patient (client) waits 5 minutes and repeats administration of NTG. Patients (clients) know that after three administrations of NTG (at 5-minute intervals) and the symptoms are still not resolved, they need to go to the emergency room.

When the patient's symptoms of ischemia amplify (instead of abating) after the exercise or activity stopped, the patient needs to be assisted to a position of comfort and emergency medical services need to be alerted.

If the patient (client) is alone ascending stairs and the symptoms of ischemia appear, he or she must stop, take a few easy deep breaths, and wait for the symptoms to abate. Then the patient (client) can descend stairs slowly to the first available help.

As a safety precaution in cases of ischemia in an inpatient facility, the PTA should follow the facility's guidelines by seeking immediate nursing personnel help. The facility may administer to the patient oxygen, EKG, and/or NTG or other anti-ischemic medication.

Table 5-59   Strength Training in Cardiac Rehab After MI

Strength training is a recent exercise addition in cardiac rehabilitation. As per research studies, it is considered safe and effective. Strength training can start with light resistance using light elastic bands or weights (1 to 3 pounds) for 12 to 15 repetitions. The resistance can be gradually increased to the patient's comfort level.

Strength training should begin at approximately 5 weeks after MI or 8 weeks after CABG surgery.

Strength training guidelines include: (1) use patient's large muscle groups before small muscle groups; (2) stress exhalation with exertion; (3) avoid sustained tight grip; (4) use slow controlled movements; (5) focus on Borg RPE 11 to 13; (6) stop exercises with any warning of patient acquiring uncomfortable signs and symptoms.

When starting and during cardiac strength training, the PTA should have the immediate availability of the PT (in the event of an emergency).

Congestive Heart Failure Intervention Patterns

Table 5-60   Basic Physical Therapy Goals for CHF Interventions (Included in the APTA's Guide to Physical Therapist Practice)[9]

To improve physiological response to increased oxygen requirements

To improve patient's self management of symptoms; to increase patient's awareness in regard to use of community resources

To increase capability of performing independent ADLs and physical tasks

To acquire behaviors that promote wellness, healthy habits, and prevention

To reduce disability associated with acute or chronic illness

To reduce risk of secondary impairments

Table 5-61   Exercise Guidelines for CHF

Low-level exercises can start when the patient's functional status of the cardiac system (hemodynamic system) is stable. Exercises should consider patient's systemic conditioning, peripheral endurance training, low-level resistance training, and respiratory muscle training.

During exercises, the patient needs to be monitored for oxygen saturation (using pulse oximetry with finger probe), vital signs (BP, HR, RR), observation, auscultation, and recording the RPE (Borg RPE scale). Also, the patient needs to be observed for orthostatic hypotension caused by exertion and significant dysrhythmias.

The exercise intensity should be low; the duration of exercise can be gradually increased as per patient's tolerance. The exercise HR should be below 115 bpm. Considering patient's medications (and that the exercises do not increase the HR more than 10 to 20 bpm), the best method for monitoring patient's exercise intensity is the RPE scale.

For patients who are deconditioned, light calisthenics in sitting position are recommended to begin the exercise program. Also, the exercises need to start with a prolonged warm up and end with a prolonged cool down. Isometrics are contraindicated.

Resistance training can start with elastic bands (yellow) or light weights for upper and lower extremities.

Chronic Obstructive Pulmonary Disease (COPD) Intervention Patterns

Table 5-62   Basic Physical Therapy Goals for Pulmonary Interventions (Included in the APTA's Guide to Physical Therapist Practice)[9]

To improve patient's (patient family's) understanding of disease process, expectations, goals, and outcomes

To increase strength, power, and endurance of peripheral and ventilatory muscles; to increase cardiovascular endurance; to improve independence in airway clearance; to decrease the work of breathing

To increase capability of performing physical tasks and ADLs/IADLs

To improve decision making capability in regard to the use of health care resources

To enhance patient's self-management of the symptoms and of the pulmonary disease

Table 5-63   COPDs General Intervention Patterns

Patient education includes: (1) topics such as smoking cessation (if patient continues to smoke); (2) types of exercises and activities (including effects, contraindications, and adherence); (3) monitoring the use of bronchodilators (before engaging in activity/exercise)—bronchodilators are medications that expand the bronchi by relaxing bronchial muscles; (4) monitoring the use of antibiotics; (5) relaxation techniques; (6) use of home humidifier (to increase moisture content of

continues

Cardiopulmonary Intervention Patterns   **401**

Table 5-63 (continued)

the air); (7) for asthma, avoidance of allergens or other environmental triggers; (8) for cystic fibrosis, educate family and patient to perform chest physical therapy and postural drainage (on a regular schedule either BID, QID, or PRN).

Secretions removal and postural drainage techniques

Breathing techniques (diaphragmatic and pursed-lip breathing) and activity pacing; monitor breathing pattern with exercises and activities

Cough techniques

Exercises: shoulder shrugs, arm circles, chest mobility exercises, postural exercises to increase expansibility of the lungs, endurance training

Table 5-64 COPD Patient Education Topics (Delivered by the Entire Rehabilitation Team)

Anatomy and physiology of respiratory disease
Nutritional guidelines
Airway clearance techniques
Stress management and relaxation techniques
Energy saving techniques
Benefits of being smoke free
Use of medications
The effects of environmental factors on COPD
Oxygen delivery systems
Psychosocial aspects of COPD
Management of COPD
Community resources

Intervention Patterns: Chronic Restrictive Lung Diseases, Atelectasis, and Pulmonary Edema

Table 5-65 General Intervention Patterns: CRLDs, Atelectasis, and Pulmonary Edema

CRLDs from surgical procedures—preoperatively physical therapy interventions assist patient following surgery with deep-breathing exercises, incentive spirometer, coughing techniques with proper incisional splinting, secretions removal, bed mobility training, patient education, ankle pumps to decrease DVT.

CRLDs from surgical procedures—postoperatively physical therapy interventions assist patient with monitoring vital signs, use of incentive spirometer, monitoring sputum production, patient education for deep breathing and coughing techniques, proper splinting techniques for the incisional line, ankle pumps to decrease DVT and increase blood flow, transfers to the edge of the bed, early post-op ambulation.

Atelectasis (pulmonary disorder due to collapse of one or more lobes of the lungs) interventions: postural drainage with percussion, segmental breathing exercises, use of incentive spirometer, and patient education for proper splinting with coughing or movement.

Pulmonary edema (effusion of serous fluid into the alveoli and interstitial tissue of the lungs, can be caused by failure or weakening of the left ventricle) interventions: deep breathing and coughing techniques, and paced activity with pursed-lip breathing.

CARDIOPULMONARY
INTERVENTIONS

Review of Cardiopulmonary System Anatomy and Physiology

Overview of the Heart

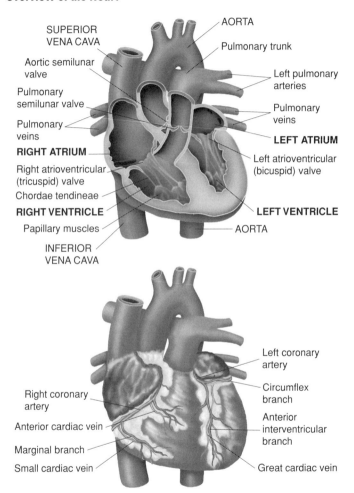

Figure 5-2 Anatomy of the Heart: From Anatomy of the Heart. From Anatomy and Physiology: Understanding the Human Body by Robert K. Clark, page 293, Figure 16.4 "Anatomy of the Heart."

CARDIOPULMONARY
INTERVENTIONS

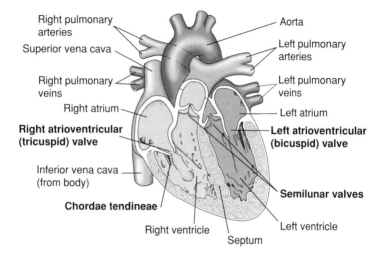

Right pulmonary arteries

Superior vena cava

Right pulmonary veins

Right atrium

Right atrioventricular (tricuspid) valve

Inferior vena cava (from body)

Chordae tendineae

Right ventricle

Septum

Aorta

Left pulmonary arteries

Left pulmonary veins

Left atrium

Left atrioventricular (bicuspid) valve

Semilunar valves

Left ventricle

Figure 5-3 Heart Valves. From Human Biology: Fifth edition by Daniel D. Chiras, page 111, Figure 6.4(a) "Heart Valves."

Table 5-66   Heart Tissue, Chambers, and Valves and Their Functions

Heart tissue	Heart Chambers: Pumps Working in Sequence	Heart Valves: One-Way Flow of Blood
Pericardium: protective tissue that surrounds the heart	Right atrium: receives deoxygenated blood from the body through superior and inferior vena cava; occurs in the systolic phase; blood is sent to right ventricle; it is separated from left atrium by the interatrial septum (wall)	Atrioventricular valves: prevent backflow of blood into the atria during ventricular systole (close when ventricular walls contract). Atrioventricular valves are: tricuspid valve (right heart valve); bicuspid or mitral valve (left heart valve)
Epicardium: inside layer of pericardium	Right ventricle: pumps blood to lungs for oxygenation via pulmonary artery; it is separated from left ventricle by an interventricular septum (wall) that is ticker than interatrial septum	Semilunar valves: prevent backflow of blood from the aorta and pulmonary arteries into ventricles during diastolic phase. Semilunar valves are pulmonary valve (prevents right backflow) and aortic valve (prevents left backflow)
Myocardium: heart muscle; the major portion of heart	Left atrium: receives oxygenated blood from the lungs (during the systolic phase); blood is sent to left ventricle	
Endocardium: smooth lining of the inner surface and the heart cavities	Left ventricle: pumps blood throughout entire systemic circulation via the aorta; it is stronger than right ventricle; has thicker walls than right ventricle to pump the blood throughout the entire body.	

See Figure 5-2 and Figure 5-3.

CARDIOPULMONARY INTERVENTIONS

Arteries of the Body

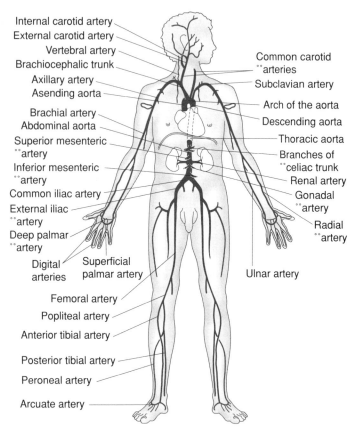

Internal carotid artery
External carotid artery
Vertebral artery
Brachiocephalic trunk
Axillary artery
Asending aorta
Brachial artery
Abdominal aorta
Superior mesenteric
°°artery
Inferior mesenteric
°°artery
Common iliac artery
External iliac
°°artery
Deep palmar
°°artery
Digital
arteries
Superficial
palmar artery
Femoral artery
Popliteal artery
Anterior tibial artery
Posterior tibial artery
Peroneal artery
Arcuate artery

Common carotid
°°arteries
Subclavian artery
Arch of the aorta
Descending aorta
Thoracic aorta
Branches of
°°celiac trunk
Renal artery
Gonadal
°°artery
Radial
°°artery
Ulnar artery

Figure 5-4   Arteries of the Body. From Anatomy and Physiology: Understanding the
Human Body by Robert K. Clark, page 304, Figure 16.17 "Overview of the
arteries."

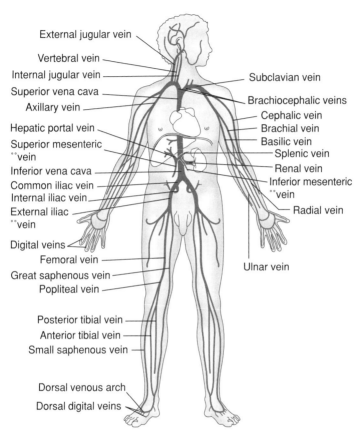

External jugular vein
Vertebral vein
Internal jugular vein
Superior vena cava
Axillary vein
Hepatic portal vein
Superior mesenteric
°°vein
Inferior vena cava
Common iliac vein
Internal iliac vein
External iliac
°°vein
Digital veins
Femoral vein
Great saphenous vein
Popliteal vein
Posterior tibial vein
Anterior tibial vein
Small saphenous vein
Dorsal venous arch
Dorsal digital veins

Subclavian vein
Brachiocephalic veins
Cephalic vein
Brachial vein
Basilic vein
Splenic vein
Renal vein
Inferior mesenteric
°°vein
Radial vein
Ulnar vein

Figure 5-5 Veins of the Body. From Anatomy and Physiology: Understanding the Human Body by Robert K. Clark, page 306, Figure 16.19 "Overview of the veins."

Overview of the Coronary Circulation (Hemodynamics)

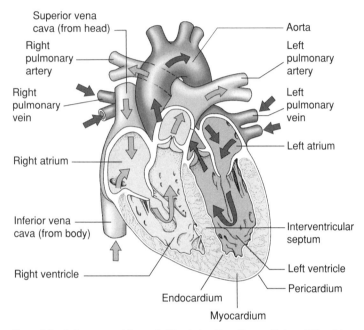

Figure 5-6 Pulmonary and Systemic Circulation. From Human Biology: Fifth edition by Daniel D. Chiras, page 109, Figure 6.2 "Blood Flow Through the Heart."

Table 5-67   Coronary Circulation

1. Deoxygenated blood from the superior and inferior vena cava enters the heart into the right atrium.
2. Blood passes down through the tricuspid valve from the right atrium to the right ventricle.
3. Blood passes through the pulmonary valve from the right ventricle into the pulmonary artery and pulmonary capillaries.
4. The gas exchange takes place in the pulmonary alveoli.
5. Oxygenated blood from the pulmonary veins passes to the left atrium.
6. Oxygenated blood passes down through the bicuspid (mitral) valve into the left ventricle.
7. Oxygenated blood goes down to the apex of the heart, and during the heart's systole, it is moved from the apex of the heart to the left ventricle outflow tract and through the aortic valve into the aorta.

See Figure 5-6.

Blood Supply to the Heart

Table 5-68   Right Coronary Artery (RCA) and Left Coronary Artery(LCA) (Has Left Anterior Descending [LAD] Artery and the Circumflex Artery)

RCA supplies: right atrium; right ventricle; inferior wall of left ventricle; atrioventricular (AV) node; Bundle of His; sinoatrial (SA) node (60% of the time)

LCA supplies: most of the left ventricle

LAD artery supplies: left ventricle; right ventricle; interventricular septum; inferior area of the apex of the heart; inferior areas of right and left ventricles

Circumflex artery supplies: lateral and inferior walls of the left ventricle; portion of the left atrium; sinoatrial (SA) node (40% of the time)

Overview of the Electrical Conduction of the Heart

Table 5-69   Conduction of the Heartbeat

The heart has specialized conduction tissue that allows rapid transmission of electrical impulses in the myocardium (called normal sinus rhythm [NSR]). The specialized conduction tissue is Purkinje fibers (specialized conduction tissue in both ventricles); nodal tissue.

Sinoatrial (SA) node initiates the electrical impulse being the main pacemaker of the heart. SA node is located at the junction of the superior vena cava and the right atrium. SA node has sympathetic and parasympathetic innervations affecting the heart rate and the strength of the contraction.

Atrioventricular (AV) node merges with Bundle of His. AV node is located at the junction of the right atrium and right ventricle. AV node has sympathetic and parasympathetic innervations.

Contraction of the heart tissue is called systole.

Relaxation of the heart tissue is called diastole.

The conduction of the heartbeat starts in the SA node. The electrical impulse spreads throughout both atria (that contract together). The impulse stimulates AV node. The impulse is transmitted down the Bundle of His to the Purkinje fibers. The impulse spreads throughout both ventricles (that contract together).

Table 5-70   Myocardial Fibers and Metabolism

Myocardial fibers are muscle tissue made of striated muscle fibers with many mitochondria. The myocardial fibers contract as a functioning unit.

Myocardial metabolism is essentially aerobic. It is sustained by continuous oxygen delivery from the coronary arteries. Coronary arteries have smooth muscle tissue inside their walls.

The Autonomic Nervous System Influences on the Heart

Table 5-71   Parasympathetic and Sympathetic Stimulation

Parasympathetic stimulation via the Vagus nerve: slows the heart rate and the force of myocardial contraction and decreases myocardial metabolism. It also causes vasoconstriction of the coronary arteries.

Sympathetic stimulation (located on the sinus node and within the myocardium): causes an increase in heart rate and the force of myocardial contraction and increases myocardial metabolism. It also causes vasodilation of the coronary arteries.

Overview of the Pulmonary Anatomy, Including the Respiratory Muscles

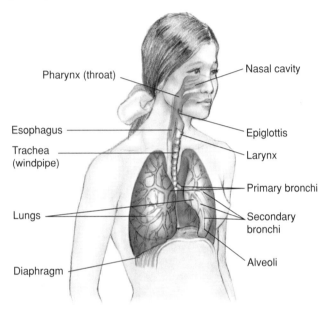

Pharynx (throat)

Nasal cavity

Esophagus

Epiglottis

Trachea (windpipe)

Larynx

Primary bronchi

Lungs

Secondary bronchi

Diaphragm

Alveoli

Figure 5-7   Respiratory system. From Anatomy and Physiology: Understanding the Human Body by Robert K. Clark, page 320, Figure 17.1 "The respiratory system."

Oxygenation

UPPER BODY

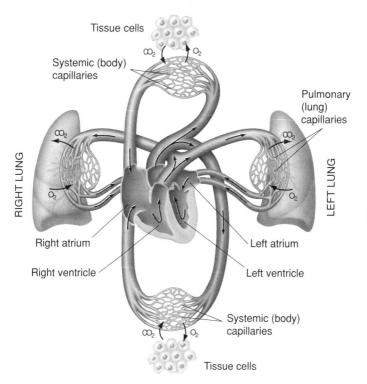

CARDIOPULMONARY
INTERVENTIONS

LOWER BODY

Figure 5-8 Oxygenation. From Anatomy and Physiology: Understanding the Human Body by Robert K. Clark, page 326, Figure 17.6 "The lungs receive the entire output of the right ventricle."

Table 5-72   Pulmonary Anatomy

Nose: organ of smell; entrance to the nasal cavities; starting point of the respiratory system; nose function is to filter, humidify, and warm the air

Pharynx: musculomembranous tube extending from the base of the skull to the level of C6 vertebrae, where it becomes continuous with the esophagus; contains nasopharynx, oropharynx, and laryngopharynx; nerves are Vagus and Glossopharyngeal; is a passageway for air from the nasal cavity to the larynx; is also a passageway for food from the mouth to the esophagus; functions are to be used for respiratory and digestive systems and to participate in speech as a resonating cavity.

Larynx: musculocartilaginous organ situated at the upper end of the trachea; contains extrinsic and intrinsic muscles; is lined with ciliated mucous membrane (part of the airway); connects the pharynx with trachea.

Trachea: cylindrical cartilaginous tube that goes from the larynx to the primary bronchi; extends from the C6 vertebrae to the T5 vertebrae, where (at carina) it divides into two bronchi; one bronchus goes to the right and the other to the left lung; it is a conducting airway; function is to transport air (not for gas exchange).

Respiratory unit made of: bronchi (two main branches from trachea to lungs; bronchi provide a passageway for air); bronchioles (smaller subdivisions of the bronchial tubes); alveolar ducts (branch of a respiratory bronchiole that leads to the alveolar sacs of the lungs); alveolar sacs (terminal portion of an air passage within the lung; the site of gas exchange); alveoli (air sacs of the lungs; perform gas exchange; blood and inspired air are separated by the cell of the alveolus and that of the pulmonary capillary).

Right lung has three lobes; each lobe has ten bronchopulmonary segments (upper lobe: apical, anterior, and posterior segments; middle lobe: lateral and medial segments; lower lobe: superior, anterior basal, lateral basal, posterior basal, and medial basal segments); each lobe has between 50 to 80 terminal bronchioles.

Left lung: has two lobes; each lobe has eight bronchopulmonary segments (upper lobe: apical-posterior, anterior, superior lingula, and inferior lingual segments; lower lobe: superior, anterior medial basal, lateral basal, and posterior basal segments); each lobe has between 50 to 80 terminal bronchioles.

See Figure 5-7.

Table 5-73   Respiratory Muscles

Muscles of inspiration: diaphragm (main muscle); accessory muscles (assist with inspiration during deeper inhalation and in the course of diseases): scalenes, sternocleidomastoid, serratus muscles, trapezius, and pectoral muscles.

Muscles of expiration: exhalation is passive when the inspiratory muscles relax; muscles that assist with forced expiration are: quadratus lumborum, intercostals, abdominal muscles, and triangularis sternum.

References

1. Dreeben, O. Introduction to Physical Therapy for Physical Therapist Assistants. Sudbury, MA: Jones and Bartlett Publishers; 2007.
2. Venes, D. (ed.) Taber's Cyclopedic Medical Dictionary: Edition 20 Illustrated in Full Color. Philadelphia: F.A. Davis Company; 2005.
3. O'Sullivan, SB, Schmitz, TJ. Physical Rehabilitation, 5th ed. Philadelphia: F.A. Davis Company; 2007.
4. Rothstein, JM, Roy, SH, Wolf, SL, Scalzitti, DA. The Rehabilitation Specialist's Handbook, 3rd ed. Philadelphia: F.A. Davis Company; 2005.
5. Sutherland, JA. The Little Black Book of Cardiology, 2nd ed. Sudbury, MA: Jones and Bartlett Publishers; 2007.
6. Centers for Disease Control and Prevention. Physical Activity for Everyone: Measuring Physical Activity Intensity: Perceived Exertion (Borg Rating of Perceived Exertion Scale). Centers for Disease Control and Prevention Web site. Available at http://www.cdc.gov. Accessed December 2006.
7. Kendrick KR, Baxi SC, Smith RM: Usefulness of the Modified 1-10 Borg Scale in Assessing the Degree of Dyspnea Patients With COPD and Asthma. Available at http://www.ac6v.com/karlaz2.htm. Accessed December 2006.
8. Lavietes MH, et al. The perception of dyspnea in patients with mild asthma. Chest 2002;120-122.
9. The American Physical Therapy Association. Guide to Physical Therapist Practice, 2nd ed. Alexandria, VA: APTA; 2001; Revised 2003.

CARDIOPULMONARY INTERVENTIONS

Part VI

Integumentary Interventions

INTEGUMENTARY INTERVENTIONS

Integumentary Data Collection

Burn Classification

Table 6-1 Burn Classification[1]

Superficial burn (epidermal burn): damage occurs only to epidermis (such as the classic sunburn or a brief scald). The skin is red and erythematous (because of epidermal damage and dermal irritation). The skin has slight (minimal) edema. There are no blisters, and the skin is dry. Pain and tenderness to touch will appear later. In 2 to 3 days, the injured epidermis will peel off (desquamate), and the skin will heal on its own without any scaring.

Superficial partial-thickness burn: damage occurs to epidermis and the papillary layer of the dermis (such as scalds or flash flame burn). The epidermis is destroyed completely, and the dermal layer is inflamed with mild to moderate damage. The skin is bright pink or red (or mottled red), with blanching and capillary refill (when pressure is exerted against the tissue). There are intact blisters, and the skin surface is moist. When blisters are removed (evacuated to speed up the healing), the skin is weeping. Extreme pain and skin sensitivity are present with light touch and changes in temperature or exposure to air (because of nerve endings involvement). If infection is present, the patient (client) will have fever. Edema is moderate. This burn will heal on its own in approximately 7 to 10 days without surgical intervention. After healing, there is a possibility of minimal scarring.

Deep partial-thickness burn: damage occurs to epidermis and dermis deep to the reticular layer of dermis (such as scalds or flash flame burn). This burn starts to resemble a full-thickness burn. Because most of the dermis is destroyed, the nerve endings, hair follicles, and sweat ducts are also injured. The skin is mixed red and waxy white with blanching and very slow capillary refill (when pressure is exerted against the tissue). The deeper the damage, the more white the blanching appears. There are broken blisters and the skin surface is very moist (because of leakage of plasma fluid). There is also water loss (through evaporation) because of vascular destruction. Patient (client) has no pain or sensitivity to light touch or gentle pin prick. There is sensitivity to pressure (because of the location of Pacinian corpuscles in the deep reticular dermis). Edema is very distinct. The wound may need a few days to stage itself as a deep partial-thickness and clearly differentiate from a full-thickness burn. Typically, the dead tissue will begin to slough, and preservation of hair follicles and new hair growth will indicate a deep partial-thickness and spontaneous healing. The healing is slow (usually in 3 to 5 weeks without infection) with new tissue that appears dry and scaly, easily abraded, and itchy. The burn needs to be kept free of infection. Creams need to lubricate the new surface of the skin artificially. After healing, there is excessive scarring. There is possibility of hypertrophic and keloid scars. A hypertrophic scar is a firm raised scar within the boundaries of the burn wound. A keloid scar spreads beyond the borders of the original burn and is made of collagen and fibroblasts. It appears shiny and rubbery.

Full-thickness burn: complete damage to all the epidermal and dermal layers (such as flame or contact with hot objects burn). The subcutaneous layer may also be damaged to some extent. This burn is white (without blood supply) and has a hard, charred, parchment-like eschar that covers the area. Eschar is dead tissue with crusty or scabbed black (deep red or white) material. White eschar indicates total ischemia (deficiency of blood) of the tissue. Red eschar indicates hemoglobin from the destroyed red blood cells. There will be no blanching of the skin. Bodily hair will pull out because of complete damage to hair follicles. Nerve endings will be destroyed, and the wound will have anesthesia. There is also damage to the peripheral vascular system that leaks fluid into the interstitial spaces (under the eschar), constricting the deep blood circulation (and possibility of blood flow occlusion and necrosis). An escharotomy may be necessary to improve the peripheral blood flow. This burn heals only with surgical skin grafting because all the epithelial cells are destroyed. There will be a large amount of scarring and the necessity of plastic surgery.

Subdermal burn: complete destruction of all tissue from the epidermis to the subcutaneous tissue. The burn is charred. The wound is anesthetic with muscle and nerve damage. Excessive surgical management using skin grafting is necessary.

Electrical burn: a different type of burn occurring from the passage of electrical current through the body after the skin made contact with an electrical source. Usually the bone offers the most resistance to electricity, whereas muscles and nerves offer the least resistance. The wound of the initial contact is charred, and the skin is yellow and ischemic. The exit wound is dry with damaged tissue (appearing as an explosion out of tissue). An area that may be viable becomes necrotic in a few days. The blood supply is altered and may have necrosis of the vascular wall. Other problems of electrical burn are cardiac arrhythmias, ventricular fibrillations, renal failure, acute spinal cord damage, or vertebral fracture.

Burn Wound Zones

Table 6-2   Burn Wound Zones

Zone of hyperemia: minimal site damage; the tissue can recover within several days; no long lasting effects.

Zone of stasis: injured cells that may die within 24 to 48 hours without treatment; infection, wound dryness, and inadequate perfusion can result in complete

continues

Table 6-2   (continued)

damage and necrosis of the tissue (that could have initially been saved); splints and compression bandages should not be placed too tightly (not to compromise the tissue).

Zone of coagulation: irreversible cell damage and skin death; similar to a full-thickness burn; requires skin graft to heal; increased risk of infection due to eschar; patient needs care in a specialized burn center.

Rule of Nines and Lund-Browder Burn Classifications

Table 6-3   Rule of Nines and Lund-Browder Burn Classifications

Rule of Nines burn classification is a formula for estimating percentage of body surface area, judging the portion of the skin that has been burned. For the adult, the head represents 9%. Each upper extremity is 9%. The anterior trunk is 18% (each half of the anterior trunk is 9%). The posterior trunk is 18% (each half of the posterior trunk is 9%). Each lower extremity is 18% (anterior lower extremity is 9%, and posterior lower extremity is 9%). The perineum is 1%.

Lund-Browder burn[2] classifications are more accurate, especially for children because they estimate the burn size based on the patient's age and changes that occur during normal growth. For newborns, each surface of the head is 9.5. Each surface of the thigh is 2.75. Each surface of the leg is 2.5.

For children 1 year old, each surface of the head is 8.5. Each surface of the thigh is 3.25. Each surface of the leg is 2.5.

For children 5 years old, each surface of the head is 6.5. Each surface of the thigh is 4.0. Each surface of the leg is 2.75.

For children between 10 and 14 years old, each surface of the head is 5.5. Each surface of the thigh is 4.25. Each surface of the leg is 3.0.

For children 15 years old, each surface of the head is 4.5. Each surface of the thigh is 4.5. Each surface of the leg is 3.25.

See Figure 6-1.

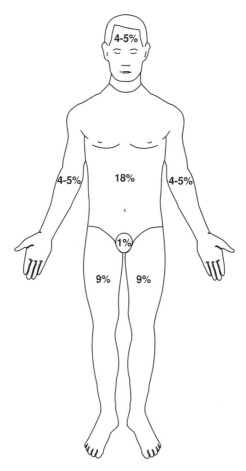

Figure 6-1 Rule of nines for the adult.

Complications of Burn Injury

Table 6-4   Systemic Complications of Burns

Complications caused by infections: risk of developing infection is very high secondary to exposed tissue. There are various types of bacteria. The two most powerful bacterial strains are *Pseudomonas aeruginosa* and *Staphylococcus aureus*. When the burn is infected, the wound (or the drainage) is discolored. The healing is delayed, and necrosis and tissue death can take place.

Respiratory system complications: respiratory system shock or inhalation injury (can be caused by exposure to smoke inhalation and fire). Inhalation injury is a life-threatening complication especially in those who have suffered facial burns. Other (early or late) respiratory system complications of burns are pulmonary edema, airway obstruction, respiratory failure, restrictive lung disease, pneumonia, and/or dyspnea.

Metabolic system complications: weight loss, decreased energy, and negative nitrogen balance (or equilibrium). Negative nitrogen balance: decreased nitrogen amount in the body because of an increased amount of nitrogen eliminated mostly through the skin sweat (also eliminated in feces and urine).

Cardiac and peripheral vascular systems complications: decreased or absent pulses, fluid and plasma loss that can lead to decreased cardiac output, increased pain with AROM, and numbness and tingling.

Urinary system complications: urine is red (indicating blood) or dark brown (indicating infection, ketone bodies, blood, bacteria, or pus).

Gastrointestinal system complications: ileus (intestinal obstruction) with distended abdomen, abdominal cramps, and abdominal collapse; gastric ulcer.

Burn Healing

Table 6-5   Burn Healing

Wound healing of the burn is dependent on the patient's age, size of the burn, type of the burn, area of the burn, trauma, nutrition, blood flow, medications, infection, and stress.

Epidermal healing includes epithelialization of the viable cells. The intact epithelial cells grow and proliferate, and then they cover the wound. The epithelialization can occur in the partial-thickness burn that has intact hair follicles and glands. When there is damage to the sebaceous glands causing dryness and itching of the wound, the therapist should teach the patient to apply moisturizing cream (to lubricate the newly healed tissue).

Dermal healing includes scar formation over the burn wound. Scar formation is divided into three phases: inflammatory, proliferative, and maturation.

Dermal healing—the inflammatory phase: begins at the time of injury and ends in about 3 to 5 days; characterized by redness, edema, warmth, pain, and decreased ROM. Physiologically, when the blood vessel is ruptured, the vessel wall contracts to decrease blood flow (vasoconstriction) to the area. Then, platelets go together and fibrin is deposited to form a clot over the area. The role of fibrin is that it partially retains body fluids, provides a firm coagulated clot, protects the underlying cells from destruction, and helps the blood cells to heal the wound. After a short vasoconstriction, there is vasodilation (increased blood flow to the wound) and increased permeability of the blood vessels bringing plasma into the interstitial space. This process of healing causes edema formation. Leukocytes clean the area of contamination, whereas macrophages clear the debris and attract fibroblasts to the wound.

Dermal healing—the proliferative phase is characterized by fibroblasts that synthesize scar tissue (made of collagen and protein polysaccharides), formation of granulation tissue (made of macrophages, fibroblasts, collagen, and blood vessels), and wound contraction (to close the wound). In this phase, skin grafting can help to decrease wound contraction and prevent scarring.

Dermal healing—the maturation phase includes remodeling of the scar tissue that can last up to 2 years. During this phase, there is a reduction in the number of fibroblasts and a remodeling of collagen (parallel alignment of collagen fibers). When the ratio of collagen production equals or exceeds breakdown, hypertrophic or keloid scars will result. Keloids scars form at the site of the wound. For African American patients (clients), keloids appear on a wound highly elevated and irregular continuing to enlarge.

Normal Physiology of Wound Healing

Table 6-6 Wound Healing Phases[1]

Wound healing is a continuous process, and its phases are not distinct but overlap with each other. Wound healing is dependent on the patient's (client's) age, size of wound, trauma, nutrition, blood flow, medications, infection, and stress.

Phase I—Inflammation: a normal immune system reaction to injury. Phase I can last from the beginning of injury to approximately day 10. Phase I healing rate is affected by the blood supply, extrinsic environment, and available nutrients. Interrupted or delayed phase I can cause chronic inflammation (months to years).

continues

INTEGUMENTARY INTERVENTIONS

Table 6-6 (continued)

Phase I events: (1) injury, (2) temporary repair (coagulation, short-term decreased blood flow), (3) necrosis (of injured cells), (4) slow spread of pathogens (debris and bacteria are attacked by a host of cells; pus may be formed), (5) oxygen delivery (increased blood flow to keep phagocytic cells working), (6) permanent repair facilitation (wound becomes clean to set the stage for re-epithelialization).

Phase II - Proliferation: new tissue fills in the wound. Phase II can last from the third day after the injury to approximately day 20. Phase II healing rate is affected by blood supply, extrinsic environment, and available nutrients. New scar tissue formed in this phase needs to be protected. Interrupted or delayed phase II can cause a chronic wound.

Phase II events: (1) fibroblasts secrete collagen, (2) new blood vessels grow from endothelial cells, (3) capillary buds grow into the wound bed, (4) new reddish (slightly bumpy) granulation tissue is formed, (5) epithelial cells differentiate into type I collagen, (6) collagen synthesis occurs and new fragile scar tissue is formed.

Phase III - Maturation/Remodeling: granulation that began in the proliferative phase continues. Phase III can last from approximately day 9 after injury to approximately 2 years. Phase III healing rate is affected by blood supply, extrinsic environment, and available nutrients.

Phase III events: (1) epithelial cells continue to differentiate into type I collagen, (2) new skin acquires tensile strength (15% of normal strength), (3) scar tissue is rebuilding (80% of original tensile strength), (4) granulation tissue is replaced by less vascular tissue, (5) in deep wounds, dermal appendages (such as hair follicles, and sebaceous and sweat glands) are replaced by fibrous tissue, (6) scar tissue matures and changes appearance (from red to pink to white and from raised and rigid to flat and flexible).

Pressure Ulcer Staging

Table 6-7   Pressure Ulcer Staging As Per the National Pressure Ulcer Advisory Panel (NPUAP)[3]

Stage I—characterized by nonblanchable erythema of intact (unbroken) skin. The wound presents clinically with redness and warmth (or coolness) that would not resolve in 30 minutes. In darker skin tones, this wound may appear persistent red, blue, or purple. Stage I wound can heal with intervention. The wound will heal using pressure relief techniques (turning and positioning), protection (cushions, protective pads, and specialty bed), improvement in patient's nutritional status (such as increase in vitamin C, proteins, and fluids), and prevention (not to worsen).

Stage II—characterized by partial-thickness wound involving the epidermis and/or part of the dermis (but not through the dermis). The wound is superficial and presents clinically as a blister (either broken or unbroken), abrasion, or a shallow crater. The base of the wound is pink and painful, but has no necrosis. Stage II wound will heal using wound care, protection, pressure relief techniques, improvement in patient's nutritional status, and prevention. Decubitus ulcer wounds in stage II are usually a result of inadequate interventions in stage I.

Stage III—characterized by full-thickness wound involving tissue loss through the dermis to subcutaneous tissue (but not through the fascia). The wound presents clinically as a crater (unless is covered with eschar), has sinus tract formation, exudate, and may have necrotic tissue. Stage III wound is a primary site for a serious infection. This wound will heal using aggressive wound care, improvement in patient's nutritional status, and infection prevention.

Stage IV—characterized by full-thickness wound involving tissue loss with extensive destruction through muscles and bone. The wound presents clinically as a deep crater with necrotic tissue, sinus tract formation, exudate, and infection (can be a life-threatening infection). There is damage to muscles and tendons and possibly to bone. The wound base is not painful. This wound will heal using aggressive wound care and/or surgical care and improvement in patient's nutritional status. In some situations, amputation may be necessary.

Warning: wounds that are covered by necrotic tissue may be staged as IV or full-thickness wounds.

In regard to documentation, the NPUAP states[3] that reverse staging is based on erroneous assumptions about the healing process, having negative clinical, regulatory, and reimbursement consequences. Reverse staging is a misconception that, for example, a healing stage IV pressure ulcer becomes first stage III and then stage II. As the pressure ulcer heals, subcutaneous tissue, bone, and muscle destroyed by a stage IV ulcer will never be replaced with the same tissue (subcutaneous tissue, bone, and muscles) but with granulation tissue and new epithelium.

Wound Characteristics

Table 6-8　Wound Characteristics (To Be Documented Throughout Wound Healing Phases)

Location: location of the wound on the patient's body.

Size: depth, width, length.

Shape: distinct or irregular.

Edges: shape of the wound edges, evidence of premature healing.

Tunneling, undermining, and sinus tracts: presence of these and the depth.

Base of the wound: characteristics of the base of the wound (compared with sides of the wound and edges of the wound); exudate (amount of exudate, the color of exudate, and the odor); granulation tissue (has or does not have granulation tissue, amount of granulation tissue, location of granulation tissue); necrosis, eschar, slough (including the amount, the texture and color, and the adherence to the wound bed); epithelialization (has or does not have epithelialization; is epithelialization on schedule or is premature); other structures exposed to the wound (bone, tendon, ligament).

Wound drainage signs: (1) serous (clear, shiny exudate; can have a slightly yellow appearance)—signifies a healthy wound; (2) seropurulent (brighter yellow drainage; slightly thicker exudate than the serous drainage; slightly malodorous)—signifies a contaminated or infected wound; (3) sanguineous (red or bloody drainage)—signifies a healthy wound; (4) serosanguineous (pinkish, red colored exudate)—signifies a healthy wound; (5) purulent or pus (thick, cloudy or opaque exudate; malodorous)—signifies infected wound.

Clinical signs of wound infection: (1) erythema (redness)—can present as a red periwound border or can present as a darker border in darker skin; (2) edema (describe volume, girth, quality, fluctuance, pitting, or nonpitting); (3) induration[4] (a raised swollen area of the periwound—commonly found in chronic infected wounds).

Periwound area: has or does not have edema, induration, and maceration.

Bacteria: is or is not present in the wound; the amount.

Pain: patient's pain level.

Wound Closure

Table 6-9　Wound Closure Terms[1]

Primary intention: healing after the wound was closed using surgery (the edges were brought together with staples, sutures, glue, and/or skin grafts or skin flaps).

Primary intention wound healing goes through the stages of healing but on a smaller scale. Dehiscence (bursts open): process by which the wound healed through primary intention opened up again because of infection or maceration. Dehiscence can happen mostly in surgical abdominal wounds. In cases of dehiscence wound, the surgeon is immediately informed. The wound needs to be covered with sterile dressing or towel moistened with warm sterile physiological saline solution.

Secondary intention: healing when the wound is left to heal on its own. The wound closes through contraction and re-epithelialization or a combination of these two. During secondary intention wound healing, contact inhibition (inhibition of cell division caused by the close contact of similar cells) can happen. In case of contact inhibition, wound healing may need to continue for several years (although the wound is closed). Also, the clinician may have to use different interventions to allow the wound to heal. Factors affecting wound closure by secondary intention are wound depth (if the wound is shallow the closure can be quicker), wound shape (linear wounds contract most rapidly; circular wounds contract slowly), superficial wounds (close by re-epithelialization), partial-thickness wounds (close by re-epithelialization with minimal contraction), full-thickness wounds (close by contraction and scar formation; however, epithelial cells migrate from the wound edges to assist in wound closure if the environment is homeostatic), wound location (areas with least pressure close more rapidly than areas with most pressure), wound etiology (least traumatic wound such as a surgery wound closes more rapidly than traumatic wound such as pressure ulcer wound).

Tertiary intention (delayed primary): wound is allowed to heal by secondary intention and then is closed by primary intention (as the final treatment).

Signs of Potential Wound Infection

Table 6-10   Potential Infection Signs

Change in wound drainage (amount, color, and odor)

Redness or warmth of the periwound areas (it is less obvious in darker skin; may need to palpate the area)

Swelling

Increase in pain and/or tenderness

Patient has fever, nausea, fatigue, loss of appetite

Change in the quality of granulation tissue or failure to produce good quality tissue; for example, granulation tissue that is soft, pale, or easy to break

No measurable wound contraction within 2 to 4 weeks

Factors Contributing to Abnormal Wound Healing

1. Intrinsic factors (internal factors): inadequate blood flow and oxygen; decreased moisture; decrease in elasticity, and collagen, and mast cell production; decrease in vascularity; and the underlying disease (such as diabetes, cancer, circulatory insufficiency, HIV infection, and/or connective tissue diseases).

2. Extrinsic factors (environmental factors): chemotherapy or radiation effects; incontinence; smoking; medications; recreational drugs; alcohol intake; malnutrition; dehydration; infection (bioburden infection, when healing is slowed by pathogens, granulomas, or necrotic tissue); and patient's stress.

3. Tatrogenic factors: injury or illness that occurs as a result of medical care (such as poor wound care because of inappropriate dressings or lack of moisture; sheer injuries such as skin tears during transfers and repositioning; inadequate or absent pressure relieving devices causing ischemia).

Arterial/Venous Insufficiency and Ulcers

Table 6-11   PVD and Ulcerations

Arterial or venous insufficiency causes peripheral vascular disease (PVD). PVD includes any condition that causes partial or complete obstruction of the flow of blood to and from the arteries or veins outside the chest. PVD includes atherosclerosis of the carotid, aortoiliac, femoral, and axillary arteries as well as deep venous thrombosis of the limbs, pelvis, and vena cava.

Venous insufficiency is a failure of the valves of the veins to function, which interferes with venous return to the heart, and may produce edema. Chronic venous insufficiency (CVI) is venous insufficiency that persists for a long period of time. The majority of patients who are diagnosed with PVD also have CVI. Eighty percent of all leg ulcers are caused by venous insufficiency disease. In addition to venous insufficiency, many patients with ulceration also have deep vein thrombosis (DVT). Clinical signs of venous insufficiency are: (1) swelling of unilateral or bilateral lower extremities; (2) itching, fatigue, aching, and heaviness in the involved limb(s); (3) skin changes (hemosiderin staining having iron–containing pigment on the skin); (4) fibrosis of the dermis; (5) increase in skin temperature of the lower legs; (6) wounds on the lower extremities (proximal to medial malleolus;

wounds are not painful; minor dull leg pain of the wound; granulation is present in the wound bed; tissue is wet from excessive draining exudates); (7) may have lymphedema of lower extremities.

Factors that lead to PVD from arterial insufficiency are hypertension, cardiac disease, diabetes, smoking, renal disease, and elevated cholesterol and triglycerides. Contributors to PVD from arterial insufficiency are obesity and sedentary lifestyle. Ten to twenty-five percent of lower extremity ulcers are caused by the PVD from arterial insufficiency disease. Clinical signs of arterial insufficiency are: (1) ulcers located on the lower extremities (at lateral malleoli, dorsum of feet, and toes); (2) abnormal nail growth with thick toenails; (3) decreased or absent leg and foot hair; (4) dry and shiny skin of the lower extremities; (5) pale skin of the lower extremities (in Caucasian people); (7) skin that is cool on palpation; (8) wounds that are painful; (9) patients who have pain in the legs and/or feet (due to intermittent claudication—during exercises muscles do not receive enough blood supply for normal function); (10) wound base of the ulcer that is necrotic and pale without granulation; (11) skin around the wound that is black and may have gangrene (dry); (12) lower extremities pulses that are decreased or absent; (13) lower extremity that is pale on elevation; (14) rubor (redness) of the lower extremity that is observed in dependent position. Patients with clinical signs of arterial insufficiency may also have diabetes.

Neuropathic Ulcers (Caused by Diabetes)

Table 6-12   Neuropathic Ulcers

Neuropathic ulcers:[4] ulcers caused by neuropathy. Neuropathy is any disease of nerves including peripheral and cranial nerves and/or autonomic nervous system. The most common disease process with neuropathy is diabetes mellitus. Diabetic neuropathy affects mostly lower extremity characterized by foot insensitivity and ulcerations. Diabetic neuropathy also called diabetic sensory neuropathy affects feet, lower extremities, and sometimes hands (late in the course of the disease). Usually with diabetic sensory neuropathy, the patient is unable to sense pain and pressure, and there is a risk of skin breakdown without patient being aware of it. Mechanical, repetitive stresses are main causes of neuropathic ulcers. Sometimes patients with diabetic sensory neuropathy may have also foot drop, claw toe or hammer toe deformities, decreased or absent skin sweat and oil production (dry and inelastic skin), heavy callus formation, arterial disorders, and increased vulnerability to skin breakdown.

continues

INTEGUMENTARY INTERVENTIONS

Neuropathic ulcers are most frequently found on the plantar weightbearing surface of the foot and/or at sites of bony prominences (or any other sites on the lower extremity). The wound can be deep, circular in shape, without any pain (secondary to sensory loss), and bleeding easily (except for associated arterial insufficiency). Skin adjacent to the neuropathic ulcer wound is regularly healthy but has also sensory deficits.

Classification of Edema

Table 6-13   Edema Classification

Edema: a local or generalized condition in which the body tissues contain an excessive amount of tissue fluid. Causes of edema are: (1) increased permeability of the capillary walls; (2) increased capillary pressure caused by venous obstruction or heart failure; (3) lymphatic obstruction; (4) disturbances in renal function; (5) reduction of plasma proteins; (6) inflammatory conditions; (7) fluid and electrolyte disturbances (caused by sodium retention); (8) malnutrition; (9) starvation; (10) bacterial toxins, venoms, histamine, or caustic substances.

Types of edema: (1) pitting—edema of the extremities (usually); when pressed firmly with a finger, the skin maintains the depression produced by the finger (1+ indentation is barely detectable; 2+ slight indentation visible when skin is depressed but returns to normal in 15 seconds; 3+ deeper indentation when pressed but returns to normal within 30 seconds; 4+ indentation lasts for more than 30 seconds); (2) nonpitting edema—when pressed firmly with a finger, the skin immediately rebounds to its original contour; (3) brawny[5]—chronic nonpitting edema that is golden brown in color; (4) fibrosis[5]—chronic edema containing fibrous tissue; (5) transudate—mild edema that is part of the inflammatory process; contains clear fluid made of water and dissolved electrolytes; (6) exudate—edema in a more extreme stage of inflammation; appears as pus-like or milky fluid; contains leukocytes; (7) inflammatory—edema associated with inflammation due to damage to the capillary endothelium; it is localized, nonpitting, red, tender, and warm; (8) anasarca[4] (or dropsy)—severe, generalized edema indicating a serious systemic problem such as heart failure or renal disease; (9) lymphedema—an abnormal accumulation of tissue fluid (potential lymph) in the interstitial spaces; can be caused by an impairment in the normal uptake of tissue fluid by the lymphatic vessels or by the excessive production of tissue fluid caused by venous obstruction (that increases capillary blood pressure); common clinical causes of lymphedema are neoplastic obstruction of lymphatic flow (such as in metastatic breast cancer), postoperative interference with lymphatic flow (such as in the axillary dissection), infectious blockage of lymphatics, and radiation damage to lymphatics (such as post treatment of breast or pelvic cancer).

Lymphedema classification: (1) stage I—reversible; is an accumulation of protein rich fluid; elevation of the affected part can reduce the swelling; may have pitting with pressure; (2) stage II—spontaneously irreversible; proteins stimulate fibroblast formation and proliferation of connective and scar tissue; minimal pitting even with moderate swelling; (3) stage III— lymphostatic elephantiasis; the dermal tissue becomes hard; the skin has papillomas and elephant-like looks.

Grading of Arterial Pulses

Table 6-14   Grading

Zero = no pulse
1+ = weak pulse (difficult to palpate)
2+ = diminished pulse (palpable but not normal)
3+ = normal pulse (easy to palpate)
4+ = bounding pulse (very strong; may imply an aneurysm or other pathological condition)

Terms Related to Integumentary Lesions

Table 6-15   Terms Related to Integumentary Lesions

Blisters (swellings) are caused by a breakdown between cells and the primary layers of the skin. A blister is a collection of fluid below or within the epidermis. Blisters can be caused by burns, friction, irritants. Blisters can be elevated (or raised), flat, depressed, ulcer, and fissure.

Elevated (raised) blisters are classified in papule (less than 1 cm in diameter), vesicle (thin walled filled with fluid and less than 1 cm in diameter), plaque (greater than 1 cm in diameter), bulla (thin-walled blister filled with fluid that is larger than 1 cm in diameter), pustule (blister filled with pus), wheal (irregular shaped blister), and crust (dried blister with blood or exudate—fluid with high concentration of protein, cells, or solid debris).

Flat blisters are symmetrical with the skin surface. They can be macules (that are spots lighter or darker than the surrounding skin; examples are freckles; petechiae—small, purplish, hemorrhagic spots on the skin that may signify platelet deficiency; and vitiligo—patchy loss of skin pigment).

continues

Table 6-15 (continued)

Depressed blisters are lower than the skin surface. They can cause excoriation when the epidermis is missing and the dermis is exposed.

Ulcer blisters are crater-like openings caused by the disintegration of the skin.

Fissure blisters are linear cracks or breaks from the epidermis to the dermis.

Urticaria or hives (or wheals) are swollen, raised, red lesions caused by the fluid loss from the blood vessels. They are very itchy and usually indicate an allergic reaction. They may appear primarily on the chest, back, face, scalp, or extremities, and may last up to twenty-four hours. Urticaria can be induced by allergic reactions to cold, ice, heat, exposure to sunlight, skin irritation, or certain medications.

Rash is a local redness accompany by inflammation. It can be caused by allergic reaction, alcoholism, vasomotor disturbance, and skin diseases. It may be accompany by skin eruption and itching. Examples of skin rash are the diaper rash (contact dermatitis caused by prolonged contact with feces and/or urine) and the butterfly rash (on the cheeks and bridge of the nose in systemic lupus erythematosus or seborrheic dermatitis).

Pruritus is skin itching or skin-burning sensation that prompts a person to scratch or rub. It may be an allergic reaction (caused by excess of bilirubin in the blood as in jaundice or by emotional factors).

Xeroderma is excessive dry skin with shedding of the epidermis. It may indicate diabetes or thyroid deficiency.

Edema or swelling of the skin can be caused by anemia, inflammation, obstruction, circulatory problems, and cardiac or renal decompensation (failure of the heart to maintain adequate circulation; failure of kidneys to work properly).

Wrinkles are creases, crevices, furrows, or ridges in the skin. They occur secondary to aging, dehydration, prolonged sun exposure, cigarette smoking, or prolonged immersion in the water.

Unusual skin growths are moles, cysts, nodules (bumps), and fibromas (encapsulated connective tissue tumors that are irregular in shape and slow to grow; they have firm consistency).

Other Integumentary Signs and Symptoms

Table 6-16   Skin Characteristics: Color, Temperature, Perspiration, Soreness, Growths

Changes in skin color: red skin may indicate carbon monoxide poisoning. Yellow skin may indicate jaundice, liver disease, or increased carotene intake. For African

American patients, redness or erythema can be detected by palpation. The skin is usually warmer in the area and is tight and edematous, and the deeper tissues are hard.

Changes in skin color: pallor of the skin may indicate lack of sunlight, shock, malnutrition, vasomotor instability, or the result of hemorrhage. For African American patients, skin pallor appears yellow brown for brown-skinned patients (clients) and ashen gray for black-skinned patients (clients). In addition, mucous membranes of African American patients appear ashen, and the lips and nail beds are similar.

Changes in skin color: cyanosis of the skin (blue, gray discoloration) may be caused by lack of oxygen or increased carbon dioxide in the blood system. For African American patients, cyanosis can be seen by close inspection of lips, tongue, conjunctiva (of the eyelids), palms of the hands, and the soles of the feet. For African American patients, one method of testing for cyanosis is pressing the palms. Slow blood return indicates cyanosis. Another sign is ashen gray lips and tongue.

For African American patients, ecchymosis (that is, superficial bleeding under the skin from trauma) can be detected by swelling of the skin surface.

Brown skin with yellow spots (or liver spots) may be caused by liver malignancies, pregnancy, or aging.

Abnormal heat may indicate febrile condition, excessive salt intake, and excitement.

Abnormal cold may indicate poor circulation.

Increased perspiration may indicate drug intake, fever, exercise performance, and pulmonary condition.

Decreased perspiration may indicate dehydration.

Clinical Impairments and Functional Limitations of Integumentary Conditions

Clinical Impairments and Functional Limitations in Wounds/Burns and Ulcerations

Table 6-17   Impairments and Functional Limitations of Wounds/Burns and Ulcerations

Joint swelling, inflammation, joint stiffness, or contracture
Increased pain
Soft tissue swelling, inflammation, and stiffness
Decreased gait, locomotion, and balance
Decreased strength, power, and endurance
Decreased postural control
Decreased sensory awareness
Weightbearing difficulties
Decreased ability to perform physical actions, tasks, or activities related to self-care, home management, work (job, school, or play), community, and leisure activities
Decreased ability to perform ADLs or IADLs
Use of assistive devices and equipment during ADLs or IADLs
Decreased tolerance of positions and activities

Integumentary Conditions and Impairments (Not Related to Wounds, Burns, and Ulcerations)

Table 6-18   Integumentary Conditions and Impairments (Not Related to Wounds, Burns, and Ulcerations)

Dermatitis is inflammation of the skin caused by the following: (1) allergic reaction (due to chemical, mechanical, or biological agents, sensitivity to sunlight, or ultraviolet exposure); (2) hereditary cause; (3) psychological disorders. Impairments are itching, skin lesions (crust, plaque, fibrotic papules and nodules), redness, and skin oozing.

Cellulitis is inflammation of connective tissue or cellular tissue (such as dermis, subcutaneous layers, and tissue spaces) accompanied by infection. Impairments are edema, erythema, skin tenderness, nodules, and skin heat.

Herpes I (herpes simplex), herpes II, and herpes zoster (shingles) are caused by viral and bacterial infections. Impairments: (1) herpes I—fever blister or cold sore; (2) herpes II—vesicular genital eruption; newborns may have inflammation of the

continues

INTEGUMENTARY INTERVENTIONS

Table 6-18 (continued)

brain and its meninges; (3) herpes zoster (shingles)—pain and tingling; itching of
the corresponding dermatome; papules (fluid-filled); malaise; fever; chills; gastrointestinal disturbances; urination difficulty; pain in the affected joints; neuralgia
(constant and intermittent).

Scleroderma (systemic sclerosis): immune integumentary disorder; chronic progressive disorder of vessels and connective tissue characterized by hardening or
excessive collagen deposition in skin, joints, internal organs (such as the gastrointestinal tract, lungs, kidneys, and heart). Scleroderma can be localized or systemic and can be accompanied by the Raynaud's phenomenon (vasospastic
disease of small arteries and arterioles; unknown causes; attacks of numbness
and sensation of cold; may have throbbing and paresthesia; affects mostly the
digits of hands bilaterally). Impairments are pain in the affected areas, joint stiffness, edema of fingers and joints, skin thickening (may be limited to face and
distal extremities or may be diffuse to face, whole extremities, and trunk), and
contractures.

Psoriasis: immune integumentary disorder; inherited chronic recurrent inflammatory
condition accompanied by rash and scaly red or silvery plaques. The rash can be
found commonly on the knees, shins, elbows, umbilicus, lower back, buttocks,
ears, and the hairline. Also, pitting of the nails can occur. The severity of the disease can range from a minimal cosmetic problem to total body surface involvement. Precipitating factors are stress, pregnancy, infection, cold weather,
smoking, endocrine changes, and anxiety. Impairments are skin that shades, skin
lesions, thick and scaly skin, and grape-like skin clusters.

Eczema: immune skin disorder; common superficial inflammatory condition characterized by itchy red rash that initially weeps or oozes serum and may become
crusted, thickened, or scaly. Causes are allergies, irritating chemicals, drugs,
scratching or rubbing the skin, and sun exposure. Eczema may be acute or
chronic, and the rash may become infected. There are different types of eczema:
erythematous, herpeticum (from herpes simplex virus), lichenoid (with thickening
of the skin), nummular (with coin or oval shaped lesions), pustular (follicular,
impetiginous such as chronic squamous eczema on soles, legs, scalp), and seborrheic (with excessive secretions from sebaceous glands). Eczema is not treated in
physical therapy; however, PT/PTA should be able to recognize the condition and
check the patient's (client's) skin before and after applying modalities that use topical substances on the skin.

Lupus erythematosus: immune skin disorder (caused by an autoimmune process);
chronic, progressive inflammatory disorder of the connective tissues characterized by remission and exacerbation. Patient (client) may have scaling, red, macu-

lar rash. Systemic lupus erythematosus (SLE): chronic autoimmune inflammatory disease involving multiple organ systems and marked by periodic acute episodes. Patient has the "butterfly" rash over the nose and cheeks. SLE is most prevalent in women of childbearing age. Impairments are malaise, overwhelming fatigue, polyarthralgia, fever, arthritis, skin rash ("butterfly" rash), photosensitivity, hair loss, and Raynaud's disease (vasospastic disease of small arteries and arterioles affecting the digits of the hands bilaterally; the cause is unknown; patient has intermittent vasospastic attacks in response to cold or emotion).

Polymyositis: immune skin disorder; inflammatory disease of skeletal muscles characterized by symmetrical weakness of the proximal muscles of the extremities; evidence of muscle necrosis on biopsy; skin rash over eyelids or papules over the dorsal surface of the knuckles; rapid and severe etiology; may require ventilator and tube feeding. It is also called dermatomyositis. Impairments are symmetrical weakness of the proximal muscles of the extremities.

Types of Integumentary Interventions

Burn Rehabilitation Interventions

Table 6-19 General Interventions for Burns

Burn rehabilitation is a team work that includes many professionals.[1] PT's goals in the plan of care are devised together with the patient and patient's family. To attain the objectives of optimal long-term function, long-term goals begin at the outset of burn care. Generally, there are three principles that the PT must consider: performing ROM, splinting and antideformity positioning, establishing a long-term relationship with the patient and family members to ensure compliance with therapy goals and to increase the patient's morale for recovery.

In the intensive care unit, PROM in all planes of motion is performed twice daily considering patient's pain, anxiety, wound status, extremity perfusion, and security of the patient's airway and vascular access devices. In burn care, PROM can be timed to coincide with dressing changes and wound cleansing minimizing the patient's need for pain medications.

Burn contractures and prevention interventions: (1) axillary adduction contractures can be prevented by positioning the shoulders widely abducted at 90° with axillary splints, padded hanging troughs of thermoplastic material, or a variety of support devices mounted to the bed. (2) Elbow flexion contractures can be minimized by statically splinting the elbow in extension; elbow splints can be alternated with flexion splints to help retain a full ROM. (3) Flexion contractures of the hips and knees (particularly common in children) can be prevented by positioning the patient in extension (for the anterior hip, supine with hip and knee extended, in external rotation and abduction, with pillow under hips for increased extension—also can be positioned prone but is poorly tolerated; for the posterior knee, knees must be positioned in supine without pillow—also can use a knee immobilizer). (4) Equinus deformity (ankle plantarflexed and foot in varus) can be prevented with static splinting of the ankles in neutral position (may use an anterior ankle conformer or an AFO at 90°); use padding on the splints over the metatarsal heads or calcaneus to distribute pressure evenly. (5) Anterior neck deformity can be prevented using a neck conformer that maintains chin to chest distance and no pillow in bed. (6) Posterior neck deformity can be prevented using a neck conformer that maintains length in posterior neck, pillow in supine position (or pillow under chest in prone position). (7) Hand deformity in an "intrinsic minus position " contracture (MP joints are fixed in hyperextension and PIP joints are fixed in flexion) can be prevented by placing the MP joints at maximum flexion (90°) to maximally stretch the collateral ligaments; placing the wrist at 30° of extension (some authors indicate only 15° anterior wrist extension or 15° for posterior wrist flexion, depending

continues

Table 6-19 (continued)

on the burned area) and IP joints in full extension; thumb must be fully abducted; with massive burns and patient resuscitation in first 24 to 48 hours, the wrist can be elevated (using a volar cock-up splint) at 70° to 80° (pulls the MP and IP joints in a safe position).

The splints need to be inspected at least twice daily to check for poor fit or pressure injury.

As critical illness is reduced and wounds progressively close, the interventions concentrate on (1) PROM; (2) AROM; (3) light strengthening exercises; (4) minimizing edema (that contributes to tightness); (5) ADL training; (6) initial scar management; (7) preparing patient for work, play, or school.

During wound closure period, the patient may be ready to be discharged from the hospital. The interventions concentrate on (1) progressive PROM; (2) strengthening exercises; (3) specific postoperative therapy after reconstructive operations; (4) and scar management.

Extreme pruritus that begins shortly after the wound has healed, peaks in intensity months after injury, and then gradually subsides in most patients. Interventions are massage, frequent application of skin moisturizers or colloidal baths, vitamin E topical cream, and topical cold compresses. In some cases, pruritus can cause skin excoriation and infections of the wound (with *Staphylococcus aureus* bacteria). In these cases, patients (clients) need to see the physician and receive antibiotics or be admitted to hospital.

Burn reconstructive surgical methods: incisional release and grafting, excisional release and grafting, Z-plasty, and random flaps (may be used for chest wall or hands burns).

Elements to Effect Wound Healing

Table 6-20   Wound Healing Elements

Oxygen:[6] necessary for wound healing; important for granulation, angiogenesis, collagen deposition, and wound contraction; has antibiotic effect to resist pathogens. With wounds, oxygen has difficulty reaching tissue especially when edema, necrotic tissue, and peripheral vasoconstriction are present. Interventions such as debridement (to clean necrotic tissue) and compression (to decrease edema) are necessary to decrease the obstruction to wound oxygenation. Vasoconstriction may not always be improved. Factors contributing to improvement of oxygen levels in the wound are nutrition, hydration, keeping the wound warm, controlling pain and anxiety, avoiding smoking, and possibly using supplemental oxygen. Recent studies[6] showed that oxygen delivered directly to a localized limb chamber (called topical hyperbaric oxygen [THBO]) improved wound healing.

Moisture:[6] necessary for wound healing; represents a newer concept of wound healing. Moisture can soften eschar and create autolytic debridement (body's own enzymes dissolves the eschar under right conditions). Factors contributing to improvement of moisture levels in the wound are wound hydration, using occlusive dressing (such as hydrocolloids that can even be applied over an infected wound with systemic antibiotic regimen), limiting fluid loss from the wound surface, controlling heavy exudates, and allowing gaseous exchange.

Nutrition:[6] necessary for wound healing. Factors contributing to improvement of wound healing through nutrition include increasing levels of iron, vitamin B_{12}, folic acid, vitamin C, zinc, vitamin A, arginine (for healing and immune response), and amino acids (high protein intake) in the blood.

Integumentary Patient Education

Table 6-21   Patient Education Elements

Community resources; support groups (related to patient's diagnosis)

Counseling

Family and/or caregiver participation

Internet resources:

   http://www.lymphnet.org/ for lymphedema (see Appendix C for patient's copy for lymphedema education)

   http://www.advancingthepractice.org/index.html or http://www.apwca.org for wound care

   http://www.ameriburn.org for burn care

   http://diabetes.niddk.nih.gov/dm/pubs/complications_feet/index.htm for diabetes

Education materials such as instructional materials, multimedia information, or self-management information

Home program: (1) skin care; (2) wound care; (3) prevention (such as for patients with diabetes: to inspect the feet daily; to be aware of changes in skin color, visible skin breakdown such as cracks, fissures, blisters and abrasions; to inspect for callus formation; to keep dry and flaky skin hydrated with nonperfumed water based lotions; not to place lotions between the toes; to place lotions after cleaning first with mild soap and warm tap water; to test the water temperature with a thermometer or their elbow but never with their fingers); (4) scar management;

continues

Table 6-21 (continued)

(5) exercises; (6) compression garment or bandage wear and care; (7) pressure-relieving devices (such as beds, mattresses, overlays placed on top of mattress, or special seat cushions); (8) edema control; (9) foot care for patients with diabetes.

Patient Education for Skin Care

Table 6-22 Skin Care Education (for Diabetes)[7]

See Appendix D for patient's copy

After you wash with a mild soap, make sure that you rinse and dry yourself well. Check places where water can hide, such as under the arms, under the breasts, and between the legs and toes.

Drink lots of fluids (such as water) to keep your skin moist and healthy.

Keep your skin moist by using a lotion or cream after you wash. Ask your doctor to suggest one.

Wear all cotton underwear. Cotton allows air to move around your body better.

Check your skin after you wash. Make sure you have no dry, red, or sore spots that might lead to an infection.

Tell your doctor about any skin problems.

Patient Education for Foot Care

Table 6-23 Foot Care Education (for Diabetes)[7]

See Appendix E for patient's copy

Wash your feet in warm water every day. Make sure the water is not too hot by testing the temperature with your elbow. Do not soak your feet. Dry your feet well, especially between your toes.

Look at your feet every day to check for cuts, sores, blisters, redness, calluses, or other problems. Checking every day is more important if you have nerve damage or poor blood flow. If you cannot bend over or pull your feet up to check them, use a mirror. If you cannot see well, ask someone else to check your feet.

If your skin is dry, rub lotion on your feet after you wash and dry them. Do not put lotion between your toes.

File corn and calluses gently with an emery board or pumice stone. Do this after your bath or shower.

Cut your toenails once a week or when needed. Cut toenails when they are soft from washing. Cut them to the shape of the toe and not too short. File the edges with an emery board.

Always wear socks or slippers to protect your feet from injuries.

Always wear socks or stockings to avoid blisters. Do not wear socks or knee high stockings that are too tight below your knee.

Wear shoes that fit well. Shop for shoes at the end of the day when your feet are bigger. Break in shoes slowly. Wear them 1 to 2 hours each day for the first 1 to 2 weeks.

Before putting your shoes on, feel the insides to make sure they have no sharp edges or objects that might injure your feet.

Tell your doctor right away about any foot problems.

As your doctor to look at your feet at each checkup. To make sure your doctor checks your feet, take off your shoes and socks before your doctor comes into the room.

Ask your doctor to check how well the nerves in your feet sense feeling.

Ask your doctor to check how well blood is flowing to your legs and feet.

Ask your doctor to show you the best way to trim your toenails. Ask what lotion or cream to use on your legs and feet.

If you cannot cut your toenails or you have a foot problem, ask your doctor to send you to a foot doctor (called a podiatrist).

Wound Cleansing Methods

Table 6-24 Wound Cleansing Methods

A whirlpool[6] is not used much anymore, except for special situations when the wound needs intensive cleansing or softening of loosely adherent tissue (before sharp, enzymatic, or autolytic debridement) that cannot be done with other methods. When the whirlpool is used, it needs minimal agitation of water for 5 to 10 minutes to limit the negative effects of temperature and pressure changes. Iodine povidone or chlorine can be added to the water only if infection is present. Also, wounds that need stimulation of peripheral circulation may benefit from the whirlpool. When the whirlpool is used with PVD, the temperature should not exceed 1°C (or 33.8°F) above skin temperature. The whirlpool water temperature ranges from 33.5°C to 35.5°C (or 92°F to 96°F). When cardiopulmonary conditions exist, the whirlpool temperature should not exceed 38°C (or 100.4°F). In general, the whirlpool is contraindicated for clean granulating wounds, epithelializing

continues

Table 6-24 (continued)

wounds, migrating epidermal cells, new skin grafts, new tissue flaps, venous ulcers (and venous insufficiency), nonnecrotic diabetic ulcers, wound maceration, and dry gangrene.

Pulsatile lavage with suction (PLWS): also called forceful irrigation is a form of cleaning the wound and performing debridement. PLWS can remove the irrigation fluid, wound exudates, and loose debris using the pulsed irrigation and the simultaneous suction. PLWS can also deliver antiseptics, topical antibiotics, and antibacterial solutions to the wound and can treat tunneling and undermining wounds (using special cannula tips). PLWS is a better method than the whirlpool because it requires less treatment time and less staff, and can be performed at the bedside or at the patient's home. Patient's family or visitors are not allowed in the room during the procedure. The disadvantages of PLWS are risk of trauma to newly formed tissue (because of the plastic tips or the suction) and risk of overuse with clean, granulating wounds.

Nonforceful irrigation is another form of cleaning the wound using minimal pressure or force. Nonforceful irrigation can be accomplished using: package saline for wound cleansing, single-dose sterile saline, and spray containers (at gentle pressure) with saline. Nonforceful irrigation can be used for infected wounds, clean wounds with new tissue growth (to remove excess fluids or residue from dressings), and necrotic wounds or debris (may need a few sessions of nonforceful irrigation or the PLWS).

Wound Debridement Methods

Table 6-25   General Debridement Methods

Debridement: removal of foreign material and dead or damaged tissue.

Nonselective mechanical debridement: removal of all tissue (necrotic and living tissue). Uses dressings such as (1) wet to dry dressings (wet gauze applied to the wound bed that debrides the wound by being pulled away when it dries; used for moderate amounts of necrotic tissue; may traumatize healthy or healing tissue; can be painful to the patient; the research is controversial about benefits and disadvantages); (2) pulsatile lavage with suction (PLWS is mentioned previously here); (3) whirlpool (mentioned previously here; biggest disadvantage is tissue maceration; waterborne pathogens that can cause contamination or infection; disinfecting additives that may be cytotoxic).

Chemical (enzymatic) selective debridement: removal of necrotic tissue (usually in large amounts) and eschar using topical agents containing enzymes. Some enzymatic debriders are selective and some are not. The dressings are prescribed by a physician. Enzymatic debridement: (1) is fast acting; (2) causes minimal or no damage to healthy tissue with proper application; (3) is expensive; (4) needs to be applied and performed carefully and only to the necrotic tissue; (5) may require a specific secondary dressing; (6) may cause inflammation or discomfort. A type of enzymatic selective debridement is the autolytic debridement that uses the body's own enzymes and moisture to rehydrate, soften, and liquefy hard eschar and slough. With this type of debridement, only necrotic tissue is liquefied. Types of autolytic debridement dressings are occlusive or semiocclusive dressings (such as hydrocolloids, hydrogels, and transparent films).

Enzymatic debriders include two general types of enzymatic debriding agents. The first type contains papain and urea in a cream base (or in a formulation of chlorophyllin and copper) that may need once or twice a day application. The second type is made of collagenase in a petroleum base that may need to be applied once daily. Examples of enzymatic dressing: (1) proteolytic enzyme dressing—uses topical enzyme (digest and liquefy necrotic tissue in the wound bed; dressing should be left in place for 2 to 3 days; when dressing is removed, the wound should be irrigated with normal saline solution to remove liquefied debris; requires multiple applications; is pain free and less stressful to the patient; is not appropriate for infected wounds; (2) collagenase—water-soluble proteinase that specifically attacks and breaks down collagen; digests undernatured collagen fibers allowing the necrotic plug to be removed; is more selective than proteolytic enzyme; studies[8,9] showed that granulation and epithelialization proceeded faster than was expected in chronic dermal lesions (ulcers and pressure ulcers); good for maintenance debridement also; decreases bacterial capability.

Sharp selective debridement: type of debridement when the clinician uses surgical instruments to remove the necrotic tissue from the wound. In physical therapy, PTs (as per the APTA) are the only individuals allowed to use sharp debridement (with scalpels, scissors, or forceps) and only in the presence of necrotic tissue (PTA to check the state's practice act). Surgeons may also use surgery (and laser) for this method of debridement. The biggest challenge in this type of debridement is to differentiate yellow slough from tendons. Usually, sharp debridement would be recommended for infected wounds with systemic sepsis or necrotizing fasciitis. Caution should be used in patients with clotting disorders or taking anticoagulants (because uncontrolled bleeding may occur). Sharp debridement is painful to the patient and is costly if the operating room and surgery are required.

Types of Wound Dressings

Table 6-26   Wound Dressings

Wound dressing choice is dependent on the following wound characteristics: necrosis, drainage, infection, granulation tissue, epithelialization, periwound area, cavities and tunneling, friction, wound odor, and incontinence.

Primary dressing: applied directly to the wound. Secondary dressing: dressing applied over the primary dressing.

Gauze dressing can be used as secondary dressing, especially if changed frequently. Gauze dressing should not be used as primary dressing because leaves contamination fibers, is adherent to wound, is permeable to bacteria, can cause wound desiccation, releases excessive amounts of bacteria, and causes pain on removal. Gauze ribbon can be used to maintain an opening for drainage in a tunneling wound. Wounds cavities should not be packed very full to allow flow of oxygen and nutrients to the wound, a place for granulation tissue, and epithelial cells survival. A type of gauze, called impregnated gauze (also called petrolatum gauze), can be used as the primary dressing (because does not stick to the wound, is minimally absorptive, can create a greasy wound bed, and offers minimal protection).

Transparent films are made of transparent membrane with acrylic adhesive layer. Films do not allow bacteria or moisture into the wound and assist with skin protection from shearing, friction, or contamination (from incontinence). Films removal can cause skin tears (with frail or aging skin). Films are semiocclusive and trap moisture, allowing autolytic debridement of necrotic wounds and creating a moist healing environment for granulating wounds. Films[10] can be used as a protective dressing and as a topical treatment for stage I and stage II pressure ulcers, minimally draining or nondraining surgical wounds, lacerations and abrasions, partial thickness wounds, noninfected wounds, and wounds with necrosis or slough.

Application of film dressing: clip excess hair around the wound site (to ensure proper adhesion). Clean the wound and periwound skin with normal saline solution (or other cleaner). Dry the skin well so that the film can adhere to it. Apply the film dressing over the wound, smoothing it into the place. Remove the film's delivery systems (such as window, frame, or paperback release) before applying it. Do not use tension when applying it (can tear the skin). Remove it as per manufacture's instructions.

Hydrogels can be amorphous (liquid-like gel) or sheets (thin, flexible sheets with 90% water). Hydrogels increase moisture[11] in a dry wound bed, and soften necrotic tissue. They may require a secondary dressing to be contained in the wound. This feels very soothing for the patient.

Foams: highly absorbent pads, sheets, or packing of polyurethane; available with or without adhesive backing; can be used as primary or secondary dressings; create an occlusive environment; should not be used alone on a dry wound.

Hydrocolloids: most occlusive of the moisture retentive dressings; also are available as less occlusive or semipermeable; are available in various styles and shapes; work the best on moderate to mild exudating wounds. Three types of hydrocolloids are available: pastes, powders, and sheets. Pastes and powders can be used as wound fillers but should not protrude above the level of the surrounding skin. The hydrocolloid sheets usually cover the pastes and powders. Hydrocolloid dressings[12,13] react with wound drainage and swell or "melt out," leaving a residue in the wound with a malodorous smell (from product breakdown, not necessarily from infection). The residue needs to be removed by cleaning gently with a wound cleanser.

Hydrocolloid application: hydrocolloids adhere best at body temperature. To increase adherence, the therapist should place his or her hand over the dressing after applying it to the wound. The heat from the therapist's hand will assist in molding the dressing to the wound and facilitate adherence. Hydrocolloid dressings with thick edges may "roll up" and adhere to patient's clothing or bed linen, decreasing the dressing's wear time. Thinner hydrocolloid dressings with tapered edges adhere better to the periwound skin without rolling up; when the dressing is removed, be careful with patient's skin (can tear).

Type of hydrocolloid dressing: 3M-Tegasorb (studies[12,13] showed that it had better adherence than ConvaTec's Granuflex; it can be used on all stages of wound healing from black necrotic tissue to the epithelializing wound).

Alginates are fibrous products derived from brown seaweed and are available in nonwoven sheets and ropes. Alginic acid (main component from alginates) is converted into calcium salts (that are water insoluble) and sodium salts (that are water soluble). Alginates can be used for wounds with moderate to heavy drainage. They form a gel when they come in contact with wound fluid. Alginate dressing can absorb up to 20 times its weight in fluid. Alginates can be used in infected and noninfected wounds. They should not be used with dry wounds or wounds with minimal drainage because they could dehydrate the wound delaying the healing process.

Alginate dressing application: alginate dressing is packed into the wound bed as the primary dressing. Then a secondary dressing is added to hold the alginate in place and maintain the moist healing environment; petrolatum gauzes or foams can secure the alginate and keep it from drying out. If the wound is infected, the secondary dressing should be nonocclusive (not to harbor bacteria and to allow the wound to be monitored). When the secondary dressing is removed, hydration of

continues

INTEGUMENTARY INTERVENTIONS

Table 6-26 (continued)

the alginate should be assessed. If the alginate has absorbed wound exudates[13,14] (as intended), it will be in a gelled state and easy to remove from the wound. If the alginate is difficult to remove or if fibrous material adheres to the wound base, the wound is drying out. In that situation, the alginate may not be needed to maintain hydration, and another dressing appropriate for a wound with little or no exudates may be used.

New type of dressing: composite dressing that has multiple layers dressing that can be used as primary or secondary dressings. They are appropriate for wounds with minimal to heavy exudates, healthy granulation tissue, necrotic tissue (or moist eschar), or a mixture of granulation and necrotic tissue. Some composite dressing cannot be used on infected wounds (check the manufacture's instructions). Composite dressings should be used cautiously if the patient is dehydrated or has fragile skin. Also, some insurers may not reimburse a facility or provider if a composite dressing is used as secondary dressing with a hydrogel or impregnated gauze. Most composite dressings have three layers: (1) a semi-adherent or non-adherent (touches and protects the wound from adhering to other material, allows dressing to be removed without disturbing new tissue, and when applying an antibiotic ointment, it will not stick to it); (2) absorptive (wicks drainage and debris from wound's surface, prevents skin maceration and bacterial growth, maintains a moist healing environment, and helps to liquefy eschar and necrotic debris—autolytic debridement); (3) bacterial (outer layer of the composite dressing that allows moisture vapor to pass from the wound to the air, keeps bacteria and particles out, and maintains a moist environment). Examples of composite dressings are Alldress, Covaderm Plus, Telfa, Ventex, Viasorb, and Tegaderm with absorbent pad.

New type of dressing: bioengineered tissue,[15–17] that is, tissue-engineered biological dressing. Bioengineered tissue can be used for burns, chronic venous or pressure ulcers, donor site and other surgical wounds, blisters, and skin desquamations. Bioengineered tissue can deliver growth factors and extracellular matrix components to the wound. Bioengineered tissue is controversial[15] in wound care because it does not match a treatment modality to an underlying pathology. Clinical effect is modest[16,17] and not necessarily justifiable from a cost benefit perspective. Examples of bioengineered tissue products are Dermagraft, Apligraf, and Cultured Epidermal Autograft (Epicel, or a newer one called OrCel). Research studies[16,17] showed that bioengineered tissue such as Dermagraft and Apligraf had suffered commercial setbacks in recent years, although the clinical trials proved the efficacy of these products. The reasons for the setbacks were high costs and restricted healthcare resources; however, new products such as OrCel or older ones such as AlloDerm acellular dermal matrix or Integra Bilayer Matrix Wound Dressing (BMWD) are finding niche applications where clinical utility is high and the cost can be defended.

Patient's Safety Precautions During Wound Interventions

Table 6-27   Precautions in Wound Interventions

Monitor patient's vital signs at all times. Some facilities may use the Ankle Brachial Index (ABI) pulse monitoring that measures patient's blood pressure (BP) at two sites (the ankle and the brachial artery) at rest and after 5 minutes of treadmill walk and then divide the highest BP at the ankle by the highest BP at the brachial artery. The normal resting ABI = 1 or 1.1 (the BP at the ankle is the same or greater than the BP at brachial artery; there is no narrowing or blockage of blood flow). Resting ABI of less than 1 is abnormal (ABI of less than 0.95 = narrowing of one or more blood vessels in the legs). Pain in the leg, foot, or buttock during exercises and ABI of less than 0.8 = intermittent claudication with exercises or activity. ABI of less than 0.4 = patient exhibits symptoms of intermittent claudication at rest. ABI of less than 0.25 or below = severe PAD is present.

During wound interventions, be aware of infection signs and symptoms and immediately inform the PT (and the nursing staff when necessary). Infection signs and symptoms are: (1) increase or decrease in BP; (2) fever; (3) a decrease in red blood cell count; (4) an increase in white blood cell count; (5) wound development signs such as the appearance and development of odor (or worsening of odor).

Be aware of excessive wound bleeding that will not coagulate (especially if debridement is included in interventions).

Pressure Ulcers and Interventions

Table 6-28   Pressure Ulcers and Interventions

Pressure ulcers: ulcers located at areas of tissue compression and inadequate perfusion. Pressure ulcers commonly occur in patients who are bed or chair bound. These patients (clients) can be: (1) patients with sensory and mobility impairments (such as spinal cord injury, stroke, or coma); (2) patients (clients) who are malnourished; (3) patients with peripheral vascular disease; (4) older patients who are hospitalized; (5) nursing home residents; (5) patients (clients) who are incontinent.

continues

INTEGUMENTARY
INTERVENTIONS

Table 6-28 (continued)

The most common sites of skin breakdown where pressure sores can occur are the bony prominences (such as elbows, scapulae, sacrum, ischial tuberosities, malleoli, greater trochanter, and heels). The combination of pressure shearing forces, friction, and moisture may lead to tissue injury and occasionally necrosis. The pressure ulcer can progress rapidly from a red patch of skin to erosion into the subcutaneous tissues and extending to muscle or bone. Deep ulcers can get infected with bacteria and develop gangrene. For staging of pressure ulcers see the above sections.

Prevention: the most important principle of therapy for pressure ulcers is prevention. Prevention includes the following: (1) regular skin inspection, (2) frequent turning of immobile patients (considering potential areas of breakdown), and (3) application of pressure relieving devices (PRDs) (such as skin protectors to bony body parts, and use of specialized air–fluid beds, waterbeds, or beds with polystyrene beads). Other prevention measures are: (4) always cleanse and dry the skin; (5) apply skin lubricants and emollients; (6) maintain clean, dry linen and clothing; (7) eliminate mechanical forces; (8) encourage early ambulation and appropriate use of assistive devices; (9) encourage ROM exercises.

Pressure ulcers interventions: (1) Use interventions with minimal skin friction (when the skin becomes ischemic, the reddened areas of the skin should never be massaged because it can damage ischemic deep layers of tissue; the skin should be thoroughly cleansed, rinsed, and dried, and emollients should be gently applied by minimizing force and friction especially over bony prominences). (2) Patients who are able to sit in a chair should be placed on a low pressure cushion and helped to shift their weight every 15 minutes. Sitting time should be limited to less than 2 hours to reduce pressure over the ischial tuberosities. (3) Patients who are not able to position themselves need to be repositioned every 1 to 2 hours to prevent tissue hypoxia (from compression). (4) A turning schedule is necessary. (5) A turning sheet or a pad can be used to turn patients (using minimal skin friction). (6) The head of the bed should not be elevated higher than 30° (except for short periods of time) to reduce shearing forces on the skin and subcutaneous tissues overlying the sacrum. (7) Early ambulation and ROM exercises should be encouraged as well as high-protein, nutritious meals. (8) Doughnut-type cushions should not be used because they decrease blood flow to tissues resting in the center of the doughnut.

When pressure ulcers occur, they need to be cleansed and debrided depending on the institution's protocol (or prescription) and the PT's Plan of Care (POC).

Other Integumentary Interventions for Lymphedema, Edema, and Wounds

Table 6-29   Other Lymphedema/Edema/Wound Interventions

Manual lymphatic drainage (MLD): specialized manual therapy technique that affects primarily the superficial lymphatic circulation. The benefits of MLD are improvement of lymph transport capacity, redirecting lymph flow toward collateral vessels, increasing the frequency of lymphangion contractions, anastomoses, and mobilization of excess lymph fluid (that overwhelms a body segment). MLD requires specialized education to be able to perform.

External compression pump (ECP): indicated for patients who have congenital lymphedema or acquired lymphatic dysfunctions (to prevent pain and infection, decrease possibility of skin breakdown, and increase function). Newest research[6] is contradictory about the use of ECP for edema or lymphedema. However, ECP can be used for: (1) chronic edema in patients with decreased mobility (creates a pumping effect in patients who have decreased muscle pump capability due to paralysis or weakness); (2) venous stasis wound (can remove edema and prevent venous pooling allowing the wound to heal); (3) residual limb shrinkage (for amputations to prepare for prosthetic fitting); (4) prevention of thrombophlebitis, tissue healing and scar management for wounds and burns; (5) arterial insufficiency (to increase venous return and provide more blood flow in arterial circulation). Types of ECP[5] include intermittent pneumatic compression (IPC) unit (air pumps), IPC units with additional features (such as the Wright linear pump, the Huntleigh sequential system, the NormaTec pneumatic compression pump, and the Jobst Cryo/Temp unit), and a small portable unit for home (Jobst Cryo/Temp unit for ankle, foot, knee, hand, wrist, and elbow injury intervention since it contains a cooling unit). Contraindications of ECP: HTN (BP of 140/90), pulmonary edema, CHF, DVT and obstructed venous vessels, unstable fracture, acute local infection, and severe peripheral arterial occlusive disease.

ECP intervention method precautions: (1) pressure on UE not to exceed 40 to 60 mmHg; (2) pressure on lower extremity not to exceed 40 to 70 mmHg; (3) pressure lower than 30 mmHg is not recommended. For postmastectomy lymphedema:[5] pressure should be 30 to 50 mmHg; two 3-hour treatments per day; 80 to 100 sec on and 25 to 35 sec off. For peripheral edema and venous stasis ulceration: pressure should be 85 mmHg; one 2.5-hour treatment, three times per week; 80 to 100 sec on and 30 sec off. For lower extremity edema: pressure should be 30 to 60 mmHg; two 3-hours treatments per day; 80 to 100 sec on and 25 to 35 sec off.

continues

INTEGUMENTARY INTERVENTIONS

Table 6-29 (continued)

Other lymphedema/wounds interventions: (1) extremity elevation (to control mild and acute swelling; may be a precursor to compression pump); (2) Unna's boot (application of zinc paste impregnated gauze; good for venous wounds); (3) four-layer bandage system (using Profore; for leg ulcers closure; can be left in place for a week; manufacturer claims that provides 40 mmHg of pressure at the ankle); (4) long stretch and short stretch bandages (for edema control and for lymphedema); (5) lymphedema bandaging (highly specialized form of bandaging using multiple layers of unique padding materials and short stretch bandages; the PT/PTA needs to learn different techniques for different body areas); (6) compression garments (garments used to assist venous flow; used for arterial wounds, venous wounds, neuropathic ulcers, lymphedema, and edema; are also used for burns and surgical scars; contraindicated for DVT, acute local infection, CHF, acute dermatitis, and cor pulmonale; provide support to venous circulation; prevent reaccumulation of fluid in the lymphedema; should not be used to remove excess fluids from an extremity; should be customized to each individual).

Prevention interventions: (1) positioning (to prevent or support pressure ulcers, wounds, edema, lymphedema, and vascular disorders); (2) pressure-relieving devices (PRD)—check Web sites for information and experts on PRD; (3) exercises (PT/PTA to make a customized exercise prescription for the patient depending on patient's needs and medical status; recommended exercises/activities are aquatic exercises and ambulation activities); (4) scar management (can use compression garments, stretching exercises, orthotics, positioning, silicone gel sheets, topical oils, creams and ointments, and specific massage techniques).

Orthotics: (1) can use resting splints; dynamic splints; total contact cast and posterior walking splints for neuropathic ulcers on plantar surface of foot; (2) can use neuropathic walker made from a removable customized AFO; (3) can use cast shoes or postoperative shoes for wound off loading; (4) can use extra depth shoes with room for the toes and deep sole for shock absorption; (5) for distal aspects of foot, can use wedge shoes such as Ortho Wedge.

Electrotherapeutic modalities: (1) high-voltage pulsed current (HVPC) (used at frequency of 100 pps for 60 minutes, 5 days/week promotes healing of dermal ulcers; method is applying one electrode over the wound using a saline-moistened gauze interface and the other electrode some distance from the wound; for debridement or epithelialization, use positive electrode; for all, others use negative electrode); (2) ultrasound (US) (pulsed 2 milliseconds on and 8 milliseconds off at a frequency of 1 or 3 MHz depending on the tissue depth, with intensity of 0.5 watts/cm^2 are best for dermal tissue).

Immunocompromised Patients and Infection Control

Table 6-30   Immunocompromised Patients and Infection Control

Patients with burns and wounds may have a compromised immune system. The altered immune system can affect: endogenous normal flora; gastrointestinal system; genitourinary system; respiratory system; mucous membrane function; skin breakdown. Immunocompromised patients vary in their susceptibility to nosocomial infections, depending on the severity and duration of immunosuppression. They are at increased risk for bacterial, fungal, parasitic, and viral infections from both endogenous and exogenous sources.

PTs/PTAs should use standard precautions for all patients and transmission-based precautions for specified patients to reduce the acquisition by these patients of institutionally acquired bacteria from other patients and environments.

For CDC standard precautions and transmission-based precautions, see Part I.

Infection control strategies during wound/burn interventions: (1) use proper hand-washing techniques; (2) use standard precautions; (3) use clean and sterile techniques when handling wounds or burns; (4) use masks for respiratory diseases; (5) sterilize and disinfect equipment used in wound/burn interventions; (6) maintain patient's (client's) skin integrity. (7) Remember the modes of transmission of infection: direct transmission (through hands and broken skin), indirect transmission (through tubes, needles, dressings, catheters, equipment), droplet transmission (cough or sneeze), and vehicle transmission (blood).

Infectious agents: exogenous and endogenous bacteria, fungi, and viruses.

Opportunistic agents: *Pseudomonas aeruginosa* (bacterial), tuberculosis, pneumocystis carinii pneumonia (protozoan), cytomegalovirus (viral), candida albicans (fungal).

SECTION 6-4

Integumentary Intervention Patterns

APTA's Guide to Physical Therapist Practice—APTA's Integumentary Intervention Patterns

Table 6-31   Therapeutic Exercises[18]

1. Strength, power, and endurance training for head, neck, limb, pelvic floor, trunk, and ventilatory muscles (such as active assistive, active, and resistive exercises, including concentric, dynamic, isotonic, eccentric, isokinetics, isometric, and plyometric; standardized, programmatic, complementary exercise approaches for task-specific performance training).
2. Flexibility exercises (such as muscle lengthening, range of motion, and stretching).
3. Balance, coordination, and agility training (such as developmental activities training; motor function training and retraining such as motor control and motor learning; neuromuscular education and reeducation; perceptual training; posture awareness training; standardized, programmatic, complementary exercise approaches for task-specific performance training).
4. Body mechanics and postural stabilization (such as body mechanics training, posture awareness training, postural control training, and postural stabilization activities).
5. Gait and locomotion training (such as developmental activities training; gait training; implement and device training; perceptual training; standardized, programmatic, complementary exercise approaches for wheelchair training).
6. Aerobic capacity and endurance conditioning and reconditioning (such as walking and wheelchair propulsion programs, aquatic programs, and gait and locomotor training).

Table 6-32   Functional Training in Self Care and Home Management Including ADL and IADL[18]

1. ADL training (such as bathing, bed mobility and transfer training, developmental activities, dressing, eating, grooming, and toileting).
2. IADL training (such as caring for dependents, home maintenance, household chores, shopping, structured play for infants and children, and yard work).
3. Injury prevention or reduction (such as injury prevention education during self-care and home management, injury prevention or reduction with use of devices and equipment, and safety awareness training during self-care and home management).

Table 6-33 Prescription, Application, and as Appropriate, Fabrication of Devices and Equipment (Assistive, Adaptive, Orthotic, Protective, Supportive, and Prosthetic)[18]

1. Adaptive devices (such as environmental controls, raised toilet seats, seating systems, and hospital beds)
2. Assistive devices (such as canes, crutches, long-handled reachers, power devices, static and dynamic splints, walkers, and wheelchairs)
3. Orthotic devices (such as braces, shoe inserts, and splints)
4. Prosthetic devices (such as lower extremity and upper extremity prostheses)
5. Protective devices (such as braces, cushions, and protective taping)
6. Supportive devices (such as compression garments, corsets, elastic wraps, neck collars, serial casts, slings, and supportive taping)

Table 6-34 Functional Training in Work (Job/School/Play), Community, and Leisure Integration or Reintegration Including IADL, Work Hardening, and Work Conditioning[18]

1. IADL training (such as community service training involving instruments, school and play activities training including tools and instruments, and work training with tools).
2. Injury prevention or reduction (such as injury prevention education during work at job, school, or play, community, and leisure integration or reintegration; injury prevention or reduction with use of devices and equipment; safety awareness training during work at job, school, or play, community, and leisure integration and reintegration).

Table 6-35 Manual Therapy Techniques (Excludes Joint Mobilization)[18]

1. Massage (such as connective tissue massage and therapeutic massage)
2. Soft tissue mobilization
3. Manual lymphatic drainage

Table 6-36 Physical Agents and Mechanical Modalities[18]

1. Physical agents (such as cryotherapy—cold pack, ice massage, vapocoolant spray; hydrotherapy—pools, whirlpool tanks, contrast baths, and pulsatile lavage; sound agents—phonophoresis and ultrasound; thermotherapy—dry heat,

diathermy, hot packs, paraffin baths; and light agents—laser and ultraviolet).

2. Mechanical modalities (such as compression therapies—compression bandaging, taping, contact casting, compression garments, total contact casting, and vasopneumatic compression devices; gravity-assisted compression devices—tilt table; mechanical motion devices—CPM).

Table 6-37   Electrotherapeutic Modalities[18]

Electrical muscle stimulation (such as EMS, TENS, and HVPC).

Table 6-38   Patient/Client-Related Instruction[18]

Instruction, education and training of patients/clients and caregivers regarding current condition (pathology; pathophysiology—disease, disorder, or condition; impairments, functional limitations, or disabilities); enhancement of performance; health, wellness, and fitness; plan of care; risk factors (for pathology; pathophysiology—disease, disorder, or condition; impairments, functional limitations, or disabilities); transitions across settings; and transitions to new roles.

Table 6-39   Integumentary Repair and Protection Techniques[18]

1. Dressings (such as wound coverage, hydrogels, and vacuum-assisted closure).
2. Topical agents (such as cleansers, creams, moisturizers, ointments, and sealants).
3. Nonselective debridement (such as enzymatic debridement, wet dressings, wet to dry dressings, and wet to moist dressings).
4. Selective debridement (such as debridement with other agents such as autolysis, enzymatic debridement, and sharp debridement).
5. Oxygen therapy (such as supplemental or topical oxygen).

INTEGUMENTARY INTERVENTIONS

Other Integumentary Intervention Patterns (Not Related to Wounds, Burns, and Ulcerations)

Table 6-40   Other Integumentary Intervention Patterns for Integumentary Conditions*

Dermatitis intervention patterns: (1) patient education about the disorder/disease awareness, healthy lifestyle, and risk reduction; (2) patient education on skin care

continues

Table 6-40 (continued)

(irritants); (3) patient education on exacerbating factors (precautions should be applied to physical therapy modalities and topical agents containing alcohol that may exacerbate the condition). The PTA should monitor patient's skin before and after application of interventions. The PTA should inform the supervising PT if the patient has an adverse reaction to any intervention.

Cellulitis intervention patterns: (1) wound care for open wounds; (2) muscle-setting exercises; (3) and positioning.

Herpes I (herpes simplex), herpes II, and herpes zoster (shingles) intervention patterns: relaxation exercises and techniques. Ultrasound and heat modalities are contraindicated because of the possibility of increasing symptoms. Standard precautions should be followed (extra caution for therapists who have not had chicken pox).

Scleroderma (systemic sclerosis) intervention patterns: (1) ROM and stretching exercises (to increase skin and joint flexibility and blood flow, to prevent contractures); (2) splints and orthotics (for joint contracture and joint protection); (3) BP monitoring; (4) precautions about cryotherapy (because of increased sensitivity to cold), cuff weights (that can increase stress on the joints), and patient's anxiety (caused by pain).

Psoriasis intervention patterns: whirlpool baths (with Aveeno or Balnetar bath oil), ROM exercises to affected extremities, mobility training, and ultraviolet light therapy (administered by the PT; PTA to check the state's practice act).

Lupus erythematosus intervention patterns: (1) gradual return of function (after acute exacerbation); (2) patient education about activity pacing; (3) patient education about relaxation exercises and techniques; (4) patient education about the disease, healthy lifestyle, and coping ability. Precautions should be applied to side effects of corticosteroids medications (that patient is taking), edema, hypertension, weight gain, acne, bruising, increased susceptibility to infection, osteoporosis, diabetes, gastric irritation, low potassium, purplish stretch marks, myopathy, and tendon rupture.

Polymyositis intervention patterns: heat, whirlpool, gentle massage, graded exercises, and aquatic therapy. When patient is in bed and cannot move needs positioning and splinting (to prevent pressure ulcers and contractures). Precautions should be applied to not giving too much exercises, and the side effects of corticosteroids.

---

*Interventions are dependent on PT's specific recommendations in the POC.

SECTION 6-5

Wound Documentation

Wound Documentation Elements

Table 6-41 Wound Documentation Elements

Wound measurements (in centimeters): trace wound edges on a clear acetate film (plastic sheet) using a fine point indelible ink marker. Measure length and width of the wound. Depth can be measured with a cotton swab into the base of the wound (place in the wound, withdraw, and measured with a tape measure). Depth can also be measured by filling a syringe with saline solution, injecting the solution into the wound cavity until filled, and subtracting the volume of liquid remaining in the syringe from the original amount. The wound surface area can also be determined by multiplying the greatest length and width of the wound. If there is access to computer[6] and software, the tracing can be digitized and area computed electronically (very accurate). Measurements (in centimeters) can also be described as linear by the clock, 12:00 to 6:00 and 3:00 to 9:00. Photographic assessments can be used in addition to measurements.

Describe wound drainage: nondraining or draining (amount—minimal, moderate, maximum; strike through of exudates; saturation of dressing; amount of time dressing was in place).

Describe types of drainage (color, viscosity, and amount): sanguineous (bloody), serous (clear), serosanguineous (clear with blood), purulence versus necrotic debris, and liquefied eschar.

Describe wound odor: foul, mild, typical of dressing type, sweet, and none.

Wound description: presence of nonviable tissue (slough or eschar), granulation (or hypergranulation), granulation buds, neoepithelium, skin buds, skin graft, undermining (measured around the area in centimeters such as 1.2 cm at 4:00), tunneling or tracts (depth and direction such as 5.8 at 7:00), exposed tendon muscle or bone, and exposed foreign body (fixators, prosthesis, screws, and stitches).

Describe wound healing for skin changes: black (necrotic), pink (sufficient vascular supply), and hard or callus formation (requires debridement).

Describe the surrounding tissues: intact healthy skin; color and pigmentation; scratches, tape injury, or rash; excoriated skin; feel and texture of the skin; neoepithelium; and maceration of the skin.

Edema circumferential measurements: measured above and below the wound site using a tape measure; areas where measurements were taken need to be described.

Describe patient's pulses (taken by palpation or by Doppler ultrasound): common pulses to assess are dorsalis pedis and posterior tibialis.

Document progress in relation to wound size, granulation, and wound drainage.

Review of Integumentary System Anatomy

Skin Anatomy

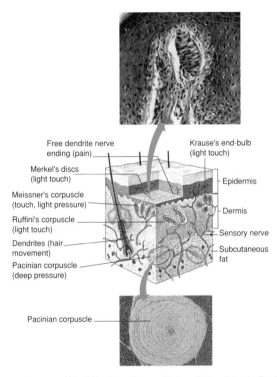

Figure 6-2   Anatomy of the Skin. From Human Biology: Fifth edition by Daniel D. Chiras, page 200, Figure 11-3 "General Sense Receptors"—only the illustration.

Table 6-42   Skin—The Largest Organ in the Body

Skin function: shields the body against infection (bacteria and chemicals), dehydration, and temperature changes; first defense against pain; provides sensory information about the environment; manufactures vitamin D; excretes salts and small amounts of urea (through perspiration); maintains fluid balance.

Epidermis: outermost skin layer made of stratified epithelium; produces melanin that is responsible for skin color.

Dermis (also called the "true skin"): inner layer of the skin made of collagen and elastin fibrous connective tissues; contains lymphatic structures, blood vessels, nerves and nerve endings, and sebaceous and sweat glands. The dermis has two layers: papillary and reticular.

Subcutaneous layer: not part of the skin, beneath the dermis, made of loose connective tissue and fat tissue (that provides insulation), and supports and cushions the skin. Fasciae and muscles are below the subcutaneous layer.

Skin appendages: hair and nails. Skin can also be classified as thin and hairy and thick and hairless (glabrous). Glabrous skin does not contain hair follicles and covers the surface of the palms of the hands, soles of the feet, and flexor surfaces of the digits.

Sensory Receptors Location in the Skin to Identify Depth of the Burn

Table 6-43   Sensory Receptors Location and Function

Epidermis contains free nerve endings—function as receptors for pain and itch; Merkel's disk (also found in the epithelial root sheath of a hair)—function as touch receptor.

Dermis contains free nerve endings—function as pain receptors.

Papillary dermis contains Meissner's corpuscle—function as touch receptor (most numerous in palmar and plantar surfaces, lips, eyelids, nipples, and tip of the tongue); Ruffini's corpuscle (also in subcutaneous tissue)—function as pressure receptor (once thought to mediate the sense of warmth); Krause's corpuscle—function as cutaneous touch receptor; and Krause's end bulb (also found in cornea)—function as touch receptor.

Reticular dermis contains: Pacinian corpuscles (also found in pancreas, penis, nipple, and clitoris)—function as deep and heavy pressure (and vibration) receptors. Pacinian corpuscles are also called Vater's corpuscles.

INTEGUMENTARY INTERVENTIONS

References

1. O'Sullivan, SB, Schmitz, TJ. *Physical Rehabilitation*, 5th ed. Philadelphia: F.A. Davis Company; 2007.

2. Rothstein, JM, Roy, SH, Wolf, SL, Scalzitti, DA. *The Rehabilitation Specialist's Handbook*, 3rd ed. Philadelphia: F.A. Davis Company; 2005.

3. National Pressure Ulcer Advisory Panel (NPUAP). *Wound Classification*. National Pressure Ulcer Advisory Panel Web site. Available at http://www.npuap.org. Accessed November 2006.

4. Venes, D, ed. *Taber's Cyclopedic Medical Dictionary: Edition 20: Illustrated in Full Color*. Philadelphia: F.A. Davis Company; 2005.

5. Hecox, B, Tsega AM, Weisberg, J, Sanko J. *Integrating Physical Agents in Rehabilitation*, 2nd ed. Upper Saddle River, NJ: Pearson Education Inc.; 2006.

6. McCulloch J. *The Integumentary System: Repair and Management: An Overview*. The American Physical Therapy Association Web site. Available at www.apta.org. Accessed November 2006.

7. National Institutes of Health: National Diabetes Information Clearinghouse: United States Department of Health and Human Services. *Prevent Diabetes Problems: Keep Your Feet and Skin Healthy*. National Diabetes Information Clearinghouse Web site. Available at http://diabetes.niddk.nih.gov/dm/pubs/complications_feet/feet.pdf. Accessed November 2006.

8. Brown-Etris M, Punthello M, Shields D, et al. *A comparison clinical study to evaluate the efficacy of 80% hypertonic wound gel dressing vs. collagenase ointment for the debridement of nonviable tissue in dermal ulcers*. Abstract presented at the 11th Annual Symposium on Advanced Wound Care and Medical Research Forum on Wound Repair in Miami Beach, Florida, April 18–22, 1998.

9. Sinclair RD, Ryan TJ. Types of chronic wounds: Indications for enzymatic debridement. In: Westerhof W, Vanscheidt W (eds). *Proteolytic Enzymes and Wound Healing* 1994;7-20.

10. Harvey, C. Wound healing. *Orthop. Nursing* 2005;2:24-25.

11. Bishop SM, et al. Importance of moisture balance at the wound dressing interface. *J Wound Care* 2003;4:12-16.

12. Williams, C. An investigation of the benefits of Aquacel Hydrofibre wound dressing. *Br J Nursing* 1999;10:8-18.

13. Vowden, K, Vowden P. Understanding exudate management and the role of exudate in the healing process. *Br. J Community Nursing* 2003;8:4–13.
14. Edwards, J. Use of Exu-Dry in the management of a variety of exuding wounds. *Br J Nursing* 2001;12:10-22.
15. Ehrenreich, M, Ruszczak, Z. Update on tissue-engineered biological dressings. *Tissue Eng* 2006;9:12-21.
16. Ehrenreich, M, Ruszczak, Z. Update on dermal substitutes. *Acta Dermatovenerol Croat* 2006;3:14-17.
17. Hunziker, T. Autologous cultured skin substitutes. *Hautartz* 2004; 11:55–66.
18. The American Physical Therapy Association. *Guide to Physical Therapist Practice*, 2nd ed. Alexandria, VA: APTA; 2001; Revised 2003.

Part VII

Geriatric Interventions

Geriatric Data Collection

Theories of Aging

Table 7-1   General Concepts of Aging

Aging is developmental.

Aging occurs across the life span.

Aging changes are a result of cellular changes. Cells increase in size as a result of fragmentation of the Golgi apparatus and mitochondria. There is also a decrease in cell capacity to divide and reproduce and an arrest of DNA synthesis and cell division.

In aging, tissue changes occur due to an accumulation of pigmented materials (Lipofuscins), an accumulation of lipids and fats, and connective tissue changes. These changes are a result of decreased elastic content, degradation of collagen, and the presence of pseudoelastins.

In aging, organ changes cause a decrease in functional capacity and decrease in homeostatic efficiency.

Table 7-2   Theories of Aging

Developmental Genetic Theory:[1] aging is intrinsic to the organism being part of the normal and continuous genetic development. Genes are programmed to modulate aging changes, and there is an overall rate of progression. Individuals vary in the expression of aging changes (such as graying of hair and wrinkles). Multiple genes are involved in aging. No one person's genes can modulate the rate of development in all aspects of aging. There are premature aging syndromes (such as the progeria) that provide evidence of defective genetic programming. Some individuals exhibit premature aging changes, such as atrophy and thinning of tissues, graying of hair, and arteriosclerosis.

Hayflick Limit Theory:[1] another aging theory characterized by the doubling of the biologic clock. This process occurs in three phases. The last phase (phase III) shows a complete cessation of cell division. Termination of cell division involves a functional deterioration within cells because of a limited number of genetically programmed cell doublings (cell replication). A person's deterioration in cells is not dependent on environmental influences, but cell aging is an intrinsic (built-in) process.

The Free Radical Theory: another theory of aging stating that free radicals are highly reactive and toxic forms of oxygen produced by cell mitochondria. Free radicals can: (1) cause damage to cell membranes and DNA cell replication; (2) interfere with cell diffusion and transport, resulting in decreased O_2 delivery and tissue death; (3) decrease cellular integrity and enzyme activities; (4) result in cross-linkages such as chemical bonding of elements not generally joined together; (5) interfere with normal cell function. Free radicals can also result in an accumulation of aging pigments (such as Lipofuscins) and trigger pathologic changes such as atherosclerosis in blood vessel wall, cell mutation, and cancer. These cell mutations (intrinsic mutagenesis) are a result of errors in the synthesis of proteins (DNA and RNA) that leads to abnormal proteins and aging changes.

The Neuroendocrine and Hormonal Theories: theories of aging that indicate functional decrements in neurons and their associated hormones lead to aging changes. These theories state that the hypothalamus, pituitary gland, and adrenal gland are the primary regulators and timekeepers of aging. They maintain that thyroxine is the master rate-controlling hormone of the body for metabolism and protein synthesis. In addition, secretion of regulatory pituitary hormones influences the thyroid. The theories also indicate that decreases in protective hormones such as estrogen, growth hormone, and adrenal DHEA (dehydroepiandrosterone) contribute to aging and that increases in stress hormones (cortisol) can damage the brain's memory center the hippocampus and destroy immune cells.

The Immunity or Immunological Theory:[1] indicates that the thymus size decreases, shrivels by puberty, and becomes less functional. As a result, bone marrow cell efficiency decreases, which results in a steady decline in immune responses during adulthood. The immune cells, T-cells become less able to fight foreign organisms, and B-cells become less able to make antibodies. As a result, autoimmune diseases increase with age. This theory is categorized as a developmental genetic theory.

Environmental Theories (also called the Stochastic or Nongenetic Theories): explain that aging is caused by an accumulation of insults from the environment. Environmental toxins include ultraviolet and cross-linking agents (such as unsaturated fats, toxic chemicals such as the metal ions Mg and Zn, radiation, and viruses). Exposure to these can result in errors in protein synthesis and in DNA synthesis/genetic sequences and can cause cross-linkage of molecules with resultant mutations. Finally, the results of these insults are that the organism reaches a level incompatible with life.

The Caloric Restriction Theory or Energy Restriction: states that a lifestyle devoted to the high-nutrient and low-calorie diet, with moderate vitamin and mineral supplementation and a regular exercises regimen, is beneficial. Caloric restrictions may be effective through the neuroendocrine system. The caloric-restricted diet also states that it can influence the aging rate and disease susceptibility because the immune system is the pacemaker of aging.

Psychological Theories such as the Stress Theory: speculates that homeostatic imbalances result in changes in structural and chemical composition of the body. The general adaptation syndrome (of Selye) postulates that an initial alarm reac-

continues

Table 7-2   (continued)

tion takes place, progressing to a stage of resistance and then progressing to a stage of exhaustion (of the body and its organs). The stress theory is closely linked to the hormonal theory.

Erickson's Psychological Bipolar Theory: a psychological theory of life span development that relates to stages of later adulthood. Erickson divides these stage into two: (1) stage 1, called the integrity (in which an individual exhibits full unification of personality; life is viewed with satisfaction such as productive life, sense of satisfaction; the individual remains optimistic and continues to grow) and (2) stage 2, called the despair (in which an individual lacks ego integration; life is viewed with despair and fear of death, feelings of regret and disappointment, and missed opportunities).

There are also sociological theories that involve life experience and lifestyle influencing the aging process. Some of these are the activity theory, stating that older persons who are socially active exhibit improved adjustment to the aging process. The activity theory indicates that a continued role performance is essential for positive self-image and improved life satisfaction. There is the disengagement theory that states that the distancing of an individual or withdrawal from society affects aging. There is a reduction in social roles leading to further isolation and life dissatisfaction. There is an increasing reliance on others for meeting physical and emotional needs. The focus of sociological theories is to enhance a person's identity improving the aging process.

An integrated model of aging assumes aging is a complex, multifactorial phenomenon in which some or all of many processes may contribute to the overall aging of an individual. Aging is not adequately explained by any single theory.

Sleep Patterns in Older Persons

Table 7-3   Sleep Patterns in Older Persons[2]

Transient insomnia: poor sleep over a few nights that may be caused by stress, work, or time zone changes.

Short-term insomnia: poor sleep over less than 1 month that may be related to acute medical or psychological conditions.

Long-term insomnia that can present as problems falling asleep (of over 1-month duration that may be related to poor sleeping habits, anxiety, medications' side effects, changes in activity level, or medical problems). Long-term insomnia can also manifest as frequent awakening (that may be related to medications' side effects, depression, sleep apnea, changes in activity level, or medical problems).

Factors Contributing to Malnutrition (Protein Deficiency) in Older Persons

Table 7-4   Malnutrition (Protein Deficiency) in Older Persons

Malnutrition in older persons is inadequate intake of protein or calories or both. Malnutrition increases a person vulnerability to skin breakdown, medication toxicity, infections, gastrointestinal ulcerations, and other illnesses. Many of the symptoms associated with malnutrition such as muscular weakness and wasting may be attributed incorrectly to advanced age and underdiagnosed as a result.

Factors[2] contributing to malnutrition (protein deficiency): alcoholism, chronic infection, cancer, COPD, depression, dental or facial pathologies, dysphagia (difficulty swallowing), excessive low-fat diet, hyperthyroidism, hypercalcemia, impaired sense of taste or smell, inability to gather or prepare food, loneliness, side effects of medications, medication withdrawal, neuroendocrine tumor that causes hypertension and is difficult to diagnose called pheochromocytoma (patient has palpitations, nausea, sweating, abdominal pain, fainting spells, hyperglycemia, weakness, and anxiety), poverty, and getting full rapidly with a little food.

Physical signs[3] of malnutrition in adults are: (1) sores at the angles of the mouth, (2) red swollen lingual papillae, (3) glossitis (inflammation of the tongue), (4) papillary atrophy of tongue, (5) stomatitis (inflammation of the mouth including the lips, tongue, and mucous membranes), (6) spongy and bleeding gums, (7) muscle tenderness in extremities, (8) poor muscle tone, (9) loss of vibratory sensation, (10) increase or decrease of deep tendon reflexes, (11) hyperesthesia of the skin, (12) purpura (rash in which blood cells leak into the skin or mucous membranes, has to do with blood coagulation), (13) dermatitis (facial butterfly type, and perineal, scrotal, and vulval dermatitis), (14) thickening and pigmentation of the skin over bony prominences, (15) nonspecific vaginitis, (16) rachitic chest deformity, (17) anemia not responding to iron, (18) fatigue of visual accommodation, and (19) conjunctival changes of the eye.

Risk Factors for Hypothermia in Older Persons

Table 7-5   Risk Factors for Hypothermia[2]

Decreased heat production due to diabetic ketoacidosis, hypoglycemia, hypopituitarism, malnutrition or starvation, myxedema (infiltration of the skin by mucopolysaccharides giving a waxy appearance, caused by hypothyroidism), and hypothyroidism.

continues

Table 7-5 (continued)

Increased heat loss due to arteriovenous shunt, inflammatory dermatitis (caused by psoriasis or exfoliation), Paget's disease, alcohol-induced vasodilation, cold exposure, and reduction in subcutaneous fat (caused by malnutrition).

Impaired thermoregulation due to neuropathy, alcoholism, diabetes, head trauma, polio, stroke, subdural hematoma, subarachnoid hemorrhage, systemic diseases (affecting hypothalamus), carbon monoxide poisoning, and uremia (body's accumulation of metabolic byproducts that are normally excreted by the kidneys; may also be caused by renal failure).

Diminished activity due to PD, parkinsonism, arthritis, dementia, a fall or other injury, and paralysis or stroke.

Age-Related Impairments and Functional Limitations and Suggestions for Interventions

Muscular Impairments and Functional Limitations and Suggestions for Interventions

Table 7-6   Muscular Impairments and Functional Limitations and Interventions

Muscular impairments and functional limitations are caused mostly by decreased activity levels (hypokinesis) and disuse atrophy than from the normal aging process.

There is a normal loss of muscular strength, which peaks at 30 years old, remains fairly constant until age 50, after which there is an accelerating loss. There is a 20% to 40% muscular strength loss by age 65 in the nonexercising adults.

A normal loss of muscular power (force/unit time) that occurs may be due to losses in speed of muscle contraction and changes in nerve conduction and synaptic transmission.

A normal loss of skeletal muscle mass (atrophy) occurs. This is due to a decrease in both size and number of muscle fibers. By age 70, there is a loss of 33% of skeletal muscle mass. Changes occur in muscle fiber composition with a selective loss of type II fibers (fast twitch fibers) important for rapid high force production. There is a proportional increase of type I fibers (slow twitch fibers) important for low force production.

There are age-related changes in muscular endurance. Muscles fatigue more readily. There is decreased muscle tissue oxidative capacity and decreased peripheral blood flow affecting oxygen delivery to the muscles.

There is a normal altered chemical composition of muscle with decreased myosin ATPase activity and glycoproteins and contractile protein. There are collagen changes, with denser collagen (an irregularity because of cross-linkages), and loss of water content and elasticity. These affect tendons, bones, and cartilages. The clinical implications of these changes are that movements become slower with increased complaints of fatigue.

Age-related changes of the connective tissues: are becoming denser and stiffer. As a result, there is an increased risk of muscle and tendon strains, and ligaments sprains.

As a result of connective tissue changes, there is also a loss of range of motion that is highly variable by joint and individual, with an accompanying loss in activity level.

There is an increased tendency for fibrous adhesions and contractures.

Functional limitations occur with decreased functional mobility as a result of movement impairments. Gait changes are: (1) gait becomes stiffer with fewer automatic movements; (2) gait has a decreased amplitude and speed, and slower cadence; (3) there is evidence of shorter steps, a wider stride, increased double support to insure safety and compensation for decreased balance; and (4) decreased trunk rotation and arm swing are shown. Gait may become unsteady because of changes in balance, strength, and the increased need for assistive devices. *There is a clinical risk of falls.*

Intervention strategies to slow or reverse muscular impairments and functional limitations are (1) patient (client) to see the physician (to improve medical health that may include correction of medical problems that may cause weakness such as hyperthyroidism, excess adrenocortical steroids, Cushing's disease, use of steroids, or hyponatremia), (2) patient (client) to see the dietician (to improve nutrition such as correcting hyponatremia), (3) recommendation to address the possibility of alcoholism, (4) increase patient's (client's) levels of physical activity by stressing functional activities and organized activity programs (with a gradual increase in intensity of activity to avoid injury; adequate warm ups and cool downs; appropriate pacing and rest periods), (5) provide strength training (using isometric and progressive resistive exercise regimes; high-intensity training programs such as 70% to 80% of one-repetition maximum [1 RM] produce quicker and more predictable results than moderate intensity programs), (6) improve functional abilities (use flexibility and range of motion exercises; use slow, prolonged stretching, maintained for 20 to 30 seconds; heat tissues before stretching; maintain newly gained range by incorporation into functional activities), and (7) increase mobility activities (gains are usually slower with older adults).

Skeletal Impairments and Functional Limitations and Suggestions for Interventions

Table 7-7   Skeletal Impairments and Functional Limitations and Interventions

Skeletal impairments and functional limitations can occur from skeletal age-related changes (such as the cartilage changes that are a result of decreased water content with cartilage becoming stiffer, fragmented and eroding by age 60; more than 60% of older adults have degenerative joint changes and cartilage abnormalities).

There is a normal loss of bone mass and density. Peak bone mass occurs at age 40. Between the ages of 45 and 70, bone mass decreases (for women, by about 25%, and for men, 15%). There is also another 5% decrease of bone mass by age 90.

There is a normal loss of calcium and bone strength, especially trabecular bone. Osteoporosis can occur as a pathological manifestation of aging.

continues

Table 7-7 (continued)

There is a normal decrease in bone marrow red blood cell production.

The intervertebral disks flatten and become less resilient because of loss of water content. There is a 30% loss by age 65 with loss of collagen elasticity.

The trunk length and overall height are decreased. As a result, postural changes are observed, such as forward head, kyphosis of the thoracic spine, and flattening of the lumbar spine. With prolonged sitting, there is a tendency to develop hip and knee flexion contractures.

Intervention strategies to slow or reverse skeletal impairments and functional limitations: (1) reduce the risk of contractures (using positioning, exercises, orthotics); (2) reduce the risk of falls (use patient/caregiver education); (3) use postural exercises stressing components of good posture; (4) use weightbearing (gravity-loading) exercises (that can decrease bone loss in older adults); (5) use walking, stair climbing, weight belts (to increase load); (6) patient (client) to see the dietician and social worker (for help with meals on wheels) to improve the nutritional and hormonal status.

Neurologic Impairments and Functional Limitations and Suggestions for Interventions

Table 7-8   Neurological Impairments and Functional Limitations and Interventions

Age-related atrophy of nerve cells in the cerebral cortex causes an overall loss of cerebral mass/brain weight of 6% to 11% between the ages of 20 and 90. There is accelerating loss after age 70. Changes in brain morphology are: gyral atrophy, with accompanying narrowing and flattening of gyri and widening of sulci; ventricular dilation; generalized cell loss in the cerebral cortex, especially in the frontal and temporal lobes with association areas of the prefrontal cortex and visual tracts; presence of lipofuscins (insoluble fatty pigments found in aging cells), senile or neuritic plaques and neurofibrillary tangles (NFTs); and significant accumulations of plaque associated with pathology of Alzheimer's dementia.

Age-related selective cell loss[1] is found in basal ganglia (substantial nigra and putamen), cerebellum, hippocampus, and locus ceruleus (depression in the floor of fourth ventricle of the brain). The brain stem is minimally affected.

Normal decrease of cerebral blood flow and energy metabolism is evident.

Normal changes in synaptic transmission take place due to decreased synthesis and metabolism of major neurotransmitters (acetylcholine and dopamine).

Age-related slowing of many neural processes is shown, especially in polysynaptic pathways (multiple synapses nerve pathways).

Age-related changes occur in spinal cord/peripheral nerves as a result of neuronal loss and atrophy. These changes are manifested in a 30% to 50% loss of anterior horn cells. There is a 30% loss of posterior roots (sensory fibers) by age 90.

Normal loss of motoneurons results in an increase in the size of the remaining motor units. There is development of macro motor units.

Slowed nerve conduction velocity is observed with greater slowing in sensory fibers than in motor fibers.

A normal loss of sympathetic nerve fibers may account for diminished autonomic stability with an increased incidence of postural hypotension in older adults.

Age-related tremors (essential tremors) occur as an isolated symptom, particularly in hands, head, and voice. These tremors are characterized as postural or kinetic and rarely occur at rest. They are usually benign and slowly progressive, although they may limit function in late stages and are exaggerated by movement and emotion.

Clinical neurologic impairments effect function such as the patient's (client's) movement. Overall speed and coordination are decreased with increased difficulties with fine motor control. There is slowed recruitment of motoneurons that contributes to loss of strength. Both reaction time and movement time are increased.

Older adults are also affected by the decreased speed/accuracy of movements. The simpler the movement, the less the change. More complicated movements require more preparation. There are longer reaction and movement times. Faster movements have a decreased accuracy with an increase in movement errors.

There is a general age-related slowing of neural processing of learning. The memory may be affected. There are problems in homeostatic regulation. Stressors (heat, cold, and excess exercise) can be harmful, even life-threatening.

Intervention strategies to slow or reverse neurological impairments and functional limitations are: (1) recommendations for patient (client) to see the physician (for correction of medical problems such as to improve cerebral blood flow); (2) patient education to improve general health (such as diet and smoking cessation); (3) increase levels of physical activity (may encourage neuronal branching, slow the rate of neural decline, and improve cerebral circulation); (4) provide effective strategies to improve motor learning and motor control (to allow for increased reaction and movement time during activities that will improve also motivation and accuracy of movements; to allow for limitations of memory by avoiding long sequences of movements; to allow for increased cautionary behaviors by providing adequate explanations and demonstrations when teaching new movement skills; to stress familiar, well-learned skills and repetitive movements; for more information on basic motor learning strategies, see Part IV).

Age-Related Impairments and Functional Limitations **483**

Sensory Visual Impairments and Functional Limitations and Suggestions for Interventions

Table 7-9   Visual Impairments and Functional Limitations and Interventions

Older adults experience a normal loss of function of the senses. The loss alters the quality of life and the ability to interact socially and with the environment. This may lead to sensory deprivation, isolation, disorientation, confusion, and give the appearance of senility. This can also strain social interactions and lead to decreased functional mobility. As a result of decreases in sensory function, there is also an increased risk of injury.

Visual impairments because of vision changes are the largest sensory impairments in older adults. Visual impairments result in a general decline in visual acuity. There is a gradual decline before the sixth decade and a rapid decline between ages 60 and 90. Visual loss may be as much as 80% by age 90.

The visual changes include presbyopia,[1] which results in a visual loss in middle and older ages. Presbyopia is characterized by the inability to focus properly and blurred images. This is due to the loss of accommodation and the elasticity of the lens. Presbyopia is also manifested through a decreased ability to adapt to dark and light. There is an increased sensitivity to light and glare, a loss of color discrimination, especially for blues and greens.

Another visual impairment is a decreased sensitivity of the corneal reflex with greater proclivity to eye injury or infection. Oculomotor responses are diminished with resultant restricted upward gaze and reduced pursuit eye movements. Ptosis (difficulty or inability to raise the eyelid) may also develop.

Additional vision impairment may be caused by a visual pathology (such as cataracts), causing visual opacity with the clouding of the lens due to changes in lens proteins. The impairments produced by cataracts can cause a gradual loss of vision, central vision first and then peripheral. There are increased problems with glare, a general darkening of vision, loss of acuity, and accompanying distortion.

Other impairments such as early loss of peripheral vision (tunnel vision) that may progress to total blindness can be caused by glaucoma (that is characterized by increased intraocular pressure, degeneration of the optic disc, and atrophy of the optic nerve). Another visual impairment such as loss of central vision that may progress to blindness can be caused by senile macular degeneration (that is characterized by age-related degeneration of the macula compromised by decreased blood supply or abnormal growth of blood vessels under the retina).

Other central vision impairment is caused by diabetic retinopathy (that is characterized by damage to retinal capillaries, growth of abnormal blood vessels, and hemorrhage leading to retinal scarring and finally retinal detachment).

A pathological visual impairment (caused by CVA) is homonymous hemianopsia, resulting in loss of half of the visual field in each eye (nasal half of one eye and temporal half of the other eye). This condition produces an inability to receive information from right or left side. The defect corresponds to the side of the sensorimotor deficit.

Side effects of certain medications may also cause vision impairments (such as decreased or fuzzy vision). The medications that may cause vision impairments are antihistamines, tranquilizers, antidepressants, and steroids.

Intervention strategies to slow or reverse sensory visual impairments and functional limitations are: (1) physical therapist examination and evaluation of visual impairments (such as acuity, peripheral vision, light and dark adaptation, depth perception, diplopia, eye fatigue, eye pain); (2) maximize visual function by assessing the use of glasses and need for environmental adaptations; (3) increase sensory thresholds by allowing extra time for visual discrimination and response; (4) patient (client) education (to work in adequate light, reduce glare, avoid abrupt changes in light and when going from light to dark); (5) proper communication and interaction with the patient or client (such as the therapist to stand directly in front of the patient at the same eye level; to assist the patient in color discrimination; to use warm colors such as yellow, orange, or red for identification and color coding; to provide other sensory cues when vision is limited such as, verbal descriptions to new environments, touching to communicate that you are listening to the patient); (6) provide safety education to reduce risk of fall; and (7) report all new findings to the physical therapist for appropriate changes to the plan of care if warranted.

Sensory Hearing Impairments and Functional Limitations and Suggestions for Interventions

Table 7-10   Hearing Impairments and Functional Limitations and Interventions

Normal aging changes in hearing can occur as early as the fourth decade. These changes affect a significant number of older individuals (23% of individuals aged 65 to 74 have hearing impairments). Forty percent (40%) of those over age 75 have hearing loss. The rate of hearing loss in men is twice the rate than in women. The hearing loss in men also starts earlier than in women.

Conductive hearing loss is common in older men. This type of hearing loss (hearing loss in the outer ear) is a result of buildup of cerumen (ear wax) obstructing the external auditory meatus.

continues

Table 7-10 (continued)

Conductive hearing loss is also a mechanical hearing loss from damage caused by trauma or disease to the external auditory canal, the tympanic membrane, or the middle ear ossicles. Conductive hearing loss can affect all sound frequencies. Tinnitus (ringing in the ears) may also be present.

Hearing changes as a result of aging process can occur in the inner ear. These changes may be significant in sound sensitivity affecting the understanding of speech. There may also be changes in the vestibular mechanism of the inner ear affecting equilibrium. The hearing changes may result with degeneration and atrophy of cochlear and vestibular structures with an accompanying loss of neurons.

Sensorineural hearing loss is a (permanent or temporary) loss affecting cochlear and peripheral structures in the inner ear. Some causal factors of sensory hearing loss can be noise exposure, acoustic or mechanical trauma, disease, drugs, and arteriosclerosis.

Presbycusis is a term describing normal loss of hearing due to aging. It is a type of sensorineural hearing loss associated with middle-aged and older adults. It is generally characterized by bilateral hearing loss, especially at high frequencies (above 3 kHz affecting reception of consonant sounds in the speech range). It can eventually affect all frequencies pertinent to speech reception. There is poor auditory speech discrimination and comprehension. This is especially prevalent in the presence of background noise. Often there is accompanying tinnitus.

Central hearing loss is a type of hearing loss that results from disorders affecting neural tracts and structures from the cochlea of the inner ear and eighth cranial nerve pathways to the auditory receptors of the brain.

Some additional hearing loss associated with pathology is otosclerosis (a condition caused by a bony overgrowth immobilizing the stapes [ankylosis of the stapes] in the middle ear with resulting conductive loss). If untreated, otosclerosis may result in eventual intrusion into the otic capsule affecting sensory function of the inner ear. When treated early, this pathology is generally amenable to surgical intervention (stapedectomy). Otosclerosis is not necessarily a type of hearing loss related to aging because it can also occur in younger individuals.

Paget's disease (osteitis deformans) is a pathology of older individuals affecting the middle and eventually, if untreated, inner ear. Paget's disease is characterized by thickening and hypertrophy of the long bones and deformity of the flat bones. It may respond to medical intervention through use of medication.

Hypothyroidism is another pathology (inadequate levels of thyroid hormone in the body) affecting hearing sensitivity and acuity.

Intervention strategies to slow or reverse sensory hearing impairments and functional limitations are: (1) recommendation for professional audiological assessment of hearing for speech acuity, word discrimination/comprehension, presence of tinnitus, cochlear recruitment, dizziness, vertigo, and pain; (2) recommendations for audiological assessment by a professional audiologist and perhaps the use of amplification (hearing aid) to improve speech discrimination and help communication; (3) improve communication by minimizing auditory distractions; (4) when communicating with a patient exhibiting hearing impairments, the therapist should speak slowly and clearly; be directly in front of the patient at the eye level; use nonverbal communication (such as gesture or demonstration) to reinforce the message; and orient the patient (client) away from topics of conversation he or she cannot hear to reduce feelings of paranoia and isolation.

Vestibular and Balance Sensory Impairments and Functional Limitations and Suggestions for Interventions

Table 7-11   Vestibular and Balance Impairments and Functional Limitations and Interventions

There are inherent changes occurring with aging in regard to the mechanism involving control of balance. These are degenerative changes in the otoconia of the utricle and saccule within the vestibular segments of the inner ear located in the temporal bone of the skull. There is a normal age-related loss of vestibular hair-cell receptors and a decreased number of vestibular neurons. This loss is accompanied by a decrease in the vestibular ocular reflex (VOR). The condition begins at age 30, with an accelerating decline at ages 55 to 60, resulting in diminished vestibular sensation. This diminished acuity results in delayed reaction times and longer response times. The reduced function of the VOR affects retinal image stability with head movements, and produces blurred vision.

As a result of altered sensory organization in the inner ear and the eye, the older adults depend more on somatosensory inputs for balance.

Older adults are less able to resolve sensory conflicts when presented with inappropriate visual or proprioceptive inputs due to vestibular losses.

Postural response patterns for balance are disorganized. This is characterized by diminished ankle torque, increased hip torque, and increased postural sway.

There are additional vestibular and balance impairments caused by pathology. These impairments are tinnitus and dizziness, and a sensation of fullness in the

continues

Table 7-11   (continued)

ear (caused by Meniere's disease) and sensorineural hearing loss (usually low frequency, also caused by Meniere's disease). Severe manifestations of Meniere's disease, if unresolved through medical intervention, may require surgical intervention.

Benign paroxysmal positional vertigo (BPPV) also causes vestibular and balance impairments characterized by brief episodes of vertigo (less than 1 minute) associated with position change. This is the result of degeneration of the utricular otoconia that settle on the cupula of the posterior semicircular canal. This condition is common in older adults.

Intervention to slow or reverse vestibular and balance sensory impairments and functional limitations are: (1) improve balance and coordination; (2) decrease incidence of falls in older adults (see somatosensory balance interventions next); (3) patient and patient's family safety education (to identify risks and modify the environment—see somatosensory balance interventions next).

Somatosensory Balance Impairments and Functional Limitations and Suggestions for Interventions

Table 7-12   Somatosensory Balance Impairments and Functional Limitations and Interventions

With normal aging changes, there is a decrease in the sensitivity of touch associated with a decline of peripheral receptors and atrophy of afferent fibers. The lower extremities are more affected than upper extremities.

There are normal proprioceptive losses with increased thresholds in vibratory sensibility, beginning around age 50. These losses are greater in lower extremities than upper extremities (greater in distal extremities than proximal).

There is a loss of joint receptor sensitivity with losses more evident in the lower extremities. Cervical joints may also contribute to loss of balance. Cutaneous pain thresholds are increased with greater changes in upper body areas (upper extremities and face) than for lower extremities. There is additional sensation impairment caused by pathology. The sensation impairment may be caused by diabetes (peripheral neuropathy), CVA (central sensory losses), and peripheral vascular disease (peripheral ischemia).

Intervention strategies to slow or reverse somatosensory balance impairments and functional limitations are: (1) physical therapist examination and evaluation for increased thresholds to stimulation and to sensory losses; (2) allow extra time for patient's (client's) responses with increased thresholds to stimulation; (3) use touch to communicate with the patient (client); (4) maximize proprioceptive inputs by using facilitation interventions such as rubbing and stroking; (5) highlight and enhance naturally occurring intrinsic feedback during movements by using stretch and tapping; (6) provide augmented feedback through appropriate sensory channels (for example, walking on carpeted surfaces may be easier than on smooth floor); (7) teach compensatory strategies to prevent injury to anesthetic limbs and to prevent falls; (8) provide assistive devices as needed for fall prevention; (9) use biofeedback devices as appropriate such as a limb load monitor (that offer a visual load signaling to prevent a fall).

Taste and Smell Impairments and Functional Limitations and Suggestions for Interventions

Table 7-13 Taste and Smell Impairments and Functional Limitations and Interventions

Aging changes in taste and smell are a gradual decrease in taste sensitivity and decreased smell sensitivity.

There is additional loss of sensation (sensitivity) with smokers, and also as a result of chronic allergies and respiratory infections.

Use of dentures contributes to loss of taste and smell as well as a CVA with involvement of the hypoglossal nerve.

Intervention strategies to slow or reverse taste and smell impairments and functional limitations are: (1) patient education for compensatory strategies for identification of odors, tastes (sweet, sour, bitter, salty), and somatic sensations (temperature, touch); (2) patient education to use taste enhancers (such as salt and sugar) to help with patient's diet and nutrition (because decreased taste and enjoyment of food leads to poor diet and nutrition); (3) environmental assessment (home or nursing facility) and use of safety monitors especially for home safety (because there is a decrease in home safety with a diminished capacity to detect gas leaks or smoke).

Cognitive Impairments and Functional Limitations and Suggestions for Interventions

Table 7-14   Cognitive Impairments and Functional Limitations and Interventions

In regard to age-related cognitive changes, there is no uniform decline in intellectual abilities throughout adulthood. Changes do not typically show up until the mid 60s. Significant declines affecting everyday life do not show up until the early 80s.

The most significant cognitive impairments (in measures of intelligence) occur in the years immediately preceding death. The condition is termed terminal drop.

Tasks involving perceptual speed show early declines by age 39 when longer times are required to complete tasks.

Numeric abilities (tests of adding, subtracting multiplying) peak in the mid 40s and is well maintained until the 60s.

Verbal ability peaks at age 30 and is well maintained until the 60s.

Memory impairments are typically noted in short-term memory. Long-term memory is retained.

Memory impairments are also task dependent. Deficits are primarily with novel conditions and with new learning.

All age groups can learn. Learning in older adults is affected by increased cautiousness, anxiety, and the pace of learning. Fast pace is problematic. There may also be interference from prior learning.

Intervention strategies to slow or reverse cognitive impairments and functional limitations are: (1) patient education to use different strategies for learning (for example, context-based strategies versus memorization work better in young adults); (2) stressing the relationship and the importance of learning for functional skills; (3) improvement of general health by recommendations to seek medical personnel and correct medical problems (for example, imbalances between oxygen supply and demand to the CNS can be present in cardiovascular disease, hypertension, diabetes, and hypothyroidism); (4) recommendations to seek medical personnel for pharmacological changes (such as drug re-evaluation and decreased use of multiple drugs); (5) monitoring the patient (client) for drug toxicity; (6) recommendations for reduction or cessation in the use of tobacco and alcohol; (7) recommendations for correction of nutritional deficiencies; (8) increased physical and mental activity (older adult should keep mentally engaged through playing chess, doing crossword puzzles, and having a high level of reading); (9) patient education to increase a lifestyle that stresses social activity through clubs, travel, and work; (10) recommendations for cognitive training activities (providing written instruction because the auditory processing may be decreased); (11) recommendations

for a stimulating, "enriching" environment for the patient (client) because hospitalization or institutionalization may produce disorientation and agitation in some
older patients (clients); (12) recommendations for counseling and family support
(to help to reduce stress).

Cardiopulmonary System Impairments and Functional Limitations and Suggestions for Interventions

Table 7-15   Cardiopulmonary Impairments and Functional Limitations and Interventions

Age-related impairments and functional limitations of the cardiovascular system are
due more to inactivity and disease than aging.

Some of the cardiovascular pathological changes[1] are degeneration of the heart
muscle with accumulation of lipofuscins (characterized by mild cardiac hypertrophy of the left ventricular wall), decreased coronary blood flow, thickening of the
cardiac valves, changes in the conduction system (loss of the pacemaker cells in
SA node), blood vessel changes (such as thicker and less distensible arteries),
slowed exchange in capillary walls and increased peripheral resistance,
increased resting blood pressure (systolic is greater than diastolic), decreased
blood volume and hemopoietic activity of bone, and increased blood coagulability.

The cardiac clinical impairments and functional limitations to consider during exercises are: (1) resting blood pressure increases, (2) cardiovascular responses to
exercise are weakened (such as a decrease in heart rate and heart rate acceleration and decrease in maximal oxygen uptake), (3) reduced exercise capacity, and
(4) increased recovery time after exercises.

There is also a decreased stroke volume due to decreased myocardial contractility.
The maximum heart rate declines with age. The cardiac output decreases 1% per
year after age 20. This is due to decreased heart rate and stroke volume.

Other clinical impairment is orthostatic hypotension (due to reduced baroceptor sensitivity and vascular elasticity) and increased fatigue.

Anemia and systolic ejection murmur are common in the elderly patients. There are
possible EKG changes with loss of normal sinus rhythm, longer PR & QT intervals,
wider QRS, and increased arrhythmias.

Age-related impairments and functional limitations in regard to the pulmonary
system are chest wall stiffness with declining strength of respiratory muscles that
results in increased work of breathing, loss of lung elastic recoil with decreased

continues

Age-Related Impairments and Functional Limitations   **491**

Table 7-15 (continued)

lung compliance, and changes in lung parenchyma (such as the alveoli enlarging, become thinner, and there are fewer capillaries for delivery of blood).

Other impairments relate to: the pulmonary blood vessels (that they thicken and become less distensible); decreased in total lung capacity and vital capacity; increased in residual volume; decreased in forced expiratory volume; altered pulmonary gas exchange (such as the oxygen tension falls with age, at a rate of 4 mmHg per decade; the partial pressure of oxygen in arterial blood [PaO_2] at age 70 is 75 mmHg, versus 90 mmHg at age 20).

There is a decrease in the homeostatic response and the immune response (caused by the decreased ciliary action to clear secretions, and the decrease of the secretory immunoglobulins and alveolar phagocytic function).

The pulmonary clinical impairments and functional limitations to consider during exercises are: (1) increased ventilatory rate during work; (2) greater blood acidosis; (3) increased likelihood of breathlessness; (4) increased perceived exertion in response to higher intensity exercises (no impairments with low and moderate exercises); (5) reduced signs of hypoxia; (6) impaired cough mechanism; (7) decreased gag reflex; (8) increased risk of aspiration.

Recovery from respiratory illness is prolonged in older patients. There are significant changes in function especially with chronic smoking, and exposure to environmental toxic inhalants.

Intervention strategies to slow or reverse cardiopulmonary impairments and functional limitations are: (1) comprehensive cardiopulmonary assessment by the physical therapist before commencing an exercise program; (2) appropriate selection of an exercise tolerance testing protocol (ETT) (considering that many older patients cannot tolerate maximal testing; therefore, submaximal testing is commonly used); (3) testing and exercise training modes should be similar; (4) an individualized exercise prescription developed by the physical therapist (considering that the choice of training program is based on fitness level, presence or absence of cardiovascular disease, musculoskeletal impairments and limitations, and the patient's goals and interests; the exercise prescription elements should include frequency, intensity, duration, mode); (5) an aerobic training program developed by the physical therapist (may include walking, chair and floor exercises, and modified strength/flexibility calisthenics that are well-tolerated by most older patients); (6) pool programs (safer for bone and joint impairments); (7) multiple modes of exercise may be used such as circuit training on alternate days (to reduce likelihood of muscle injury, joint overuse, pain, and fatigue); (8) increase the physiologic benefits of the patient due to the aerobic training program (these can be decreased heart rate at a given submaximal power, improved maximal oxygen uptake, improved peripheral adaptation and muscle oxidative capacity, improved recovery heart rates, decreased systolic blood pressure, increased maximum ventilatory capacity, and reduced breathlessness); (9) increase the psychologic benefits of the patient due to the aerobic training program (improved sense of well-being and self-image; improvement in functional capacity); (10) increase the overall daily activity levels for independent living; (11) patient education (about the lack of exercise as an important risk factor in the development of cardiopulmonary diseases and contributing to problems of immobility and disability in the older population).

Integumentary, Gastrointestinal, and Renal Impairments

Table 7-16   Integumentary, Gastrointestinal, and Renal Impairments

Age-related integumentary impairments are changes in skin composition (the dermis becomes thinner with a loss of elastin; there is decrease in vascularity; vascular fragility that results in easy bruising; decreased sebaceous activity; decline in integumentary hydration; skin appears dry, wrinkled, yellowed, and inelastic; aging spots appear; aging spots are clusters of melanocyte pigmentation that increases with exposure to the sun).

There is a normal general thinning and graying of the hair because of vascular insufficiency and decreased melanin production.

Nails grow more slowly and become brittle and thick.

There is a loss of integumentary efficiency as a protective barrier (the skin grows and heals more slowly; the skin is less able to resist injury and infection; the skin inflammatory response is slower; there is decreased sensitivity to touch and perception of pain and temperature; there is an increased risk for injury from concentrated skin pressures or excess temperatures).

Decreased sweat production with loss of sweat glands results in decreased temperature regulation and homeostasis.

There are gastrointestinal impairments: decreased salivation, taste, and smell. These impairments are exacerbated by the possibility of inadequate chewing because of tooth loss and/or poor fitting dentures.

Poor swallowing reflex may lead to poor dietary intake and nutritional deficiencies. There is reduced motility and control of the lower esophageal sphincter with possible acid reflux and heartburn. Hiatal hernia is common in older adults.

In the stomach, there is reduced motility and control of the lower esophageal sphincter, delayed gastric emptying, decreased digestive enzymes and hydrochlo-

continues

Table 7-16 (continued)

ric acid, and decreased digestion and absorption. Indigestion is common in older adults.

There is decreased intestinal motility with constipation common.

In the kidneys, there is a loss of mass and total weight with nephron atrophy. There is decreased renal blood flow and decreased filtration. The blood urea rises. There are decreased excretory and reabsorptive kidneys capacities.

Bladder Impairments and Interventions (for Incontinence)

Table 7-17 Bladder Impairments and Interventions (for Incontinence)

In the bladder, muscle weakness impairments result in decreased capacity causing urinary frequency. There is difficulty with emptying the bladder causing increased urinary retention. Urinary incontinence is common, affecting over 10 million adults. Over half of nursing home residents and one third of community-dwelling older persons are affected. Urinary incontinence affects older women with pelvic floor weakness and older men with bladder or prostate disease. There is an increased likelihood of urinary tract infections.

Incontinence interventions for older women are: isometric exercises for pelvic floor awareness training and strengthening. These exercises are used to treat or prevent incontinence and a "leaky bladder," which may occur with coughing, sneezing, laughing, or other straining activities. Instruct the patient (client) to use these exercises and to practice sphincter control by attempting to stop her urine flow intermittently when using the bathroom. Patient position: (1) supine or side-lying positions are the easiest in which to begin; progress to sitting or standing. (2) Instruct the patient (client) to tighten the pelvic floor as if attempting to stop urine flow. (3) Patient to hold the contraction for 3 to 5 seconds and to relax. The bladder should be empty when performing this exercise.

Caution during the exercises: the pelvic floor muscles are highly fatigable. Contractions should not be held longer than 5 seconds and with a maximum of 10 repetitions per session. When fatigued, substitution of the gluteals, abdominals, or hip adductors may occur.

Geriatric Disorders/Diseases and Intervention Patterns

Osteoporosis and Intervention Goals

Table 7-18   Osteoporosis and Intervention Goals

Osteoporosis[4] is a disease process that results in reduction of bone mass caused by failure of bone formation (osteoblast activity) to keep pace with bone reabsorption and destruction (osteoclast activity). More bone is reabsorbed than laid down. The skeleton loses some of the strength derived from its intact bone trabeculation. Aging process causes type II osteoporosis (that used to be called senile osteoporosis). Type I osteoporosis (also called involutional bone loss) occurs as a result of the protective effects of estrogen on bone. Type I osteoporosis takes place at menopause.

The National Osteoporosis Foundation (NOF) estimates that 10 million Americans[4] have osteoporosis. From these, 8 million are women, and 2 million are men. Eighty percent (80%) of individuals affected by osteoporosis are women. Twenty percent (20%) of non-Hispanic, white and Asian women aged 50 and older are estimated[4] by the NOF to have osteoporosis and 52% to have low bone mass. Seven percent (7%) of non-Hispanic and Asian men aged 50 and older are estimated by the NOF to have osteoporosis and 35% to have low bone mass.

Etiologic factors[4] are (1) hormonal deficiency (estrogen in women and testosterone in men); (2) nutritional deficiency (inadequate calcium, impaired absorption of calcium, excessive alcohol, and caffeine consumption); (3) decreased physical activity (inadequate mechanical loading); (4) diseases that affect bone loss (hyperthyroidism, diabetes, hyperparathyroidism, rheumatoid arthritis, liver disease, Paget's disease, and certain types of cancer); (5) medications that affect bone loss (corticosteroids, thyroid hormone, anticonvulsants, catabolic drugs, some estrogen antagonists, chemotherapy); (6) additional risk factors (family history, white/Asian race, early menopause, thin/small build, and smoking).

Osteoporosis characteristics: one third of individuals affected by osteoporosis will experience major orthopedic problems related to osteoporosis. Bone loss progresses for many years without causing symptoms. Bone loss is about 1% per year (starting for women at ages 30 to 35 and for men at ages 50 to 55). Accelerating bone loss happens in postmenopausal women (approximately 5% per year for 3 to 5 years). Structural weakening of bone can take place (decreasing ability to support loads; having a high risk of fractures; trabecular bone more involved than cortical bone). As a result of bone weakening, fractures, bone pain, and loss of mobility can occur. Also skeleton deformities such as kyphosis and loss of height occur (especially if verebral compression fractures take place).

Medications approved[4] by the FDA to prevent and/or treat osteoporosis: Alendronate and Alendronate plus vitamin D (Fosamax and Fosamax plus D), Ibandronate (Boniva), Risedronate and Risedronate with calcium (Actonel and Actonel with calcium), Calcitonin (Miacalcin), estrogens (Climara, Estrace, Estraderm, Estratab, Ogen, Premarin, and others), estrogens and progestins (Activella, Premphase, Prempro and others), parathyroid hormone (Teriparatide), and Raloxifene (Evista).

Common areas affected by osteoporosis are vertebral column (spine and ribs), femoral neck, distal radius/wrist, and humerus.

Physical therapy common assessments and reassessment in osteoporosis: dizziness, sensory integrity, vision, hearing, somatosensory system, vestibular system, sensory integration, motor function, strength, endurance, motor control, ROM and flexibility, postural deformity (such as the feet, for hammer toes and bunions leading to antalgic gait), postural kyphosis (forward head position), hip and knee flexion contractures, postural hypotension, and gait and balance.

Physical therapy intervention goals: (1) maintain bone mass using exercises and activities (such as weightbearing exercises; daily walking for at least 30 minutes; stair climbing; use of weight belts during walking to increase loading; resistance exercises for hip and knee extensors and triceps; postural/balance training; postural exercises to reduce kyphosis; and flexibility exercises); (2) functional balance exercises (such as chair rises; standing/kitchen sink exercises; toe raises; unilateral stance for hip extension and abduction; partial squats); (3) gait training; (4) safety education and fall prevention; (5) patient education (using proper shoes with thin soles and using flat shoes that enhance balance abilities); (6) assistive devices training (using cane or a walker as needed); (7) patient education for fracture prevention (such as counseling on safe activities; avoiding sudden forceful movements; avoiding twisting, standing for too long, bending over, lifting, and performing supine sit-ups).

Common Geriatric Fractures and Interventions

Table 7-19   Common Geriatric Fractures and Interventions

Fractures: associated with low bone density and multiple risk factors, especially for older patients/clients (such as age, co-morbid diseases, dementia, and psychotropic medications).

Hip fractures: most common orthopedic problem[5] of older adults in the United States. The mortality rate for hip fractures is associated mostly with post-fracture complications. Most of the hip fractures occur in the femoral neck or intertrochanteric area of the femur. Preoperatively, Buck's traction may be used for a short period of time to alleviate muscle spasms. Most of the hip fractures are treated surgically

continues

Table 7-19   (continued)

using an open reduction internal fixation [ORIF] (to realign the bone ends). A femoral prosthesis may be used for femoral neck or femoral head fractures. In older patients, bone healing takes from 6 to 12 weeks.

Interventions for hip fractures may include: positioning; progressive weightbearing (as per MD/DO) and gait training; assistive devices for ambulation training; transfer training; ROM, strengthening, and conditioning exercises; and balance activities.

Other types of fractures: vertebral compression fractures (occur in lower thoracic, lumbar regions at T8-L3; may result from routine activities such as bending, lifting, or rising from a chair). Patient's chief complaints are immediate, severe local spinal pain that increases with trunk flexion. Vertebral compression fractures may lead to the following: shortening of spine, progressive loss of height, and spinal deformity (kyphosis) that can progress to respiratory compromise.

Vertebral compression fracture intervention goals: (1) acute phase: patient education for horizontal bed rest (being out of bed for 10 minutes every hour); patient education for proper posture (such as keeping the spine in extension in sitting, standing, or sleeping; bending forward is contraindicated); isometric extension exercises in bed; (2) chronic phase: patient education (extension exercises; avoidance of flexion activities); postural training; modalities and physical agents for pain relief; patient education for safety and modification of the environment; decrease vertebral loading; and the use of soft-soled shoes.

Other types of fractures: stress fractures (are fine, hairline fractures without soft tissue injury). Stress fractures are common in the pelvis, proximal tibia, distal fibula, and metatarsal shafts.

Stress fracture intervention goals: (1) rest, (2) correction of exercise excesses or faulty exercise program, (3) reduction of vertical loading, and (4) the use of soft-soled shoes.

Other types of fractures: upper extremity fractures such as the humeral head and the Colles' fractures (for interventions, see Part III).

Clinical implications of geriatric fracture interventions: fractures heal more slowly. Older adults are prone to complications such as pneumonia and decubitus ulcers. Mental status complications may occur with hospitalization. Rehabilitation may be complicated or prolonged by lack of support systems. Co-morbid conditions exist (such as decreased vision and poor balance).

Degenerative Joint Disease and Interventions

Table 7-20   Degenerative Joint Disease and Interventions

Degenerative joint diseases (osteoarthritis—O/A): a noninflammatory, progressive disorder of joints, typically affecting hips, knees, fingers, and the spine. The incidence of O/A increases with age. O/A can cause moderate to severe limitations in functional daily activities.

O/A characterization: pain, swelling, and stiffness; worse early in the morning or with overuse; may have knee pain, hip pain, muscle spasm, loss of range of motion, mobility deficits, crepitus, bony deformity, and muscle weakness secondary to disuse atrophy.

O/A intervention goals:[5] (1) reduction of pain and muscle spasm (using modalities and physical agents, and relaxation exercises); (2) therapeutic exercises and activities (to maintain or improve ROM; correct muscle imbalances; strengthening exercises to support joints; exercises to improve balance and ambulation); (3) aerobic conditioning; (4) walking programs (associated with decreased joint symptoms, improved function, and sense of well-being); (5) aquatic programs (such as walking in the pool and pool exercises); (6) aerobic conditioning (the Arthritis Foundation suggests an excellent aerobic program); (7) patient education (about disease, taking an active role in the care, joint protection, and energy-conservation strategies); (8) assistive device and equipment training (for ambulation and activities of daily living); (9) promotion of healthy lifestyle; (10) weight reduction (to relieve stress on the joints).

O/A general physical therapy interventions: joint protection, modalities, and physical agents for pain control and decreasing edema and adhesions, conditioning exercises, ROM and strengthening exercises, gait training, orthotics as necessary, and assistive devices during ambulation as necessary (for more interventions, see Part III).

Stroke and Parkinson's Disease and Interventions

Table 7-21   Stroke and Parkinson's Disease and Interventions

Cerebrovascular Accident (CVA): sudden, focal neurologic deficit resulting from ischemic or hemorrhagic lesions in the brain; most common cause of adult disability in the United States. Possible impairments: homonymous hemianopsia, impaired sensory and motor function on the affected side, decreased or lost sensation, hypertonicity, increased reflexes, synergy patterns, hemiplegia or hemi-

continues

Table 7-21 (continued)

paresis, incoordination, motor programming deficits, speech and language disorders with lesions involving the dominant hemisphere, perceptual disorders with lesions of the parietal lobe of the nondominant hemisphere, cognitive and behavioral changes, bladder and bowel dysfunction, and oral and facial dysfunction. Possible functional limitations: decreased mobility skills, impaired gait, impaired postural control and balance, and impaired activities of daily living (ADLs) and instrumental (ADLs).

CVA general physical therapy interventions may include gait training, transfers, positioning, orthotics (AFO), ROM and strengthening exercises, facilitation and inhibition techniques, locomotion training, balance and coordination training, FES, and family and patient education (for more interventions, see Part IV).

Parkinson's disease (PD): chronic, progressive disease of the nervous system. Possible impairments: rigidity, bradykinesia, and resting tremor and impaired postural reflexes. Possible functional limitations: decreased mobility skills, difficulty initiating movements and freezing episodes, slowed movements, gait deficits (such as shuffling gait, festinating gait, and/or loss of arm swing and reciprocal trunk movements), impaired postural control and balance (such as flexed, stooped posture, and/or impaired balance reactions), impaired speech, oral-motor deficits, impaired handwriting, and deficits in ADLs and IADLs.

PD general physical therapy interventions may include gait training (without assistive device), stretching exercises, breathing exercises, relaxation exercises, facilitation and inhibition techniques, balance and coordination training, and functional training (for more interventions, see Part IV).

Clinical implications of geriatric neurologic interventions: older adults are prone to complications (such as contractures, deformities, decubitus ulcers, and mental status complications. Interventions may take longer time or be complicated by lack of support system, co-morbidities, sensorimotor deficits, and/or poor balance. Focus should be on the improvement of function. Compensatory treatment strategies should be used when impairments cannot be remediated (such as environmental modifications and the use of assistive devices and equipment for home).

Cognitive Disorders and Intervention Goals

Table 7-22   Cognitive Disorders and Intervention Goals

Delirium is an acute, reversible state of agitated confusion. Delirium may be potentially irreversible. Delirium produces temporary confusion and loss of mental function. It is characterized by: acute onset (often at night); intervals of lucidity;
hypoalertness or hyperalertness; impaired orientation; memory deficits (affecting
immediate and recent memory); illusions and/or hallucinations; worst symptoms at
night; lasts hours to weeks; disorganized thinking; incoherent speech; disrupted
sleep and wake cycles. Delirium may not necessarily happen in patients 65 years
or older. Delirium can be caused by drug and alcohol withdrawal, drug toxicity
and/or systemic illness, oxygen deprivation to brain (hypoxia), environmental
changes and sensory deprivation, recent hospitalization or institutionalization
(and infections such as sepsis or surgery), and electrolyte and acid base imbalances.

Delirium intervention goals: (1) Provide supportive care by minimizing unanticipated,
frightening, or invasive procedures. (2) Integrate orienting statements into normal
conversation. (3) Do not try to convince the patient (client) that their perception is
distorted. (4) Speak in a calm, clear voice, and maintain eye contact. (5) Encourage patient participation in ADLs. (6) Provide complementary interventions such
as music therapy, massage, and shared activities.

Dementia: progressive, irreversible decline in intellectual functions and memory
causing diminished social, occupational, and intellectual abilities. Criteria for
dementia characterization: (1) intellectual impairments (such as impoverished
thinking, impaired judgment, disorientation, confusion, and impaired social functioning); (2) higher cortical functions impairments (such as aphasia as language
impairments, apraxia as a motor skill impairment, agnosia as a perception impairment); (3) memory impairments (such as loss of recent and long-term memory); (4)
personality impairments (such as alteration or accentuation of premorbid traits
and behavioral changes); (5) fragmented sleep (alertness may be normal). Types
of most common dementias: (1) reversible dementia; (2) primary dementia associated with Alzheimer's disease (can be presenile dementia of the Alzheimer's
type—PDAT, that begins in middle age and results from cerebral arteriosclerosis
or Alzheimer's disease, and senile dementia of the Alzheimer's type—SDAT); (3)
multi-infarct dementia—MID (resulting from multiple small strokes).

Reversible dementia:[1] 10% to 20% of dementias. Reversible dementia has multiple
causes: caused by (1) medications such as sedatives, hypnotics, antianxiety, antidepressants, antiarrhythmics, antihypertensives, anticonvulsants, antipsychotics

Geriatric Disorders/Diseases and Intervention Patterns   **501**

Table 7-22   (continued)

and/or drugs with anticholinergic side effects; caused by (2) nutritional disorders such as B-6 deficiency, thiamine deficiency, B12 deficiency and pernicious anemia, and/or folate deficiency; caused by (3) metabolic disorders such as hyper/hypothyroidism, hypercalcemia, hyper/hyponatremia, hypoglycemia, kidney or liver failure, Cushing syndrome, Addison's disease, hypopituitarism, and/or carcinoma; caused by (4) psychiatric disorders such as depression, anxiety, and/or psychosis; caused by (5) toxins such as air pollution and/or alcohol ingestion.

Primary dementia associated with Alzheimer's disease: 50% to 70% of dementias; affects a very large amount of individuals; very costly; may need institutionalization of the patient. Primary dementia can be presenile dementia of the Alzheimer's type—PDAT, and senile dementia of the Alzheimer's type—SDAT. Etiology includes multiple interacting causes: genetic risk factors (such as evidence of chromosomal abnormalities, family history, and/or Down's syndrome); environmental agents (such as viruses, traumatic brain injury, aluminum toxicity, and/or minor strokes). PDAT: starts between 40s and 60s; affects women more than men; has rapid onset; is less gradual and more severe than SDAT; progresses rapidly; has poor prognosis; is diffuse and generalized; has a mean survival of 4 years; death may occur and be caused by general systemic failure or infection; may have occasional seizures. SDAT starts after 60 (average age 75); affects women more than men; varies months to years; mean survival can be between 7 to 11 years; has gradual onset; can progress slowly or rapidly; prognosis is poor (moderate to severe cases); death may occur and be caused by general systemic failure or infection; may have rare episodes of seizure. PDAT and SDAT impairments and functional limitations are: may have occasional tremors; generalized weakness; unsteady gait; increased tone; rigid postures; decreased postural reflexes; increased risk of fall; repetitive behaviors; periods of agitation, restlessness, and wandering; sundowning syndrome (when confusion and agitation increases in late afternoon); progressive disorientation; memory loss; impaired cognition; impaired judgment; impaired abstract thinking; visual and spatial deficits; apraxia; delusions; hallucinations; disorders of sleep and eating, inappropriate sexual behaviors, and apathy (in late stages); personality changes (such as egocentricity, impulsivity, irritability, and inappropriate social behaviors).

Multi-infarct dementia (MID): 20% to 25% of dementias; caused by large and small vascular infarcts in both gray and white matter of brain, and producing loss of brain function. MID is associated with a history of stroke, hypertension, and cardiovascular disease. MID has sudden onset rather than insidious; has spotty and patchy distribution of deficits; and has areas of preserved ability along with impairments. Impairments and functional limitations are: gait and balance abnormalities, muscular weakness, exaggerated DTRs, and emotional lability.

Other types of dementias: Parkinson's disease dementia (in late stages of Parkinson's disease) and alcohol-related dementia (caused by chronic alcoholism with prolonged nutritional deficiency of vitamin B1).

Dementia intervention goals: (1) provision of a safe living environment (to prevent injury, falls, and consequently further dysfunction); (2) provision of patient's safety from wandering using safety monitoring devices; (3) provision of a calming environment and reduction of environmental disturbances (reducing agitation and increasing patient's attention); (4) maintaining patient's remaining functional abilities (by retraining the patient in ADLs; by approaching the patient in a friendly, supportive manner and modeling calm behavior); (5) use of consistent, simple commands and speaking slowly; (6) use nonverbal communication (such as sensory cues, gesture, and demonstration); (7) reorient the patient as necessary (by using prompts, calendars, daily schedules, and memory aids); (8) avoid stressful tasks and emphasize familiar, well-learned skills; (9) use simple learning techniques (such as repetitions, progress slowly, and provide adequate rest time); (10) provide intellectual stimulation (such as simple, well-liked activities and games); (11) provide regular physical activity interventions (such as a walking program; balance activities for fall prevention; activities to promote body awareness and sensory stimulation); (12) family education (is a team approach).

Depression: one of several mood disorders characterized by lack of interest or pleasure in activities and living. Depression can take place with older adults living in community and in institutions. The United States Preventive Services Task Force recommends screening for depression in primary care settings. A simple means of screening for depression is to ask patients the following two questions: "Over the past two weeks have you felt, depressed, or hopeless?" "Over the past 2 weeks have you felt little interest or pleasure in doing things?"

The predisposing factors for depression may be family history, prior episodes of depression, illness, medications' side effects, hormonal, chronic conditions, a loss of physical functions, pain (especially after a stroke), a loss of vision or hearing, losses among the family or friends (death of the husband or wife or a close friend), a loss of a job, a loss of income, a loss of independence, social isolation (including lack of family support), and psychological losses (such as memory and/or intellectual functions).

Characteristics of depression: sadness, hopelessness, tearfulness, a loss of energy, persistent fatigue, persistent feelings of guilt or self-criticism, irritability and agitation, inability to concentrate, a decreased interest in ADLs and, consequently, self-neglect, changes in appetite or body weight (losing or gaining weight), insomnia or excessive sleep, recurrent thoughts of death or suicide, local and general body weakness, impaired memory, indecisiveness, and withdrawal from family and friends.

continues

Table 7-22 (continued)

Depression intervention goals: (1) PTA to report a patient's (client's) depression characteristics immediately to PT; (2) PT to recommend that patient receives medical interventions (sees a physician, psychotherapist, or behavioral therapist; receives medications; receives adequate nutrition and hydration); (3) the therapist to avoid excessive cheerfulness when working with the patient (client) and to provide support and encouragement; (4) the therapist to assist patient in the adjustment process (for losses); (5) patient education (for coping strategies); (6) the therapist to encourage activities and exercise programs (such as an aerobic training program); (7) the therapist to assist in improving and maintaining independence (by patient education for independent skills); and (8) the therapist reaching short-term goals (rather than long-term goals).

Cardiopulmonary Disorders/Diseases and Intervention Goals

Table 7-23   Cardiopulmonary Disorders/Diseases and Intervention Goals

Hypertension (BP of above 120/80): common condition affecting the cardiovascular system; one of the major risk factors for CAD, CHF, stroke, PVD, kidney failure, and retinopathy. Research shows that controlling hypertension increases longevity and helps prevent cardiovascular illnesses. Older patients taking medications for hypertension can have drug induced side effects such as dizziness, hypokalemia, depression, syncope, and confusion.

Coronary artery disease (CAD): narrowing of the coronary arteries as a result of atherosclerosis. CAD accounts for most of all hospital admissions of older persons. CAD is characterized by: (1) angina (warning: angina pain is not always a consistent indicator of ischemia in older patients; shortness of breath is a better indicator of ischemia than angina pain); (2) EKG changes (ST segment depression—may be the most reliable indicator in older patients); (3) acute myocardial infarction (clinical presentation may vary from younger adult; may present with sudden dyspnea, acute confusion, and syncope; clinical course of myocardial infarction is often more complicated in the older patients; mortality rates are higher than of the younger adults).

Congestive heart failure (CHF): inability of the heart to circulate blood effectively and meet the body's metabolic needs. Older patients having CHF may present with: shortness of breath (because of inadequate oxygen to the heart muscles); marked need for rest even after mild physical activity; rising pulse over the day with a slow and incomplete recovery during resting periods; difficult to complete ADLs;

dyspnea while lying down to rest (causing fear to go to sleep and increasing fatigue); ankle edema (that needs to be distinguished from deficit in venous return); absence of systemic BP normal increase with exercises; and slow recovery of pulse and respiration after cessation of effort.

Peripheral vascular disease may be the result of untreated hypertension, diabetes mellitus, and hypercholesterolemia. Atherosclerosis and other forms of peripheral vascular disease can lead to partial or complete obstruction of the main arterial supply to the extremities. This can cause intermittent claudication (cramping or pain in leg muscles) with a small amount of walking and skin lesions (that may lead to amputations). In older patients, an acute lack of oxygen to the working muscles (intermittent claudication) is very dangerous. The reason is that intermittent claudication associated with a minor orthopedic problem such as a hammer toe can develop an ulcer that may lead to gangrene (due to inadequate blood supply), immobility, depression, renal complications, and even death (as a result of coronary thrombosis or hemorrhage).

Chronic obstructive pulmonary diseases (COPDs) that affect older patients (clients) may be asthma (reversible obstructive airway disease with episodic increases in airway resistance due to spasm and narrowing of airways in response to infection, allergic reaction, and environmental conditions), emphysema (abnormal increase in the size of air spaces distal to the terminal bronchiole and destruction of the alveolar walls), and chronic bronchitis (chronic inflammation of the tracheobronchial tree with increased mucous secretion due to cigarette smoking, and environmental agents such as asbestos, silica, coal, and dust). Older patients (clients) may have emphysema and chronic bronchitis at the same time. The impairments of COPDs in older patients (clients) may present (as results of hypoxia or hypercapnia) as shortness of breath (dyspnea), confusion, and fatigue.

Pneumonia is an infectious pulmonary disease that requires hospitalization. Older patients do not necessarily experience high fever and productive cough (as typical symptoms) but altered mental status (confusion), alteration of sleep and wake cycles, anorexia, tachypnea, and dehydration. Early recognition of pneumonia is very important for successful medical interventions.

Cardiopulmonary intervention goals include: (1) patient education for CAD prevention (such as reduction or discontinuation of risk factors such as cigarette smoking and controlling hypertension); (2) cardiac and pulmonary interventions (see Part V); (3) cardiac exercise prescription using the exercise tolerance test (ETT); (4) maintaining consistency with medications; (5) not exceeding the target heart rate during exercises; (6) increasing the recovery time during cardiac rehab or aerobic exercises; (7) individualizing the warm-up and/or the cool-down periods (to address muscle imbalances, postural deficits, and/or flexibility problems); and (8) increasing the patient's (client's) functional level.

Integumentary Conditions/Diseases and Intervention Goals for Pressure Ulcers

Table 7-24   Integumentary Conditions/Diseases and Intervention Goals for Pressure Ulcers

Pressure ulcers (decubitus ulcers): localized area of tissue ischemia and ulcer formation; the result of prolonged pressure over an area or damage to the skin by shear forces; potentially fatal in frail older and chronically ill patients.

Risk factors for decubitus ulcers: immobility and inactivity, sensory impairments, cognitive deficits, decreased circulation, poor nutritional status, and incontinence and moisture.

Bony prominences common to decubitus ulcer formation: ischial tuberosities, sacrum, greater trochanter, heels, ankles, elbows, and scapulae.

Assessments and reassessments for decubitus ulcers: sensory deficits, cognitive impairments, hygiene (incontinence), mobility and activity level of patient, and the effective use of pressure relieving devices.

Decubitus ulcers intervention goals: (1) prevention (special attention to potential areas of skin breakdown); (2) regular skin inspection; (3) patient, patient's family, medical personnel education (about proper skin care such as cleansing and drying the skin; applying skin emollients and lubricants; eliminating mechanical forces; maintaining clean, dry linen and clothing); (4) providing wound care (see Part VI); (5) providing pressure relief (using frequent positioning changes—every 2 hours or less while lying in bed and every 15 minutes or less while sitting; turning schedules); (6) consistent use of appropriate pressure relieving device (such as air fluid beds, waterbeds, beds with polystyrene beads; using a log for pressure relieving devices schedule); (7) improve circulation and healing (using physical agents such as electrical current and ultrasound; AROM; PROM; functional mobility training through ambulation and use of assistive devices as necessary); (8) discuss patient's nutritional status with the rehab team members.

Herpes zoster (shingles): the result of an acute viral infection (varicella-zoster or chickenpox virus) and associated with inflammation of posterior root ganglia of only a few segments of the spinal or cranial peripheral nerves. Patient has intense pain (especially in older patients) and vesicular eruption. The virus may cause meningitis or affect the optic nerve or hearing.

Malignant skin tumors increase in incidence with age. Types of skin cancers: (1) basal cell carcinoma (most common human cancer found on the skin exposed to sun or other forms of ultraviolet light; it begins as a small shiny papule and enlarges to form a whitish border around a central depression or ulcer that may bleed); (2) squamous cell carcinoma (carcinoma that develops primarily from squamous cells; can be found on the skin, mouth, lungs, bronchi, esophagus, or cervix); (3) malignant melanoma (malignant tumor of darkly pigmented cells that often arises in a brown or black mole; can spread aggressively throughout the body to the brain and other internal organs; prevalent in older individuals; 90% of melanomas occur on the skin; survival depends on the depth of the lesion and whether is ulcerated and thicker).

Diabetes Mellitus and Intervention Goals

Table 7-25   Diabetes Mellitus and Intervention Goals

Diabetes mellitus (DM): disorder of carbohydrate metabolism characterized by elevated blood sugar (hyperglycemia) and sugar in urine (glycosuria). DM results from inadequate production of insulin (type 1 DM—insulin-dependent or juvenile onset diabetes). DM results from inadequate utilization of insulin (type 2 DM—non–insulin-dependent or maturity onset diabetes). Type 2 DM results partly from a decreased sensitivity of muscle cells to insulin mediated glucose uptake and partly from a relative decrease in pancreatic insulin secretion. Aging is associated with deteriorating glucose tolerance and type 2 DM (that is caused primarily by obesity and sedentary lifestyles).

Medical problems associated with long-term elevation of blood glucose: neuropathy, retinopathy and blindness, cardiovascular disease, cerebral vascular accident, peripheral ulcerations (feet ulcerations), kidney disease, reduced resistance to infections, and erectile dysfunction. Classic symptoms of DM: frequent urination, increased thirst, dizziness on arising, fatigue, nausea, weight loss, and blurred vision. Severe DM can progress to delirium coma or death.

DM intervention goals: (1) recommendations for patient's dietary assessment (low-fat diet for weight reduction); (2) exercises and activities are important (may delay disease onset, improve blood glucose control and circulation, and reduce cardiovascular risks); (3) exercise testing is recommended prior to exercise (because of increased cardiovascular risk; exercise prescription should include daily aerobic exercises); (4) response to exercise is dependent upon adequacy of disease control; (5) monitoring the patient for exercise/activity-induced hypoglycemia (anxiety, confusion, dizziness, unusual fatigue, headache, nausea, and sweating); (6) patient education about the exercise/activity induced hypoglycemia (patient should recognize symptoms of low blood sugar such as confusion, sweats, and palpitations); (7) patient education about hypoglycemia control (reducing insulin or increasing carbohydrate intake prior to or during exercise); (8) patient education about hyperglycemia (patient should recognize symptoms of high blood sugar

continues

Geriatric Disorders/Diseases and Intervention Patterns   **507**

Table 7-25 (continued)

such as excessive urination and excessive thirst); (9) patient education emphasizing skin care especially of the legs and feet (see patient education in Appendices); (10) patient education for health promotion (to reduce other atherosclerotic risk factors such as smoking cessation and control of hypertension).

Immobility and Intervention Goals

Table 7-26 Immobility and Intervention Goals

Impaired mobility and disability can result from a host of diseases and problems; limitations in function increase with age, especially in individuals over 65.

Immobility can result in additional health problems leading to complications in almost every major organ system. These immobility complications may be: pressure sores, contractures, bone loss, muscular atrophy, general deconditioning, negative nitrogen and calcium balance, impaired glucose tolerance, decreased blood plasma volume, altered drug absorption and metabolism, loss of positive self-image and depression, confusion, dementia secondary to sensory deprivation, egocentricity, and loss of independence and dependency.

Immobility can be classified in: (1) acute immobilization (due to acute catastrophic illnesses such as severe blood loss, burns, hip fracture), (2) chronic immobilization (due to long-standing problems such as CVA, amputations, arthritis, PD, low back pain, and cardiopulmonary diseases), (3) accidental immobilization (due to accidents caused by the environmental barriers in acute and chronic care settings such as bed rails accidents, inappropriate chair accidents, or physical restraints accidents), (4) immobilization due to cognitive impairments (such as depression, anxiety, or fear of falling), and (5) immobilization due to sensory changes or cancer.

Intervention goals for immobility include: (1) increase patient's (client's) optimal function (through a gradual progression of activities to resume ADLs); (2) prevention of further complications or injury; (3) establishing a supportive relationship with the patient and patient's family; (4) using a team approach of health professionals to address all aspects of the patient's problems (medical, pharmacological, nutrition, psychological, social, religious, physical, occupational, and speech therapy); (5) including the patient (and patient family) in decision making.

Falls and Intervention Goals

Table 7-27   Falls and Intervention Goals

Falls and fall injury are a major public health concern for older individuals. For the older individual, falls may result in increased caution and fear of falling, a loss of confidence to function independently, reduced motivation and levels of activity, and increased risk of recurrent falls.

Falls are the result of multiple factors:[2] (1) intrinsic factors (age-related factors, including decreased proprioception; slower righting reflexes; increased postural sway; decreased muscular tone and strength; slower gait and lower foot swing height during gait; decreased visual abilities such as depth perception, visual clarity, adaptation to dark, color sensitivity, increased sensitivity to glare, and decreased visual and spatial function); (2) extrinsic factors (such as poor lighting, furnishings that are too low or too high, slick or irregular floor surfaces, unsafe stairways, bathroom fixtures that are too low or too high, bathroom fixtures that have no arm support).

Medical conditions that may predispose an older patient to fall may include: (1) neurologic conditions (CVA, TIA, PD, delirium, seizures, cerebellar disorders, carotid sinus supersensitivity; myelopathy); (2) cardiovascular dysfunctions (MI, orthostatic hypotension, cardiac arrhythmias); (3) musculoskeletal conditions (deconditioning; muscular weakness; decreased ROM; altered postural synergies; foot deformities; arthritis; proximal limb myopathy; corns; calluses; bunions); (4) gastrointestinal problems (diarrhea; bleeding; loss of consciousness during or immediately after a bowel movement called defecation syncope; and loss of consciousness following a meal called postprandial syncope); (5) visual deficits (cataracts, glaucoma, age-related macular degeneration); (6) metabolic dysfunctions (hypoglycemia, hypothyroidism, anemia, dehydration, hypokalemia, hyponatremia); (7) genitourinary problems (incontinence, excessive urination at night called nocturia, and loss of consciousness during urination called micturition syncope); (8) vestibular disorders (Meniere's disease, benign proximal positional vertigo, hearing loss, and acute labyrinthitis); (9) proprioception impairments (caused by peripheral neuropathy from diabetes mellitus and vitamin B12 deficiency); (10) psychological disorders (depression and anxiety).

Medications that may predispose an older patient to fall may include: (1) analgesics (such as opioids) and antidepressants (such as benzodiazepines) that may cause decreased alertness; (2) antihypertensive medications (such as vasodilators, diuretics, and antiarrhythmics that may impair cerebral blood perfusion); (3) aminoglycosides (antibiotics that include gentamicin and tobramycin) and high-

continues

Geriatric Disorders/Diseases and Intervention Patterns   **509**

Table 7-27   (continued)

dose loop diuretics (to treat hypertension, CHF, and edema) that may contribute to vestibular toxicity; (4) phenothiazines (tranquilizers) that may induce extrapyramidal syndromes that exhibit tremors, chorea, athetosis, and dystonia.

Activity-related risk factors for fall: most falls occur during normal daily activity (such as getting up from bed or chair; turning the head and the body; bending, walking, and ascending and descending stairs). Descending stairs is more hazardous for falls than ascending stairs. The first and last steps are the most dangerous when ascending or descending stairs. Common sites of outdoor falls are curbs and steps. In institutions, the most common sites of falls are by the patient's bedside (during transfers in and out of bed) and in the bathroom.

Standardized tests and measures for functional balance and instability:[2] (1) Tinetti Performance Oriented Mobility Assessment (POMA)—assesses balance (balance subtest that has nine items, four static and five dynamic) and walking (gait subtest that has eight items); maximum score is 28; patients who score less than 19 are at high risk for falls; scores between 19 and 24 are at moderate risk for falls; POMA focuses on maintenance of posture, postural response to voluntary movement, postural response to perturbation, and gait mobility; (2) The Berg Balance Scale (see Appendices)—assesses functional balance (14 items), including maintenance of position (sitting, standing); postural adjustment to voluntary movements (such as sitting to standing, standing to sitting, transfers, stepping up); maximum score is 56; patients who score less than 36 are at high risk for falls; focuses on maintenance of position and postural adjustment to voluntary movement; (3) the Functional Reach Test, FR (Duncan)—assesses maximal distance a person can reach forward beyond arm's length while maintaining a fixed position in standing (single item test); functional reach normatives for adults between 41 to 69 (men, 14.9 ± 2.2; women, 13.8 ± 2.2); adults 70 to 87 (men, 13.2 ± 1.6; women, 10.5 ± 3.5); focuses on postural responses related to voluntary upper extremity movement, and examines limits of stability. An FR of less than 10 is indicative of increased fall risk. (4) The Falls Efficacy Scale (Tinetti Scale)—assesses functional performance in 10 common activities and the patient's (client's) extensive fear of falling that contributes to the functional decline.

Falls intervention goals: (1) eliminate or minimize all fall risk factors (by stabilizing the disease process and consistent use of medications); (2) improve functional mobility; (3) provide exercises to increase strength and flexibility; (4) provide sensory compensatory strategies (such as using mostly sensory systems that are not affected instead of the affected ones; for example, using visual system in ambulation instead of proprioception); (5) balance and gait training; (6) functional training (focusing on sit-to-stand transitions, turning, walking, and ascending and descending stairs); (7) ADLs modification for safety (by providing assistive devices and adaptive equipment as needed); (8) allow adequate time for activities (and instruction in gradual position changes); (9) patient safety education (such as identifying risks, providing instructions in writing, and communicating with family and caregivers); (10) modify the environment to reduce falls and instability (using the environmental checklist, ensuring adequate lighting, using contrasting colors to delineate hazardous areas, and simplifying the environment and reducing clutter).

In cases of falls: (1) Do not attempt to lift patient by yourself (get help, provide first aid, and call EMS). (2)Provide reassurance to the patient. (3) Check patient for risk factors (that may have preceded the fall). (4) Contact the supervising PT. (5) Write a report after the EMS (or help) arrives and the patient is medically stabilized.

Environmental modifications[2] to reduce falls: (1) Bathroom modifications are: eliminate slippery surfaces in the bathtub, install grab bars, eliminate unstable towel racks near the tub and the shower, check for adequate room lighting for the bathroom cabinets, check for safe distances while trying to reach objects in the bathroom cabinets, and assure that the medications stored in the bathroom cabinets have correct and legible labeling. (2) Kitchen modifications are: kitchen cabinets should be at proper height that the person does not need to reach excessively; eliminate slippery surfaces in the kitchen; appliances should be of adequate size to read all the controls; kitchen tables should have stable legs; if the kitchen table has curved legs, check that do not impede the walking path; kitchen chairs should be sturdy with arms and without leg rollers. (3) Stairs modifications are: step height on the stairs should be six inches or less; stairs should have handrails; the stair surfaces should be nonskid; stairs must have proper lighting; if there are inclines on the stairs assure that they are not too long to be managed by the person, and that there are places where someone can rest. (4) Other environmental considerations are: properly position electrical cords that could impede walking; eliminate unstable furniture; arrange furniture to minimize obstacles; assure a comfortable temperature in the house or room; eliminate throw rugs that may impede walking.

SECTION 7-4

Reimbursement Overview

Medicare Reimbursement

Table 7-28   Medicare Reimbursement[5]

Medicare: the largest provider of health services in the United States. Medicare was established in 1965 by the United States Congress as Title XVIII of the Social Security Act to provide medical coverage and health care services to individuals 65 years old or older. Medicare is administered by the Center for Medicare and Medicaid Services (CMS).

Medicare funding comes from the Social Security payroll deductions of employees, the Social Security Act contributions of persons who are self-employed, and the Social Security contributions of employers.

Medicare provides medical coverage and health care services to individuals 65 years or older, persons under 65 years old who have a long-term disability, persons under 65 years old who have chronic renal disease, and widows 50 years old or older who are eligible for disability payments.

The fee-for-service Medicare program has two major parts: Medicare Part A and Medicare Part B. Medicare Part A is the hospital insurance part, whereas Medicare Part B is the medical insurance part. Medicare Part A requires no premiums if an individual or their spouse paid Medicare taxes while working. If a beneficiary does not get premium-free Medicare Part A, they may be able to buy it (under certain conditions). If they have limited income and resources, their state may help them pay for Part A. Medicare Part B requires premiums because it is considered a supplemental medical insurance program that is purchased separately by the beneficiary. The beneficiary has to pay a monthly premium to acquire Medicare Part B coverage. In addition, every Medicare beneficiary (Part A and Part B) must pay deductibles and coinsurance.

Medicare Part A covers: (1) in general inpatient hospital services and supplies; (2) skilled nursing facility services (including rehabilitative services only after a three-day inpatient hospital stay for a related illness or injury); (3) certain home health agency services such as home health-aide services, physical therapy, occupational therapy, and speech and language pathology ordered by a physician and provided by a Medicare certified home health agency; (4) hospice care (for people with a terminal illness; less than 6 months to live; given usually in patient's home including a nursing facility if it is their home).

Medicare Part B covers: (1) physician visits (but not routine physical exams except for the one-time "Welcome to Medicare" physical exam within 6 months of being a Medicare beneficiary); (2) outpatient hospital services as part of a physician's care including outpatient physical therapy, occupational therapy, and speech and

continues

Reimbursement Overview   **513**

Table 7-28   (continued)

language pathology services; (3) outpatient laboratory tests and x-rays, MRIs, CT scans, EKGs, and other diagnostic tests; (4) prosthetic and orthotic items; (5) surgical dressings for treatment of a surgical or surgically treated wound; (6) certain home health services limited to reasonable and necessary part-time or intermittent skilled nursing care and home health aide services as well as physical therapy, occupational therapy, and speech and language pathology that are ordered by a physician and provided by a Medicare certified home health agency; (7) home health services also include medical social services, durable medical equipment (such as wheelchairs, hospital beds, oxygen, and walkers), and medical supplies for use at home; (8) kidney dialysis services and supplies (in a facility or at home); (9) hearing and balance exam (if ordered by a physician); (10) hearing aids and exams for fitting hearing aids are not covered; (11) hepatitis B shots (for people with Medicare who are at high or medium risk for hepatitis B); (12) mammogram screening (to check for breast cancer once every 12 months); (13) medical nutrition therapy services (for people who have diabetes or renal disease and for people who have kidney disease but are not on dialysis); (14) mental health care (with certain limits); and (15) smoking cessation counseling (if ordered by a physician).

References

1. Lewis, CB, Bottomley JM. *Geriatric Physical Therapy: A Clinical Approach.* Norwalk, CT: Appleton & Lange; 1994.
2. Rothstein, JM, Roy, SH, Wolf, SL, Scalzitti, DA. *The Rehabilitation Specialist's Handbook*, 3rd ed. Philadelphia: F.A. Davis Company; 2005.
3. Venes, D. (ed.) *Taber's Cyclopedic Medical Dictionary: Edition 20 Illustrated in Full Color.* Philadelphia: F.A. Davis Company; 2005.
4. National Osteoporosis Foundation. *Fast Facts on Osteoporosis.* Available at the National Osteoporosis Foundation Web site at http://www.nof.org. Accessed December 2006.
5. Dreeben, O. *Introduction to Physical Therapy for Physical Therapist Assistants.* Sudbury, MA: Jones and Bartlett Publishers; 2007.

Part VIII

Pediatric Interventions

PEDIATRIC INTERVENTIONS

Section 8-2: Pediatric Interventions

Screening for Scoliosis
Pediatric Mobility Interventions
Pediatric Orthotic Interventions
Other Types of Pediatric Physical Therapy Interventions
Pediatric Wheelchair Positioning Components

Section 8-3: Pediatric Disorders/Diseases and Intervention Patterns

Pediatric Spondyloarthropathies and Intervention Patterns
Pediatric Orthopedic Disorders/Diseases and Intervention Patterns
Other Pediatric Disorders/Diseases and Intervention Patterns

References

Pediatric Data Collection

PEDIATRIC INTERVENTIONS

Pediatric Screening Tests

Table 8-1   Pediatric Screening Tests[1]

Test	Age Range	Characteristics
APGAR	At 1 and 5 minutes after birth	Screening test performed by physicians or nurses; administered to a newborn infant twice: at 1 and 5 minutes after birth. APGAR test measures the newborn's HR, breathing function, color, muscle tone, and response to stimulation. The results determine the immediate care necessary for the newborn. A score of 7 to 10 is normal. A score of less than 7 indicates that the baby needs assistance (for example, to assist in breathing).
Neonatal Behavioral Assessment Scale (NBAS)	3 days to 4 weeks	Assesses interactive behavior, infant competence, and neurologic status. NBAS is an effective predictor of future neurologic problems and a good tool for teaching parents about infant behaviors.
Neurological Evaluation of the Newborn and Infant	Birth to 12 months	Measures reflexes and muscle tone and provides range of motion expectations.
Movement Assessment of Infants	Birth to 12 months	Assesses muscle tone, reflexes, automatic reactions, and purposeful movement.
Alberta Infant Motor Scale	Birth to age of walking	An observational tool that identifies the components of motor development. It differentiates what is atypical development and small increments that may be attributed to maturation or intervention.
Milani-Comparetti Motor Development Screening Test	Birth to 2 years	Measures functional movement, related reflex, and automatic responses. This screening test: assesses motor development in infants and young children; alerts

		clinicians to deviations in motor development; provides an overview of gross motor status by examining the integration of primitive reflexes and the emergence of purposeful movement.
Hawaii Developmental Charts (formerly Hawaii Early Learning Profile)	Birth to 3 years	Used to demonstrate approximate age ranges in motor, cognitive, language, self-help, and social skills. It is intended for use in planning intervention programs, documenting progress, and monitoring achievement of individual objectives.
Revised Gesell and Amatruda Developmental Neurological Exam	1 month to 5 years	Assesses four areas of development: motor, adaptive, language, and personal–social.
Bayley Scales of Infant Development II	Birth to 42 months	Includes a mental scale, motor scale, and behavioral record. It is scored as a developmental index and incorporates data on special populations (such as prematurity, Down syndrome, HIV, developmental delays).
Denver Developmental Screening Test	2 weeks to 6 years	Measures four domains: personal–social, fine motor adaptive, language, and gross motor. Screens children for delays and determines need for further evaluation.
Peabody Developmental Motor Scales	Birth to 83 months	Includes gross and fine motor scales. It gives standard scores and age-equivalent scores. It also identifies emerging skills. The child does not need to understand verbal language to be scored on this test.

PEDIATRIC INTERVENTIONS

continues

Table 8-1 (continued)

Test	Age Range	Characteristics
The Pediatric Evaluation of Disability Inventory	6 months to 7.5 years	Assesses functional skills: designed for rehabilitation use. It includes self-care, mobility, and social skills. Scores are based on function, amount of assistance required, and need for equipment or modification.
Miller Assessment for Preschoolers	2 years, 9 months to 5 years, 8 months	Identifies children with mild to moderate delays. It combines sensory-motor and cognitive domains and uses developmental approach.
Tufts Assessment of Motor Performance-Pediatric Clinical Version	3 years and above	Measures functional and motor performance skills to monitor child's response to treatment and to determine if treatment goals were met. Measurements include proficiency of skill and time to complete skill.
Bruininks-Oseretsky Test of Motor Performance	4.5 to 14.5 years	Assesses gross and fine motor function in order to make educational and therapeutic placement decisions. Scores are given as age equivalents.
Purdue Perceptual Motor Survey	6 to 10 years	Identifies children lacking perceptual motor abilities needed to acquire academic skills. It includes balance and postural flexibility, body image and differentiation, perceptual–motor match, ocular control, and visual achievement forms.
Test of Motor Impairment	5 to 13 years	Detects motor dysfunction problems indicative of possible neurological dysfunction. It is divided into five areas: balance, upper limb coordination, whole-body coordination, manual dexterity, and simultaneous movement.

Infant Reflexes and Possible Effects If Reflexes Persist

Table 8-2   Infant Reflexes and Possible Effects If Reflexes Persist[1]

Primitive Reflexes	Possible Negative Effects If Reflex Persists
1. Asymmetrical Tonic Neck Reflex (ATNR) Stimulus: Head position turned to one side. Response: Arm and leg on face side are extended; arm and leg on scalp side are flexed; spine is curved with convexity toward face side. Normal age of response: Birth to 6 months.	*Interferes with:* • Feeding • Visual Tracking • Midline use of hands • Bilateral hand use • Rolling • Development of crawling • If ATNR persists, can also lead to skeletal deformities (such as scoliosis, hip subluxation, hip dislocation).
2. Symmetrical Tonic Neck Reflex (STNR) Stimulus: head position, flexion, or extension. Response: When head is in flexion, arms are flexed, legs are extended; when head is in extension, arms are extended, legs are flexed. Normal age of response: 6 to 8 months.	*Interferes with:* • Ability to prop on arms in prone position • Crawling reciprocally • Sitting balance when looking around • Attaining and maintaining hands and knees position • Use of hands when looking at the object in hands (in sitting)
3. Tonic Labyrinthine Reflex (TLR) Stimulus: position of labyrinth in inner ear—reflected in head position. Response: In the supine position, body and extremities are held in extension; in the prone position, body and extremities are held in flexion. Normal age of response: Birth to 6 months	*Interferes with:* • Ability to initiate rolling • Ability to prop on elbows with extended hips when prone • Ability to flex trunk and hips to come to sitting position from supine position • Often causes full body extension, which interferes with balance in sitting or standing

PEDIATRIC INTERVENTIONS

continues

Table 8-2 (continued)

Primitive Reflexes	Possible Negative Effects If Reflex Persists
4. Galant Reflex Stimulus: touch to skin along spine from shoulder to hip. Response: Lateral flexion of trunk to side of stimulus. Normal age of response: 30 weeks of gestation to 2 months.	*Interferes with:* • Development of sitting balance • Can lead to scoliosis
5. Palmar Grasp Reflex Stimulus: pressure in palm on ulnar side of hand. Response: Flexion of fingers causing strong grip. Normal age of response: birth to 4 months.	*Interferes with:* • Ability to grasp and release objects voluntarily • Weightbearing on open hand for propping, crawling, and protective responses
6. Plantar Grasp Reflex Stimulus: pressure to base of toes. Response: Toe flexion. Normal age of response: 28 weeks of gestation to 9 months.	*Interferes with:* • Ability to stand with feet flat on a surface • Balance reactions and weight shifting in standing
7. Rooting Reflex Stimulus: touch on cheek. Response: Turning head to same side with mouth open. Normal age of response: 28 weeks of gestation to 3 months.	*Interferes with:* • Oral–motor development • Development of midline control of head • Optical righting, visual tracking, and social interaction

8. Moro Reflex

Stimulus: head dropping into extension suddenly for a few inches.

Response: Arms abduct with fingers open, then cross trunk into adduction; cry.

Normal age of response: 28 weeks of gestation to 5 months.

Interferes with:

- Balance reactions in sitting
- Protective responses in sitting
- Eye–hand coordination
- Visual tracking

9. Startle Reflex

Stimulus: loud, sudden noise.

Response: Similar to Moro response but elbows remain flexed and hands closed

Normal age of response: 28 weeks of gestation to 5 months.

Interferes with:

- Sitting balance
- Protective responses in sitting
- Eye–hand coordination
- Visual tracking
- Social interaction, attention

10. Positive Support Reflex

Stimulus: weight placed on balls of feet when upright.

Response: Stiffening of legs and trunk into extension.

Normal age of response: 35 weeks of gestation to 2 months.

Interferes with:

- Standing and walking
- Balance reactions and weight shift in standing
- Can also lead to contractures of ankles into plantarflexion

11. Walking (Stepping) Reflex

Stimulus: supported upright position with soles of feet on firm surface.

Response: Reciprocal flexion/extension of legs.

Normal age of response: 38 weeks of gestation to 2 months.

Interferes with:

- Standing and walking
- Balance reactions and weight shift in standing
- Development of smooth, coordinated reciprocal movements of lower extremities

PEDIATRIC INTERVENTIONS

Impairments and Functional Limitations of Tonic Reflexes When the Reflexes Persist

When the Tonic Labyrinthine Reflex (TLR) in supine persists, the child may have the following impairments: contractures, limited visual field, and abnormal vestibular input. Functional limitations may be: rolling from supine to prone, sitting, coming to sit, and reaching in supine.

When the TLR in prone persists, the child may have the following impairments: contractures, abnormal vestibular input, and limited visual field. Functional limitations may be: rolling from prone to supine, sitting, and coming to sit.

When the Symmetrical Tonic Neck Reflex (STNR) persists, the child may have the following impairments: contractures, deficiency in trunk rotation, and deficiency in upper and lower extremity dissociation. Functional limitations may be: creeping, walking, and kneeling.

When the Asymmetrical Tonic Neck Reflex (ATNR) persists, the child may have the following impairments: contractures, trunk asymmetry, hip dislocation, and scoliosis. Functional limitations may be: reaching, segmental rolling, and bringing hand to mouth.

Other Reflexes and Postural Reactions

Table 8-3 Other Reflexes and Postural Reactions

1. Babinski reflex:[2] stimulus—stroking lateral aspect of the plantar surface of foot. Response: extension and fanning of the toes. Normal age of response: birth to 12 months. If reflex persists, the child will have difficulty with balance in standing and weightbearing on his or her feet.
2. Flexor withdrawal reflex: stimulus—noxious stimulus (using pressure or causing pain) to sole of foot or palm of hands. Normal age of response: birth to 2 months. If reflex persists, the child may have hypersensitivity to sensory stimuli.
3. Sucking reflex: stimulus—object in mouth. Normal age of response: 28 weeks of gestation to 2 months. If reflex persists, the child may have difficulty developing more mature oral motor patterns. It is similar to the rooting reflex.
4. Traction response: stimulus—traction on upper extremities as in pull to sit. Normal age of response: 1 to 5 months. If reflex persists, the child may have difficulty grading upper extremity response to traction.

5. Landau reflex: stimulus—in a prone position, when passively flexing the head forward, the child's body flexes. The normal age of response: 3 to 18 months. If reflex persists, the child may have difficulty developing various body movements. The Landau reflex is absent in children with cerebral palsy and gross motor retardation.

6. Neonatal neck righting (neck on body [NOB]): stimulus—head turned to the side. Response: body turns to the side following the head. Normal age of response: birth to 6 months.

7. Optical righting: stimulus—body tilted with respect to upright. Response: head orients to upright position. Normal age of response: 1 month through adulthood.

8. Body righting on head (BOH): stimulus—body contact with solid horizontal surface. Response: head orients to upright position. Normal age of response: 2 months through 5 years.

9. Body righting on body (BOB): stimulus—body in contact with solid horizontal surface. Response: the body will orient itself to gravity. Normal age of response: 4 months to 5 years.

10. Labyrinthine righting: stimulus—body tilted with respect to upright with eyes blindfolded. Response: head orients to upright position. Normal age of response: 1 month through adulthood.

11. Tilting reactions in prone (start at 5 to 7 months), supine (start at 7 to 9 months), sitting (start at 8 to 11 months), quadruped (start at 9 to 12 months), and standing (start at 12 to 18 months): stimulus—instability at the base of support. Response: abduction of arm, leg, and concavity of the spine toward the upward side. Normal age of response: 5 months through adulthood.

12. Protective reactions in sitting: forward at 6 months; lateral at 7 months; backward at 9 months. Stimulus—loss of equilibrium. Response: extension of arm to support the body and keep from falling.

13. Protective reactions in standing: staggering response at 15 to 18 months. Stimulus—loss of equilibrium. Response: placement of lower extremities to reestablish equilibrium.

14. Downward parachute (or visual placing or protective extension downward): stimulus—downward momentum toward a solid surface. Response in the upper extremities: extension of shoulders and elbows to support self. Response in the lower extremities: extension of hips and knees to support self. Normal age of response: 4 months through adulthood.

Reflexes and Developmental Reactions of Childhood

Table 8-4   Reflexes and Developmental Reactions of Childhood

Reflexes and Developmental Reactions[1]	Effects on Development of Motor Skills
Birth to 1 Month Reflexes: sucking and swallowing; palmar grasp; plantar grasp; asymmetrical tonic neck; tonic labyrinthine; Galant; Moro; startle; positive support. Developmental reactions: head righting.	Infant learns vertical orientation to the world. Infant is beginning to strengthen postural muscles. Infant can lift head in prone position to clear airway.
2 to 3 Months Reflexes: traction response of arms in pull to sit is stronger. Sucking and swallowing reflexes are weaker. Galant reflex is inhibited. Stepping reflex is inhibited. Developmental reactions: optical and labyrinthine head righting develops.	Able to hold head up when held at shoulder. Infant holds head up to 90° briefly in prone position, head bobbing upright in supported sitting position, and chest up in prone position with some weight through forearms.
4 to 5 Months Reflexes: integration of asymmetrical tonic neck reflex (ATNR); integration of palmar grasp reflex. Developmental reactions: equilibrium reactions in prone position develop; protective extension forward in sitting position develops; Landau response getting stronger.	Infant rolls from prone to supine position, pivots in prone position, bears weight through extended arms in prone position, forward propping beginning in sitting position, sits alone briefly, and grasps and releases toys.
6 to 7 Months Reflexes: symmetrical tonic neck reflex develops (STNR); Moro reflex inhibited. Developmental reactions: protective extension sideward in sitting position; equilibrium reactions in supine position.	Rolls from supine to prone position, holds weight on one hand to reach for toy, gets to sitting position without assistance, and stands holding on.

8 to 9 Months

Reflexes: inhibition of plantar grasp; STNR is inhibited. Developmental reactions: protective extension backward develops in sitting position.

Gets into hands-and-knees position, moves from sitting to prone position, sits without hand support, creeps on hands and knees, and cruises along furniture.

10 to 11 Months

Developmental reactions: equilibrium responses emerge in quadruped position.

Stands briefly without support and pulls to stand using half-kneel intermediate position.

16 to 24 Months

Developmental reactions: protective extension sideways and backward in standing position.

Squats in play, kicks ball, and propels ride-on toys.

Pediatric Development of Gross and Fine Motor Skills

Table 8-5   Gross and Fine Motor Skills[1]

Newborn to 1 Month

Gross motor skills: (1) prone: physiological flexion, lifts head briefly, head to side; (2) supine: physiological flexion, rolls partly to side; (3) sitting: head lag in pull to sit; (4) standing: reflex standing and walking. Fine motor skills: regards objects in direct line of vision, follows moving object to midline, hands fisted, arm movements are jerky, and movements may be purposeful or random.

2 to 3 Months

Gross motor skills: (1) prone: lifts head 90° briefly, chest up in prone position with some weight through forearms, rolls prone to supine; (2) supine: asymmetrical tonic neck reflex (ATNR) influence is strong, legs kick reciprocally, prefers head to side; (3) sitting: variable head lag in pull to sitting position, needs full support to sit, head upright but bobbing; (4) standing: poor weightbearing, hips in flexion, held behind shoulders. Fine motor skills: can see further distances, hands open more, visually follows through 180°, grasp is reflexive, uses palmar grasp.

4 to 5 Months

Gross motor skills: (1) prone: bears weight on extended arms, pivots in prone to reach toys; (2) supine: rolls from supine to side position, plays with feet to mouth; (3) sitting: head steady in supported sitting position, turns head in sitting position,

continues

Table 8-5 (continued)

sits alone for brief periods; (4) standing: bears all weight through legs in supported stand. Fine motor skills: grasps and releases toys and uses ulnar–palmar grasp.

6 to 7 Months

Gross motor skills: radial-palmar grasp and "rakes" with fingers to pick up small objects. Fine motor skills: voluntary release to transfer objects between hands.

8 to 9 Months

Gross motor skills: (1) prone: gets into hands-and-knees position; (2) supine: does not tolerate supine position; (3) sitting: moves from sitting to prone position; sits without hand support for longer periods and pivots in sitting position; (4) standing: stands at furniture, pulls to stand at furniture, lowers to sitting position from supported stand; (5) mobility: crawls forward, walks along furniture (cruising). Fine motor skills: develops active forearm supination and radial-digital grasp, uses inferior pincer grasp, extends wrist actively, points and pokes with index finger, release of objects is more refined, and takes objects out of container.

10 to 11 Months

Gross motor skills: (1) standing: stands without support briefly, pulls to stand using half-kneel intermediate position and picks up object from floor from standing with support; (2) mobility: walks with both hands held, walks with one hand held, and creeps on hands and feet (bear walk). Fine motor skills: fine pincer grasp developed, puts objects into container, grasps crayon adaptively.

12 to 15 Months

Gross motor skills: (1) mobility: walks without support, fast walking, walks backward, walks sideways, bends over to look between legs, creeps or hitches upstairs, throws ball in sitting position. Fine motor skills: marks paper with crayon, builds tower using two cubes, turns over small container to obtain contents.

16 to 24 Months

Gross motor skills: squats in play, walks upstairs and downstairs with one hand held and both feet on step, propels ride-on toys, kicks ball, throws ball forward, picks up toy from floor without falling. Fine motor skills: folds paper, strings beads, stacks six cubes, imitates vertical and horizontal strokes with crayon on paper, holds crayon with thumb and finger.

2 Years

Gross motor skills: rides tricycle, walks backward, walks on tiptoe, runs on toes, walks downstairs alternating feet, catches large ball, and hops on one foot. Fine motor skills: turns knob, opens and closes jar, buttons large buttons, uses child-sized scissors with help, does 12- to 15-piece puzzles, and folds paper or clothes.

Preschool Age (3 to 4 Years)

Gross motor skills: throws ball 10 feet, hops 2 to 10 times on one foot, jumps distances of up to 2 feet, jumps over obstacles up to 12 inches, throws and catches small ball, runs fast and avoids obstacles. Fine motor skills: controls crayons more effectively, copies a circle or cross, matches colors, cuts with scissors, draws recognizable human figure with head and two extremities, draws squares, and may demonstrate hand preference.

Early School Age (5 to 8 Years)

Gross motor skills: skips on alternate feet, gallops, can play hopscotch, can balance on one foot, is able to control hopping and squatting on one leg, jumps with rhythm and control (jump rope), bounces large ball, kicks ball with greater control, limbs are growing faster than trunk (allowing greater speed and leverage). Fine motor skills: hand preference is evident, prints well and is starting to learn cursive writing, able to button small buttons.

Later School Age (9 to 12 Years)

Gross motor skills: mature patterns of movement in throwing, jumping, running; competitiveness increases, enjoys competitive games; improved balance, coordination, endurance, attention span; boys may develop preadolescent fat spurt; girls may develop prepubescent and pubescent changes in body shape (hips, breasts). Fine motor skills: develops greater control in hand usage, learns to draw, handwriting is developed.

Adolescence (13 Years)

Gross motor skills: rapid growth in size and strength, boys more than girls; puberty leads to changes in body proportions: center of gravity rises toward shoulders for boys, lowers to hips for girls. Fine motor skills: balance skill, coordination, eye-hand coordination, endurance may plateau during growth spurt; develops greater dexterity in fingers for fine tasks (knitting, sewing, art, crafts).

PEDIATRIC
INTERVENTIONS

Table 8-6 Social, Language, Cognitive, and Adaptive Skills of Childhood[1]

Age	Social	Language	Cognitive	Adaptive/ Self-Help
Newborn to 1 month	Eye contact; molds body when held; relaxes when held; regards the face	Crying to indicate needs; monotonous nasal cry; makes comfort sounds	Quiets when picked up; responds to voice; consoles self by sucking	Opens and closes mouth in response to food; beginning coordination of sucking, swallowing, and breathing
2 to 3 months	Watches speaker's eyes and mouth; responds with smile when socially approached; enjoys social play; vocalizes pleasure/displeasure	Coos open-vowel sounds; cries vary in pitch and volume to indicate different needs; laughs; squeals	Searches with eyes for sound; shows active interest in person or object for 1 minute; inspects and plays with own hands	Brings hand to mouth—better coordination of sucking, swallowing, and breathing; stays awake longer periods during the day; sleeps for longer periods at night
4 to 5 months	Socializes with strangers/anyone; lifts arms to mother; enjoys social play; vocalizes pleasure/displeasure	Reacts to music; reacts to own name; babbles consonant chains "bababa"; babbles to people	Looks for hidden voice; plays for 2 to 3 minutes with one toy; finds partially hidden object; works to obtain object out of reach	Holds bottle; eats pureed or strained foods; drinks from cup; naps two to three times per day; sleeps up to 12 hours at night
6 to 7 Months	Smiles at self in mirror; does not like to be separated from mother; recognizes	Babbles double-consonant "baba;" waves bye-bye; produces	Looks for family members when named; shakes toys to hear sound; plays peek-a-	Mouths solid food; feeds self cracker; bites and chews toys

Age				
	mother visually; anxious about strangers; yells to get attention; loves vigorous play	more consonant sounds when babbling	boo; plays with paper; imitates simple gestures	Finger-feeds self; chews using munching pattern; sleeps up to 14 hours at night
8 to 9 months	Lets only mother meet needs; explores environment enthusiastically; enjoys social games	Babbles single consonant "ba"; adult pattern of inflection in babbling; says "dada" or "mama" nonspecifically	Responds to simple verbal requests ("come here," "give mommy"); throws and drops objects; looks at pictures when named	
10 to 11 months	Tests parental reactions; extends toy to show, not give	Babbles monologue when alone; says "dada" or "mama" specifically; repeats sounds or gestures if laughed at; unable to talk while walking	Enjoys looking at pictures in books; stacks and unstacks rings; guides action toy manually; dances	Holds spoon; extends arm or leg for dressing
12 to 15 months	Displays tantrum behaviors; acts impulsively; enjoys imitating adult behaviors; says "no" and resists adult control; distractible	Uses exclamatory sentences ("uh-oh," "no-no"); uses words or word approximations to express self; has one- to three-word vocabulary; says "no" meaningfully; speech may plateau as child learns to walk	Enjoys messy activities such as finger painting; feeding self; recognizes individuals outside family; helps turn pages	Brings spoon to mouth; holds cup and drinks with some spilling; indicates discomfort over dirty diaper; shows pattern of elimination behavior

continues

PEDIATRIC INTERVENTIONS

Table 8-6 (continued)

Age	Social	Language	Cognitive	Adaptive/Self-Help
16 to 24 Months	Expresses affection; plays alone for short times; gets frustrated easily; displays wide range of emotions, including jealousy of a family member; parallel play; interacts with peers using gestures and vocalizations	Imitates environmental sounds; uses two-word sentences; attempts to sing songs; expressive vocabulary up to 50 words; uses own name to refer to self; uses jargon mixed with intelligible words	Can put things away; names six body parts; matches sounds to pictures of animals; sorts objects	Feeds self with spoon, with some spilling; uses rotary jaw movements to chew food; removes shoes; plays with food; helps with washing hands; turns knob to open doors; begins toilet training
2 years	Talks loudly; becomes bossy and demanding; obeys simple rules; has trouble with changes; separates easily from mother in familiar surroundings; may have tantrums; may develop fears of unfamiliar things such as animals or clowns	Child gains language quickly, up to four words per day; uses three-word sentences; frustrated when not understood; tells full name; recites simple nursery rhymes; sings phrases of songs	Matches shapes; completes a 3- to 4-piece puzzle; understands concept of two; plays house; loves being read to; sorts colors, matches some colors	Undresses/dresses with help; uses spoon and fork; uses napkin; washes and dries hands; uses toilet consistently; places clothes up on hook; blows nose with help; insists on doing things without help

Preschool-aged child (3 to 4 years)	Enjoys making friends; plays cooperatively; needs praise and guidance from adults; enjoys helping with adult activities (shopping, setting table); enjoys imitating adult behavior; fears of unfamiliar things may continue	Child talks to self at play and rest; uses rhythmic language; uses language actively; has expressive vocabulary of up to 1,000 words; learns entire songs and nursery rhymes; loves to talk	Identifies colors and shapes; able to do a 30-piece puzzle; identifies money, coins; enjoys books; has vivid imagination; may confuse fantasy with reality	Dresses/undresses independently except for back buttons; uses toilet without help; uses utensils (fork, spoon) independently; brushes teeth with supervision; may be very modest with dressing, toileting, bathing
Early school-aged child (5 to 8 years)	Prefers to play with peers rather than adults; refines social skills of giving, sharing, and receiving; cares deeply what others think of them; likes to impress peers	Uses plurals, pronouns, tenses correctly; recites or sings rhymes, television commercials, and songs; interested in new words; has a vocabulary of 2,000 to 4,000 words	Learns to read; learns basic math skills of addition and subtraction; learns concept of conservation; learns to write (printing)	May have stomach aches related to school attendance; knows likes and dislikes with food; learns to use knife for spreading, cutting; learns to tie shoes

continues

PEDIATRIC INTERVENTIONS

Table 8-6 (continued)

Age	Social	Language	Cognitive	Adaptive/Self-Help
Late school-aged child (9 to 12 years)	Increased interest in group activities; spirit of adventure high; interested in organized sports and sees athletes as heroes; interested in practicing skills to gain social approval and develop skills	Increasing vocabulary and maturity of language skills	Enjoys table games; able to think more abstractly; increased attention span; intellectually curious; reads greater variety of materials including nonfiction	Can bathe independently, wash hair with supervision; independent in daily care activities; learns to cook; takes role in household tasks
Adolescent (13 to 18 years)	Peer-oriented; self-conscious; interest in opposite sex; increase in social maturity	Expressive writing skills improve	Can develop hypotheses, theories; increased attention span; interests expand beyond self to environment, those less fortunate, etc.	Takes on greater household roles (laundry, cooking, cleaning); learns to drive

Common Surgical Procedures for the Hip in Children

Table 8-7 Common Surgical Hip Procedures[1]

Type of Surgery	Disorder/Disease	Surgical Procedure
Myotomy	Cerebral Palsy (CP)	Soft tissue releases, usually of the adductor muscles, can reduce abnormal pressures that cause subluxation and potential dislocation of the femoral head.
Fixation in situ	Slipped Capital Femoral Epiphysis	A pin is driven through the femoral neck into the femoral head to stabilize the head on the neck.
Proximal femoral derotation osteotomy	CP	The femoral head is rotated to decrease the angle of anteversion. This procedure is usually done with a varus osteotomy.
Proximal femoral varus osteotomy	Developmental Hip Dysplasia; Legg Calve Perthes Disease; CP	A wedge is cut out of the femoral neck so that the neck-to-shaft angle is reduced (the neck sticks out more from the shaft). This procedure increases stability of the femur.
Innominate pelvic osteotomy	Developmental Hip Dysplasia; Legg Calve Perthes Disease; CP	If the acetabulum faces more anteriorly and laterally than normal, the hip is not stable in a normal weight-bearing position. This procedure rotates the acetabulum so that it faces more downward and provides more stability for the femoral head during weightbearing.
Pemberton pelvic osteotomy	Developmental Hip Dysplasia; Legg Calve Perthes Disease; CP	The acetabulum is deepened and rotated downward to provide more stability to the femoral head. This procedure is used for the younger child with shallow, dish-shaped acetabulum.

PEDIATRIC INTERVENTIONS

Juvenile Rheumatoid Arthritis Medications and Possible Side Effects

Table 8-8   Juvenile Rheumatoid Arthritis Medications and Possible Side Effects[3]

Class of Drugs	Examples of Drugs	Possible Side Effects
Aspirin and nonsteroidal anti-inflammatory drugs (NSAIDs)	Naproxen, Tolmetin, Ibuprofen, Indomethacin, Fenoprofen, Aspirin	Stomach irritation, tinnitus, Reye's syndrome (aspirin only), rash, headache, dizziness, renal toxicity, edema
Slow-acting antirheumatic drugs (SAARD) Gold salts Antimalarial drugs	Hydroxychloroquine, Penicillamine, Sulfasalazine	Sepsis, rash, thrombocytopenia, kidney problems
Corticosteroids	Prednisone	Infection, osteoporosis, growth retardation, weight gain, sterility
Immunosuppressive and cytotoxic agents	Cyclosporin A Methotrexate	Liver disease, bone marrow suppression, pneumonitis

Scoliosis Classifications

Table 8-9   Scoliosis: Onset, Curve, and Location

Age of Onset	Magnitude of Curve	Direction	Location	Curve
Congenital: Birth to 3 years Juvenile: 3 years to puberty Adolescent: during or after puberty	Mild: 0° to 20° Moderate: 20° to 40° Severe: ≥ 40°	Right or left apex	Cervical, cervicothoracic, thoracic, thoracolumbar, or lumbar curves	Minor or major curve Single or double curve

Table 8-10   Types of Scoliosis

Functional (also called postural, nonstructural): no structural changes; correctable with bending or postural correction; may be related to poor posture; may be related to musculoskeletal anomalies

Structural: changes in vertebrae and supporting tissues; decreased flexibility. Usually rotation of vertebrae is present; related changes are to rib cage, pelvis, and hips. Structural scoliosis has a fixed rotational component. Vertebral bodies rotate toward the convexity of the curve. The rotation results in a posterior rib hump in the thoracic region on the convex side of the curve. Structural scoliosis can be treated with bracing and surgery.

Congenital: malformation of vertebrae at 3 to 5 weeks of gestation

Neuromuscular (paralytic): associated with neuromuscular diseases (such as cerebral palsy, muscular dystrophy, or myelomeningocele) and diseases with orthopedic manifestations (such as arthrogryposis and osteogenesis imperfecta).

Idiopathic: cause is unknown. It may be familial tendency for scoliosis. The prognosis varies with age of onset (variable); it is the most common form of scoliosis.

Traumatic onset: associated with spinal fractures, irradiation, tumors, or metabolic disorders (rickets).

Common Surgical Procedures for Scoliosis

Table 8-11   Common Surgical Procedures for Spinal Stabilization

1. Dwyer anterior fusion: requires resection of a rib and cutting through diaphragm to expose vertebrae. Screws are applied to each vertebra with wires between them to stabilize the spine. Dwyer anterior fusion is used only for low curves in thoracolumbar or lumbar areas. All procedures use bony fusion of spine with instrumentation to stabilize fusion. Most require postsurgical orthosis. Newer procedures allow children to get up within first few days of surgery and increase their activities gradually over the first year after surgery.

2. Zielke anterior fusion: same as Dwyer but a newer procedure with better screws used with rods to stabilize segments. It is used only for low curves in thoracolumbar or lumbar areas. Physical therapy post-op interventions includes teaching child and family to use postsurgical orthosis.

3. Harrington rod posterior instrumentation: older procedure not often used. Two rods are attached by hooks to posterior spinal segments: distraction rod on concave side of curve and compression rod on convex side. It cannot control sagittal

continues

Table 8-11 (continued)

plane correction. It always requires postsurgical immobilization of spine. Formerly, it was a standard procedure for spinal stabilization. Harrington procedure is infrequently used because of long rehabilitation time needed and poor correction in sagittal plane. Physical therapy post-op interventions include teaching child and family body mechanics and functional skills, including getting in and out of bed, transfers, dressing, and ambulation.

4. Cotrel-Dubousset posterior instrumentation: two rods with compression and distraction hooks are attached to pedicles or lamina of vertebrae. Normal spinal curves in sagittal plane can be obtained by contouring the rods. Children who have idiopathic scoliosis with good correction may not need spinal orthosis after surgery. It is commonly used for idiopathic scoliosis and neuromuscular scoliosis. Physical therapy postoperative interventions include the following: teaches general range-of-motion and strengthening exercises, emphasizes importance of early ambulation, monitors the fit and the use of spinal orthosis (postoperative), monitors neurologic signs postoperative, and monitors patient's skin for stability of instrumentation.

5. Luque procedure (posterior): two L-shaped rods attach to each level with wiring. Provides good stabilization and allows for lumbar lordosis and pelvic stability. It is good for children with poor bone, skin, or muscle quality. It is associated with a high risk of neurologic deficit.

Types of Developmental Dysplasia of the Hip in Infancy

Table 8-12   Developmental Dysplasia of the Hip in Infancy

1. Dysplasia: hip disorder where the acetabulum may be shallow or small with poor lateral borders. Acetabular dysplasia may occur alone or with any level of femoral deformity or displacement. Physical therapy considerations with all types of dysplasia: the hip must be kept abducted and flexed with the femoral head centered in the acetabulum. In this position, the acetabulum will continue to deepen, maintaining a correct shape, and the ligaments and joint capsule will tighten to provide extra joint stability.

2. Subluxatable dysplasia: the femoral head can be partially displaced to the rim of the acetabulum. It slides laterally, but not all the way out of the socket.

3. Dislocatable dysplasia: the femoral head is in the socket, but it can be displaced completely outside the acetabulum with manual pressure.

4. Dislocated dysplasia: the femoral head lies completely outside the hip socket but can be reduced with manual pressure.

5. Teratologic dysplasia: the femoral head lies completely outside the hip socket and cannot be reduced with manual pressure. Deformity of the joint surfaces is significant; it is usually related to another severe developmental anomaly, such as arthrogryposis or myelomeningocele. Surgery will be needed to reconstruct the joint. After surgery, the child may have pain with some hip movements and will probably have significant limitation in ROM (most likely in abduction and extension).

Spina Bifida Classification and Functional Skill Levels

Table 8-13   Spina Bifida Classification and Functional Skill Levels

Types of Spina Bifida and Innervations	Functional Skills
1. Occulta (not visible): no tissue protruding from nonfused spinous processes; no disability results from this disorder.	Functional abilities: excellent; usually no neurologic or orthopedic problems.
2. Acculta or cystica (visible) A. Meningocele: cerebrospinal fluid and superficial tissue protrudes from the spine in a sac; although tissue protrudes in a sac, neurologic tissue is rarely involved; has no disability.	Functional abilities: excellent; usually no neurologic or orthopedic problems.
B. Myelomeningocele: the meninges and parts of the spinal cord protrude from the abnormally formed spine in a sac; abnormal neural elements are part of the protruding sac; may have disability depending on the involvement level. Types of myelomeningocele: thoracic; high lumbar (L1-L2); mid lumbar (L3-L4); low lumbar (L4-L5); and sacral.	

PEDIATRIC INTERVENTIONS

continues

Table 8-13   (continued)

Types of Spina Bifida and Innervations	Functional Skills
• Myelomeningocele thoracic levels: the innervated muscles are neck, upper limbs, shoulder girdle, and trunk musculature.	No volitional lower limb movements are present. For lesions below T10, lower trunk muscles may be weak; will need to use a wheelchair for mobility (power w/c, RGO, standing frame); likely to develop hydrocephalus; no bowel or bladder control.
• High lumbar myelomeningocele: L1 to L2 levels. Innervated muscles: the same as the thoracic levels; in addition, has hip flexors; however, has weak hip flexion; may develop dislocated hips; is at risk for hip flexion contracture.	May ambulate short distances with assistive devices and orthoses; will need wheelchair for longer distances; no bowel and bladder control; likely to develop hydrocephalus.
• Mid lumbar myelomeningocele: L3 to L4 levels. Innervated muscles: the same as the L1 to L2 levels; in addition, has hip adductors, knee flexors and extensors, and some innervations in ankle dorsiflexion (L4); has no sensation in lower legs or feet.	Will need orthoses and crutches for household and short-distance community ambulation and a wheelchair for longer distances; no bowel and bladder control; likely to develop hydrocephalus.
• Low lumbar myelomeningocele: L 4 to L5 levels. Innervated muscles: the same as the L2 to L3 levels; in addition, has hip extension (weak) and abduction (weak), weak plantarflexion against gravity with eversion; sensation impaired in lower legs and feet; may have some active knee flexion and ankle dorsiflexion with stronger knee extension.	Weak hip extension and abduction; good knee flexion against gravity; weak plantarflexion with eversion and strong dorsiflexion with inversion may lead to foot deformities; can walk without orthoses but needs aids for fatigue; can ride a bicycle; may need a wheelchair for long community distances; no bowel and bladder control; less likely to develop hydrocephalus.

- Sacral myelomeningocele: Has the same innervated muscles as low lumbar myelomeningocele; in addition, has increased strength in ankle plantaflexion and dorsiflexion; has more control of intrinsic foot muscles. Sensation is impaired in feet; has good hip strength and function.

Improved hip stability leads to independent walking without support (except AFO). Weakness in hip abductors and plantarflexors lead to gait deviations; good ambulation with weak push-off and decreased stride length with rapid movement; may have impaired bladder and bowel control.

Classifications of Cerebral Palsy

Table 8-14 CP Classifications[4]

By the Muscular Tone and by the Severity	By Motor Involvement	By Brain Involvement
Muscular Tone Classification: (1) Hypotonic CP characterized by: low muscle tone; floppy, rag doll; weak DTRs; weak primitive reflexes; being overweight; impaired speech; gait deficits such as wide base of support, short stride; has poor balance. (2) Ataxic CP characterized by: poor balance; gait deficits such as wide base of support; poor visual tracking; weak DTRs; weak primitive reflexes. (3) Athetoid or dystonic CP characterized by: writhing movements; fluctuating tone; high DTRs; persistence of ATNR, STNR, TLR; impaired speech; being thin; poor balance; excessive movements in gait. (4) Hypertonic CP characterized by: high muscle tone; tight muscles; spastic, stiff, and rigid; contractures in hip adduction, IR, and flexion, knee flexion, and ankle DF; being thin; impaired speech; poor muscle control in gait; poor balance. (5) Mixed CP characterized by: hypertonicity and athetosis or hypotonicity and ataxia, or hypertonicity and ataxia.	*Body Involvement Classification:* (1) Monoplegia (one extremity involved); (2) Diplegia (both lower extremities are affected; may have less involvement of trunk and arms); (3) Hemiplegia (one arm and one leg on the same side are affected); (4) Quadriplegia or Tetraplegia (all four extremities and trunk are affected); (5) Triplegia (both legs and	*General Classification:* extrapyramidal (including basal ganglia), pyramidal (including motor tracts and multiple areas), and cerebellar.

continues

Table 8-14   (continued)

By the Muscular Tone and by the Severity	By Motor Involvement	By Brain Involvement
	one arm are affected).	
Severity Classification: Mild CP characterized by: development of independent functional skills and some language skills. Moderate CP characterized by: development of independent mobility—crawling, walking with support. Moderate CP may develop a few words of language. Severe CP characterized by: needs help for most function including mobility and feeding; has no language skills.		

Common Causes of Cerebral Palsy

Table 8-15   CP Common Causes

Prenatal (Before Birth) Causes	Perinatal* Causes	Postnatal (After Birth) Causes
Genetic; viruses (such as herpes, cytomegalovirus, rubella); infections (such as toxoplasmosis); drugs; alcohol; prescription and nonprescription drugs with teratogen effects (adversely affecting normal cellular development in the embryo or fetus).	Prematurity; low birth weight; severe jaundice; intraventricular hemorrhage; poor nutrition (of the mother); asphyxia; prolonged labor; breech birth; prolapsed cord.	Infection; trauma; motor vehicle accident; child abuse; shaken baby syndrome; asphyxia; head injury; near drowning; cardiac arrest; cerebral vascular accident; brain tumor; lead exposure; thrombosis; sickle cell anemia.

*Perinatal = from 28th week of pregnancy to 28 days after birth

Table 8-16 Clinical Signs for Hypotonic, Hypertonic, and Athetoid CP

CP	Hypotonic	Hypertonic	Athetoid
Characteristics	Low tone, floppy, "rag doll"	High tone—spastic, stiff, or rigid	Fluctuating tone, writhing, constantly moving
Distribution	Generalized, symmetrical	Generalized, often asymmetrical	Generalized, can be asymmetrical
Range of motion	Excessive, too much joint movement, stiffness caused by lack of movement in older children	Limited, contractures developing with age	Full range of motion resulting from constantly moving through range
Risk for contractures and deformities	Risk of dislocation (jaw, hip, atlantoaxial joint), risk for contractures caused by lack of movement in older children	Risks for contractures (flexor muscles), dislocation (hip joint), and deformities (scoliosis, kyphosis)	Risk for deformities (scoliosis, lordosis), risk for joint contractures if spasticity is present in addition to athetosis
DTRs	Weak	Abnormally strong	Abnormally strong
Integration of primitive reflexes	Weak display of reflexes, sometimes delayed integration	Often delayed integration of reflexes	Often delayed integration of reflexes
Achievement of motor milestones	Delayed (amount of delay correlates with severity of hypotonicity)	Delayed (amount of delay correlates with severity of hypertonicity)	Delayed (amount of delay correlates with severity of tone deviations)
Body position influence	Tone remains the same	Tone fluctuates with change in body position	Tone fluctuates with change in body position

continues

Table 8-16 (continued)

CP	Hypotonic	Hypertonic	Athetoid
Muscle consistency	Soft, doughy	Hard, rock-like	Stringy and elastic
Respiratory problems	Shallow breathing, choking because of weakness in pharyngeal muscles	Decreased thoracic mobility, limited inspiration and expiration	Decreased thoracic mobility and shallow breathing related to poor control of respiratory muscles
Speech problems	Shallow breathing, difficulty with sustaining voice sounds	Dysarthria (difficulty with motor speech) secondary to hypertonicity in oral muscles	Dysarthria secondary to poor motor control in oral muscles
Feeding problems	Weak gag reflex, open mouth and protruding tongue, poor coordination of swallowing and breathing	Abnormally strong gag reflex, tongue thrust, bite reflex, rooting reflex	Abnormally strong gag reflex, tongue thrust, poor coordination of oral muscles for chewing and swallowing

Genetic Disorders

Table 8-17   Genetic Disorders[5]

Chromosome Abnormalities (Deviation In the Number of Chromosomes)

Types: (1) Down syndrome—trisomy 21 (characteristics: facial features include flat occiput, flat face, upward slanting eyes; hypotonicity; broad, short feet and hands; protruding abdomen; mental retardation; possible cardiac anomalies); (2) Edwards syndrome—trisomy 18 (characteristics: small stature; long, narrow skull; low set ears; hypotonicity; rocker-bottom feet; scoliosis; profound mental retardation); (3) Patau syndrome—trisomy 13 (characteristics: microcephaly—abnormally small head; cleft lip and palate; polydactyly of hands and feet—having more than five fingers per hand or toes; severe to profound mental retardation).

Sex Chromosomes Abnormalities

Types: (1) Turner syndrome—XO syndrome (characteristics: congenitally webbed neck caused by fetal lymphedema; growth retardation; ptosis of upper eyelids—drooping of the upper eyelids; lack of sexual development; congenital heart and kidney disease; scoliosis; low normal intelligence); (2) Klinefelter syndrome—XXY (characteristics: long limbs; tall and slender build until adulthood when obesity becomes a problem—if no testosterone replacement therapy; small penis and testes; low average to mild mental retardation; tremors, behavior problems).

Partial Deletion Syndrome (or chromosome 9, partial monosomy 9p; or partial deletion of short arm of chromosome 9)—**Rare Pediatric Diseases**

Types: (1) Cri du chat syndrome 5p—caused by a DNA mutation of chromosome 5 (characteristics: high-pitched, catlike cry in infancy; microcephaly; low-set ears; hypotonicity; severe mental retardation; scoliosis; clubfeet; dislocated hips); (2) Prader-Willi syndrome 15—caused by absence of chromosomal material from chromosome (characteristics: low tone with feeding disorder in infancy; insatiable appetite that develops in toddlerhood; moderate mental retardation; hyperflexibility; obesity; characteristic facial features including almond-shaped eyes; small stature; small hands and feet; small penis); (3) Williams Beuren syndrome—caused by a chromosomal deletion near the elastin gene on chromosome 7 (characteristics: syndrome characteristic facial abnormalities, including prominent lips, medial eyebrow flare, and open mouth; mild microcephaly; mild growth retardation; short nails; mild to moderate mental retardation; cardiovascular anomalies).

Specific Gene Defects Autosomal Dominant

Types: (1) Neurofibromatosis (characteristics: has areas of hyperpigmentation or hypopigmentation of skin, including "café au lait" spots or axillary "freckling"; has tumors along nerves, in connective tissue, eyes, or meninges; macrocephaly—

continues

Table 8-17   (continued)

abnormally large head; short stature; may have skeletal abnormalities including scoliosis, bowing of long bones, and dislocations); (2) Tuberous sclerosis—rare genetic disease that causes benign tumors to grow in the brain and on other vital organs such as the kidneys, heart, eyes, lungs, and skin (characteristics: causes seizures and mental retardation; skin lesions on cheeks, around nose; "café au lait" spots; cyst-like areas in bones of fingers; kidney and teeth abnormalities); (3) Osteogenesis imperfecta—brittle bone disease (characteristics of most common types: type I—small stature; thin bones; bowing of bones; fractures of long bones; hyperextensible joints; kyphoscoliosis; flat feet; thin skin; deafness in adult life; blue sclerae of eyes; blue or yellow teeth; type II—prenatal growth deficiency; short limbs; multiple fractures; hypotonia; hydrocephalus; frequent early death; type III—short stature; bowing and angulations of long bones; multiple fractures; kyphoscoliosis; type IV—osteoporosis leading to fractures; variable mild deformity of long bones; normal sclerae of eyes; may have poor teeth).

Autosomal Recessive Disorders

Types: (1) Spinal muscular atrophy (characteristics: progressive muscle atrophy and weakness; normal intelligence; normal sensation; weakness may begin before birth, in early childhood, or in later childhood); (2) Sickle cell disease (characteristics: a group of diseases characterized by blood disorders related to hemoglobin defects; mostly seen in people of African or infrequently of Mediterranean descent; sickle-shaped red blood cells cause anemia, and possible blockages in veins, causing a variety of conditions including leg ulcers, arthritis, acute pain, and problems in major organ systems such as spleen, liver, kidney, bones, heart, and central nervous system; children may exhibit weakness, pain or fever and may have growth retardation); (3) Hurler syndrome (characteristics: normal or rapid growth during the first year with deterioration during second year; coarse facial features characterized by full lips, flared nostrils, thick eyebrows, low nasal bridge, and prominent forehead; stiff joints; small stature; small teeth, enlarged tongue; kyphosis, short neck; claw hand, hip dislocation and other joint deformities; mental retardation); (4) Phenylketonuria (characteristics: children cannot metabolize the amino acid phenylalanine; causes mental retardation, growth retardation, hypertonicity, seizures, pigment deficiency of hair and skin if left untreated; can be successfully treated by limiting the amount of phenylalanine in the diet); (5) Cystic fibrosis—most common single gene disorder in whites (characteristics: abnormal secretions of body fluids including unusual sweat and a thick mucous that prevents the body from properly cleansing the lungs; the mucous interrupts vital organs function leading to infections); (6) Tay-Sachs disease—fatal disorder (by age 5) causing a progressing degeneration of CNS; is caused by an absence of an enzyme hexosaminidase A, that builds up nerve cells in the body.

Sex-Linked Disorders (Affecting Only Boys)

Types: (1) Fragile X syndrome (characteristics: one of the most common causes of mental retardation in boys; characteristic facial features include elongated face, large ears, and prominent jaw; includes enlarged testicles in adulthood and prolapse of the mitral valve in the heart; mental retardation is usually in the severe range, sometimes with aggressive behaviors; some boys will have poor coordination and hypotonia); (2) Duchenne muscular dystrophy (characteristics: progressive muscular weakness beginning between 2 to 5 years of age; characteristic gait disturbances, including toe walking, abducted gait, lordosis, waddling gait; progressive weakness leads to wheelchair use, decreased independence in all areas, and finally death by respiratory or cardiac failure); (3) Lowe syndrome—X-linked genetic trait and symptoms caused by a lack of the enzyme phosphatidylinositol 4, 5-biphosphate, 5-phosphatase; it is also known as oculocerebrorenal syndrome (characteristics: rare inherited metabolic disease; lack of muscle tone—hypotonia; multiple abnormalities of the eyes and bones; the presence at birth of clouding of the lenses of the eyes—cataracts; mental retardation; short stature; multiple kidney problems; protrusion of the eyeball from the eye socket; failure to gain weight and grow at the expected rate; weak or absent deep tendon reflexes); (4) Lesch-Nyhan syndrome—inherited metabolic disease that produces an excess of uric acid because the absence of an enzyme essential in body's purine metabolism (characteristics: moderate to severe mental retardation; hypertonicity leading to dislocated hips, club foot, growth retardation, movement disorders including chorea, ballistic movements, and tremor; has self-mutilating behaviors including lip-biting and fingertip-biting).

Osteogenesis Imperfecta

Table 8-18 Osteogenesis Imperfecta Classifications

Osteogenesis imperfecta is a genetic disorder characterized by fragile bones that break easily (often without apparent causes), low bone density, and scoliosis. The characteristics of OI vary from person to person, and not all characteristics are evident in each case.

Type I: most common and the mildest type of OI; the collagen structure is normal, but the amount of collagen is less than normal; the child may have triangular shaped face and thin and smooth skin; the sclera of the eyes have a blue, purple, or gray

continues

Table 8-18 (continued)

tint; the teeth may be brittle; may have hearing loss that began in 10s or 20s; bones fracture easily; most fractures occur before puberty; the joints are loose, and the muscles are weak; bone deformity is absent or minimal.

Type II: less common; is the most severe form; collagen is improperly formed; there are numerous fractures and severe bone deformity; newborns with OI can get a fracture before birth and may die shortly after birth (because respiratory problems); children who live with this type of OI have small stature and undeveloped lungs.

Type III: least common; very severe form; collagen is improperly formed; fractures are present at birth and x-rays reveal healed fractures that occurred before birth; the child has short stature, loose joints and poor muscle development; the child has a progressive deformity of the long bones, the skull, and the spine; the child may have a barrel shaped rib cage; the child may have hearing loss and dental problems; the child may have respiratory difficulties because of severe kyphosis and scoliosis (both); the child may have hearing loss.

Type IV: is a type between type I and type III in severity; collagen is improperly formed; the child has loose and easily overstretched joints; has dental problems; has fairly short stature, triangular face, and barrel shaped rib cage; hearing loss is possible; the child may be able to ambulate.

Type V: is clinically similar to type IV; bone has a "mesh-like" appearance (when viewed under the microscope); x-rays show a dense band adjacent to the growth plate of the long bones; the fracture sites (or surgical procedures sites) have unusually large hypertrophic calluses (where new bone is laid down as part of the healing process); the membranes between the radius and ulna in the forearm are calcified restricting the forearm supination and pronation; the child has normal teeth but white sclera of the eyes.

Type VI: can be determined by a blood test and a bone biopsy (to diagnose this type with certainty); the bone appearance under the microscope has a "fish-scale" look; very few people are identified with this type; people with this type are moderately to severely affected; they have normal white or slightly blue sclera of the eyes; the teeth are not affected; they have slightly elevated alkaline phosphatase enzyme (that is important in bone formation).

Slipped Capital Femoral Epiphysis

Table 8-19   SCFE Classifications

Chronic slip SCFE: gradual onset with progression of symptoms for 3 weeks or more; most common type of onset.

Acute slip SCFE: sudden onset of severe pain; it is precipitated by the trauma.

Acute on chronic slip SCFE: symptoms build up gradually over a period of time; then a traumatic episode causes severe symptoms.

Grades of slippage for SCFE: (1) preslip (exhibits mild changes on x-rays, including a widened growth plate); grade I (mild slip; femoral head slipped less than a one third the width of the femoral neck); grade II (moderate slip; femoral head slipped between one third and one half the width of the femoral neck); grade III (severe slip; femoral head slipped more than one half the width of the femoral neck).

Signs and symptoms of SCFE: the child has intermittent limp and pain in the groin, buttock, or thigh. Mild strain (such as jumping off a step) or severe strain (such as falling off a bicycle) may start the pain. The child may lean toward the side of the pain and ambulate with an antalgic (painful) gait. The child may also exhibit a Trendelenburg gait (of the unaffected side) because weakness of the abductor musculature on the affected (involved) side. The leg may be held in external rotation. Also when attempting to flex the hip, the child will exhibit external rotation. Range of motion limitations may be found in the hip internal rotation, abduction, and flexion.

SECTION 8-2

Pediatric Interventions

Screening for Scoliosis

Table 8-20   Scoliosis Screening

Standing:

The child is standing and facing away from examiner.

1. Assess symmetry of the shoulders. Shoulder may be elevated on the convex side.
2. Assess symmetry of scapulae and posterior rib cage. Scapula may be high and rib cage may be prominent on the convex side of the curve.
3. Assess symmetry of the waist and gluteal folds. The waist may appear fuller on the convex side of the curve. Gluteal folds may be symmetrical.
4. Assess symmetry of the hips. One hip may protrude.
5. Drop plumb line from occiput to assess trunk alignment. Plumb line may fall lateral to gluteal crease. If it falls over gluteal crease, check for a compensatory curve.
6. Assess symmetry of spinous processes.

Bending Forward:

7. The child bends forward from the waist as if to touch the ground. The arms should swing freely.
8. As the child bends forward, assess symmetry of the rib cage. Rib hump may appear posteriorly on the convex side.

Pediatric Mobility Interventions

Table 8-21   Mobility Interventions: Ambulation With Assistive Devices[1]

1. Gaining the confidence of the young children before getting them up to learn to walk on crutches is important. This can be achieved by: having the child medicated prior to activity (if the child has pain post surgery); gaining the confidence of parents or caregivers whom the child trusts; sitting and talking or playing with a child for a few minutes before getting the child up; telling the child in an honest and simple way what you are planning to do and why; being firm with your expectations, yet considerate of the child's feelings; using toys, games, or music to engage the young child during the activity; and using appropriate safety equipment including a gait belt (for the child's safety and control).
2. Use appropriate assistive devices or equipment to help the child learn the skills. For example, a child younger than 5 years will probably not be able to learn to use crutches, and thus, a pediatric-sized, front-rolling, or pickup walker may be most appropriate. Crutches and walker should be fitted before getting the child up. In addition, for a child with significant pain and/or fears, progressing from parallel

continues

Table 8-21 (continued)

bars to a walker to crutches may be the most effective method to learn to use the assistive device.

3. Involve the parent or guardian in mobility interventions as much as possible. Teach the parent or guardian how to help the child get to a sitting position on the side of the bed and how to help the child stand up using crutches or walker. The parent should be able to guard the child while walking on flat surfaces, uneven surfaces, and up and down stairs using crutches. The therapist needs to demonstrate the skills with the child and then observe the parent doing it. It is very important that the parent be successful in learning these skills because the child may need help for several days after discharge (from the hospital) until the skills are mastered. In addition, if the child is frightened and uncooperative with the therapist, teaching the parent, grandparent, or sibling to help the child learn the skill is an alternative strategy.

4. Measuring crutches or walker. The height of the crutches should be two finger widths shorter than the child's axillae. The height can be estimated and then fine tuned when the child first stands. The handpads of the crutches should be placed so that child's elbows are slightly bent when standing with the crutches. Then when the elbows are extended fully, the child will be able to lift him or herself up off the ground slightly. When measuring the walker, the walker height should be between the child's waist and the hip level. The walker's height will be dependent on the child's skills and confidence.

5. Teaching ambulation skills on even surfaces. Standing up and sitting down in a chair should be the first skill that is learned. From sitting position, a child should hold the walker or crutches in one hand and place the other on the armrest or seat of the chair. Weight should be placed through the uninvolved leg while the arm pushes off the chair. The arm holding the crutches or walker should be used for balance only. Sitting down should be accomplished using the same steps in reverse. Put the crutches or walker in one hand. Reach back for the chair with the other hand, and gently lower to sitting. Teach how to walk on flat surfaces first. The weightbearing status of the child should be considered before walking. The child should firmly grasp crutches with both hands. Elbows should be held close to sides to stabilize the crutch tops against the ribs. Weight should not be borne through the axillae but through the arms from the hands. The child needs to move the crutches forward, push down through the crutches, and swing the body either to the crutches (or through the crutches) for a longer stride. Guarding should be done from diagonally behind or next to the child. One hand (of the therapist) is on the child's shoulder closest (to the therapist), and the other is on the gait belt. The priority is to help the child regain balance before a fall (not to catch the child once a fall is imminent).

6. Teaching ambulation skills up and down the stairs. Going up and down stairs: in going up or down stairs, the therapist or the parent should guard the child diagonally from behind or next to the child in the same manner as on flat surfaces. Standing on a lower step in front of the child when the child descends (as for adults) is not safe enough for children. The involved leg and the crutches always move together. The child should go up with the "good" and down with the "bad." During ascent of stairs, the uninvolved leg moves up before the crutches and the involved leg and the crutches follow. During descent of stairs, the involved leg and the crutches move down first together. They should move only one step at a time. The therapist should not attempt to have the child take longer strides on the stairs.

Pediatric Orthotic Interventions

Table 8-22   Splints: Indications and Precautions

Indications for Splints	Precautions for Splints
Splints are indicated to prevent joint stress caused by excess motion; prevent or correct contractures and deformity; maintain range-of-motion gains achieved by casting, manipulation, or surgery; rule out undesirable joint motion; support joints in optimal functional position; simplify patterns of coordination; facilitate muscle activity; and decrease agonist spasticity.	When splints are used, avoid unnecessary restriction of movement; interference with sensory input; pressure/friction over bony prominences or at splint edges; nerve compression; incorrect angle of pull; misalignment between movable splint axis and actual joint axis; improper size of splint. When the patient is wearing a splint, observe for stressing or overstretching of a joint; developing stiffness in a splinted joint; impaired circulation; and muscular weakness.

Table 8-23   Pediatric Hand and Wrist Orthotics

Static Splints

Dorsal resting hand splint and volar resting hand splint indicated for: cerebral palsy; head injury; arthrogryposis; limb deficiency; juvenile rheumatoid arthritis; burns; trauma. Benefits: lightweight; durable; attractive; comfortable; broad contact area

continues

Table 8-23   (continued)

(decreased pressure); can be easily remolded. Precautions: splint fit must be monitored as child grows to prevent skin breakdown. Prolonged use can produce joint stiffness. Static thumb index web space splint indicated for cerebral palsy, head injury, spasticity, and fisted thumb. Benefits: Inhibits spastic muscles; maintains range for thumb opposition; places thumb in a functional position. Precautions: monitor splint edges around thumb because this can be area of increased pressure.

Semidynamic Splints

Types: Sof-Splint; Joe Cool thumb splint; Good Samaritan splint; Neoprene web space splint; and Benik Corporation Thumb abduction splint indicated for marked thumb adduction; cerebral palsy; web space tightness; increased tone in hand; limited active use of thumb; excessive thumb joint mobility. Benefits: allows controlled arc of motion; stable and functional position of thumb; quick and easy to fabricate; inexpensive; allows sensory exposure of hand; elasticity prevents too much pressure. Precautions: not to be used with fixed deformity, bony changes, or strong flexion pattern at wrist. With Neoprene web space splint, skin needs to be monitored closely because it has poor ventilation.

Dynamic Splints

Orthokinetic wrist splint and MacKinnon splint indicated for spastic cerebral palsy; hemiplegia with fixed posture of upper extremity; to inhibit spastic flexor muscles; to facilitate extensor muscles; and to encourage bilateral hand use. Precautions: not recommended for children with fisted hands, cortical thumb, or severe radial or ulnar deviation.

Table 8-24   Pediatric Lower Extremity Orthotics

Dynamic ankle-foot orthosis (DAFO): indicated for neuromuscular disorders. Benefits: contoured to produce even pressure distribution; has varying degrees of ankle support; holds forefoot and hind foot in alignment. The DAFO is tolerated more easily than conventional plastic bracing, even in cases of extreme and difficult to manage spasticity. Allowing some sensation of "give" to the brace reduces the tendency of the child to "hold" forcefully against any portion of the brace. Because it is total contact, pressures are distributed much more evenly throughout the brace, reducing the tendency for skin breakdown. Skin breakdown problems are essentially nonexistent in a well-fitting DAFO, even in cases of repeated breakdown and fit problems with conventional AFOs. Precaution: splint fit must be monitored as child grows to prevent skin breakdown.

DAFO with free plantar flexion: indicated for mild or severe abnormal lower extremity tone. Benefits: allows dorsiflexion and plantar flexion; allows maximal lower leg contact during crawling; and does not interfere with balance reactions. Precautions: splint fit must be monitored as child grows to prevent skin breakdown.

Solid-back DAFO: indicated for children who are unable to do "foot flat" voluntarily during the stance phase of gait. Benefits: may eliminate hyperextension of knee; keeps heel down in splint; can prevent shortening of calf muscles. Precautions: observe for redness and poor skin tolerance.

Floor reaction AFO: indicated for crouch gait caused by weakness (secondary to myelodysplasia). Benefits: blocks ankle dorsiflexion; easy donning and doffing; encourages hip and knee extension. Precautions: poor intrinsic foot control; does not work well for children with crouch gait because of high tone (spastic diplegia).

Resting splints for night use: indicated for plantar flexion contracture not managed by daytime splinting. Benefits: prolonged stretch on soft tissues; worn at night; good also for static standing. Limitation: not for ambulation.

Foot orthotics indicated for hypotonicity and hypermobility of feet with good control of muscle activity. Types of foot orthotics: UCBL MOD (for hypermobile, flexible, pronated feet with severe transverse plane subluxation and calcaneal eversion); gait plates in toe and out toe (functional orthotics for fourth and fifth metatarsal heads); Robert Whitman (for children with excessive—but not severe—pronation at midfoot); Kiddythotics (prefabricated for beginning walkers through 4 or 5 years old depending on shoe size; for moderate pronation). Benefits: support weight-bearing surface of foot; help with balance; improve mild discrepancy in alignment. Limitations: does not control spastic foot; does not help with foot that fixes into a poorly aligned position.

Other Types of Pediatric Physical Therapy Interventions

Table 8-25 Other Pediatric Interventions

Stretching exercises: used for minor deformities or to supplement orthotics; stretching to be done to counter the deformity (such as for ankle plantarflexion, stretch the ankle into dorsiflexion); when stretching the gastrocnemius or soleus, be careful not to tear the midfoot ligaments.

Promotion of normal developmental skills through play: using creeping; rolling; cruising; pulling to stand; standing; walking.

Types of sensory input stimulation interventions: rubbing using textured material; sand playing; water playing; massage; weightbearing. To increase muscular tone

continues

Table 8-25 (continued)

(for hypotonicity) use: firm handling; tapping; vibration; brushing; quick movements; deep pressure; spinning; bouncing; swinging. To decrease muscular tone (for hypertonicity or athetosis) use rocking; rhythmic movements; firm touch; stroking; slow movements; singing; warm water; relaxing music; wrapping or swaddling; gentle handling.

To maximize function, position the child to facilitate: visual access; use of arms; child's attention; mobility.

Positioning for hypertonicity: facilitate symmetrical posture (aligned trunk, pelvis, and extremities; head in midline to minimize persistent primitive reflexes); position hips and knees at 90°; position hips and knees more than 90° if the child has a strong extensor tone; use the posterior tilt in space position (to help trunk and head upright alignment using the gravity); use static standing positioning (improves weightbearing through long bones; improves visceral function such as bowel and bladder elimination, respiration, and venous return; decreases or prevents lower extremity flexion contractures); use dynamic positioning (using supports; facilitates mobility; increases dynamic postural control; promotes weightbearing).

Improvement of functional skills: elongate shortened muscle groups; inhibit primitive reflexes; facilitate dynamic mobility; facilitate optimal muscular tone; promote weightbearing activities; improve balance; increase muscular strength (and tone); educate the child (and the parent to help the child) to learn new skills.

Positioning for contractures: facilitate positions to prevent or minimize joint deformities (especially for hip flexion contractures)—see previously positioning for hypertonicity.

Pediatric Wheelchair Positioning Components

Table 8-26   Wheelchair Components*

Head support: provides posterior, lateral, or anterior support for head; provides safety during transportation.

Lateral trunk supports: provide postural support for upright positioning and can also be used for trunk support in patients having scoliosis.

Lateral hip guides: promotes neutral positioning of lower extremities and pelvis.

Medial thigh supports: provides a neutral positioning of the thighs and should not be used as a weightbearing surface for the groin (to keep the pelvis back in the chair).

Foot supports: support lower extremities and provide neutral positioning of the lower extremities.

Wheelchair accessories

Lap tray: provides upper extremity positioning and support; assists with trunk extension; provides a surface for the upper extremity activities.

Pelvic belt: maintains pelvic positioning in the chair and provides patient's safety and prevents falling.

Butterfly strap: provides a broad surface to promote anterior chest support and helps upright positioning.

Chest strap: maintains trunk positioning; prevents falling forward and can be used as a supplement to a posterior and lateral positioning aide.

Thigh strap: promotes pelvic alignment in sitting and can be a supplement to the pelvic belt.

---

*For more postural support components, see Part III.

PEDIATRIC INTERVENTIONS

Pediatric Disorders/Diseases and Intervention Patterns

Pediatric Spondyloarthropathies and Intervention Patterns

Table 8-27   Pediatric Spondyloarthropathies and Intervention Patterns[1]

Spondylo-arthropathies	Age of Onset	Characteristics and Interventions
Ankylosing Spondylitis	Adolescence (boys > girls)	May begin with pauciarticular arthritis in childhood or back pain in adolescence and can lead to general arthritis and in severe cases to ankylosis or fusion of the spine. Medical interventions include medications (similar to those used in juvenile rheumatoid arthritis) to decrease inflammation. Physical therapy interventions include swimming and gentle exercise to maintain range of motion and strength.
Psoriatic Arthritis	9 to 10 years (girls > boys)	Arthritis that involves primarily the distal joints of the hands with psoriasis. Girls are affected more commonly than boys. It is usually a mild disease but may lead to general joint destruction. Management is similar to that of other forms of arthritis.
Reactive Arthritis	Variable	Also known as Reiter's syndrome. The syndrome includes urethritis, ocular disturbances, and arthritis. It may be a brief illness with complete recovery or may have long-term sequelae.
Inflammatory Bowel Disease	Variable	Arthritis may be the presenting complaint in children with ulcerative colitis or Crohn's disease. Abdominal cramping, diarrhea, weight loss, unexplained fever, and pauciarticular arthritis are common symptoms. Septic joints, especially the hip, can occur. Interventions vary according to symptoms.

PEDIATRIC INTERVENTIONS

Pediatric Orthopedic Disorders/Diseases and Intervention Patterns

Table 8-28 Pediatric Orthopedic Disorders/Diseases and Intervention Patterns

1. Congenital hip dysplasia is abnormal development of the hip joint resulting in hip instability and dislocation. Etiology: develops in the last trimester of pregnancy; it is believed to have some relationship to hormonal changes (affected by the female hormone called relaxin) during pregnancy or trauma at birth (improper and tight positioning in utero and breech positioning at birth); it affects girls six times more than boys. If the hip dysplasia is not recognized by the age of 18 months, more complications will occur (contractures). Clinically, the child has asymmetrical hip abduction in flexion, asymmetrical groin or buttock skinfolds, the affected hip moving in and out of the socket with manual traction, and apparent femoral shortening on the affected side. Physical therapy tests: Ortolani test (feeling a hip click with passive movement of adducted and flexed hip into abduction with traction); Barlow test (feeling a hip click with manual movement of the flexed hip from abduction to adduction). Medically, the hip will show subluxation or dislocation on the x-rays. Medical interventions: surgical or manual repositioning of the femur into the acetabulum with stabilization (using plaster spica cast from 6 to 18 months) of the surrounding structures. Physical therapy interventions: (1) bracing or splinting of affected hip in flexion and abduction (measuring and fitting the brace); (2) parent education about brace application; proper positioning of hips (in abduction and flexion); lifting and carrying the baby while maintaining the hips in flexion and abduction; (3) interventions involving sensory and motor input to promote normal growth pattern; (4) strengthening exercises (encouraging kicking in infants; encouraging movement transitions such as sit to hands and knees or pulling to stand; encouraging mobility interventions such as creeping or cruising); (5) ROM and stretching exercises (to maintain and increase ROM); and (6) promotion of developmental skills. Postsurgery interventions for dysplasia (initiated after surgery and cast removal): strengthening exercises, stretching exercises, and family education.

2. Osteogenesis imperfecta (OI) is (see types mentioned previously) a connective tissue disorder affecting the formation of collagen during bone development (fragile bones that break easily); genetic disorders causing problems with the amount and quality of collagen in the body; equal likelihood in boys or girls; the child may have low bone density or scoliosis. The child could have fractures, contractures, and deformity. Physical therapy interventions: (1) in general, must address treatment and prevention of fractures, contractures, and deformity; (2)

parent education for infants (about positioning, transfer—infants and young children need to be supported at the head and trunk, not the long bones; when rolling the child for diaper change, not to hold the infant at the ankles); (3) orthotics (splints; lower extremity orthotics; body jackets for protection); (4) strengthening exercises (against gravity; low impact endurance activities such as swimming and walking; for type IV OI may use weight training with light weights); (5) active stretching (not passive stretching due to risk of fractures and joint subluxation); (6) positioning; (7) mobility training with assistive devices (walkers or crutches); and (8) ADLs (dressing, bathing, and training for reaching device).

3. Skeletal fractures may result from genetic OI (during formation and development of bone), trauma, motor vehicle accidents, and child abuse. The characteristic of fractures in children is rapid healing (because of thicker bone periosteum and better bone blood supply than adults). In a newborn, a femur fracture can heal in 3 weeks, but in an 8 year old, it takes 8 weeks to unite the bones. Signs and symptoms of fractures: redness, pain, swelling, heat, and deformity of the extremity, muscle spasm, the child not using the extremity, and the child crying. Most common types of fractures: Buckle fracture (compression of long bone on one side of the bone); Greenstick fracture (on one side of the long bone is compression, while on the other side is distraction); Epiphyseal fracture (involves epiphyseal plate—the growth plate); Spiral fracture (caused by twisting forces on the long bone). Medical interventions: immobilization (plaster casts, splints, internal/external fixation) and medications (analgesics). Physical therapy interventions: (1) pain control (using modalities); patient education for mobility training with assistive devices (using crutches or walker—for children under age of 5); (2) strengthening and endurance exercises of the uninvolved extremity before cast removal and of the involved extremity after cast removal; (3) balance/coordination, and endurance (conditioning with treadmill, bike) exercises.

4. Osgood Schlatter disease (or Jumper's knee) is common in athletic children from osteochondritis of the epiphysis of the tibial tubercle (degenerative changes in the epiphyseal plate of bone during periods of rapid growth); it may result in aseptic necrosis of bone or gradual healing and repair of the bone. The site of pathology is patellar tendon insertion into tibial tuberosity (partial separation of bone). Patient cannot kneel on the tibia. Physical therapy interventions: in acute stage, the patient needs a splint (a felt bar; athletic tape; elastic support; or cast), and decreased loading of knee (no jumping, running); RICE; isometric quads exercises. Later interventions: patellar tendon taping; mobility training (using crutches); ROM exercises. Parent education: not to allow the child to jump or run.

continues

Table 8-28 (continued)

5. Legg-Calve-Perthe's disease (LCPD) is osteochondrosis of the femoral head. It is the most common and most serious disease of avascular conditions in children due to disturbances in blood supply to the femoral head. Causes of LCPD: genetic predisposition, trauma, anatomical variations, and generalized disorder of epiphyseal cartilage. Age of onset: 4 to 8 years, boys have a four times greater incidence than girls (older girls may get LCPD; between 9 and 16 years old). There is necrosis of the epiphyseal plate with collapse of subchondral bone. The head of femur flattens, and healing is slow (because it has less blood supply). The child will start with a limp and mild pain in the groin, medial knee, or the thigh; later the child will have limitation in gait in hip flexion, abduction, and external rotation (called psoatic limp); Trendelenburg gait (pelvis drops on one side due to opposite side gluteus medius weakness); limb length discrepancy; thigh, calf, or buttock atrophy. X-ray shows bony crescent sign. Medical interventions include immobilization in abduction in plaster cast or splints (young child of 5 years old) or femoral surgery (osteotomy for older child). Physical therapy interventions include gait deviation corrections; contracture prevention; patient and parents education (gait training, ROM, strengthening exercises, transfers, and functional skills); mobility training with assistive device on even/uneven surfaces and stairs; consulting with teachers and classroom staff to encourage and support the child and mobility in school; strengthening exercises; ROM exercises; and functional skills.

6. Scheuermann's disease (osteochondrosis of thoracic spine): spinal deformity with an autosomal dominant inheritance; occurring mostly in early adolescence; the child has a marked thoracolumbar kyphosis (called also round back). Symptoms: complaints of back pain in the affected area and complaints of poor posture or fatigue. The child may also have avascular necrosis of three to four thoracic vertebrae. The child presents with rounded shoulders while in school. Interventions in physical therapy: TLSO (Milwaukee brace) and postural awareness exercises; pain control (modalities). Operative interventions are reserved for children with significant deformity and those individuals who stopped growing.

7. Juvenile rheumatoid arthritis (JRA): inflammation of connective tissue presenting with painful and inflamed joints. Etiology is related to bacterial or viral infections (triggering an autoimmune response) and genetic predisposition. JRA presents with inflammation of joints and muscles and pain and stiffness caused by an autoimmune response (when the body's own immune system cannot distinguish normal cells from infectious or destructive antigens). The result of the disease is destruction of healthy tissue causing ankylosis of the joint. There are three kinds

of JRA: oligoarthritis, polyarthritis, and systemic. Half of patients have four to five joints affected, and the onset age is 10 years old (males more than females). Complications of JRA include iridocytis with vision impairment or blindness. Patients can have periods of exacerbation and remission. Seventy percent (70%) of systemic RA (also called Still's disease) experience remission before 16 years old. Physical therapy interventions: maintain ROM and prevent deformities (splinting of hands and fingers in extension; splinting of knee in extension); stretching exercises (to maintain soft tissue flexibility; stretching of HS, biceps, finger flexors); patient/family education (stretching; to avoid joint trauma especially during inflammation flare ups); strengthening and endurance exercises; developmental interventions (facilitation of appropriate development depending on the developmental skills and age; such as movement transitions from floor to standing, cruising, walking, or running).

8. Idiopathic scoliosis: abnormal lateral curvature of the spine (consisting of two curves, the original abnormal curve and a compensatory curve in the opposite direction). Normal curves of the spine are cervical and lumbar lordosis and thoracic kyphosis. Types of scoliosis (see types mentioned previously): most common types are structural (irreversible) and nonstructural (also called reversible; may also be functional or habitual). Nonstructural scoliosis: caused not by actual spinal deformity but by another condition such as a leg length discrepancy or a habitually improper posture or position. The scoliosis curvature is classified based on the convexity of the curve. The most common is "S" curve, right thoracic, left lumbar. A curvature greater than 10° requires physical therapy interventions. Physical therapy interventions: bracing (donning and doffing the brace); strengthening exercises; orthotic management for the shoe such as a shoe lift (if there is a leg-length discrepancy); electrical stimulation; stretching exercises of the tight muscles on the concave side of the curve (in prone, side lying, or heel-sitting positions); strengthening exercises of the weak muscles on the convex side of the curve; and trunk axial elongation (stretching vertically by "walking up the wall with both hands or hang by both arms from an overhead bar).

10. Slipped capital femoral epiphysis (SCFE)—also called coxa vara or epiphyseal hip fracture: hip deformity related to the slippage of the femoral epiphysis. Etiology: hormonal influences (interaction between sex and growth hormones) and genetic predisposition. It occurs mostly in (see types mentioned previously): boys (two to three times more often than girls); tall children with delayed skeletal maturity (obese) near the puberty (9 to 16 years old); African American or Polynesian children (less common in white children). Signs and symptoms: intermittent limp and pain in the groin, buttock, or thigh; Trendelenburg gait; trauma due to

continues

PEDIATRIC INTERVENTIONS

Table 8-28 (continued)

pain and weakness (jumping off a step or falling off a bicycle); leg held in external rotation (also when trying to flex hip goes in external rotation); and limited internal rotation and abduction. Physical therapy interventions: (1) for children without slippage—nonweightbearing with crutches (and dietary changes to lose weight—by dietician); gait or mobility interventions (crutches) and (2) post-surgery—wheelchair training; strengthening exercises; home evaluation for wheelchair accessibility; consultation with teachers regarding school mobility; parent education for home exercises, transfers, mobility.

11. Arthrogryposis multiplex congenita: nonprogressive neuromuscular disorder; present at birth; may be associated with mother having a fever during first trimester; generally includes severe joint contracture and lack of muscular development; may affect foot, hip, knee, shoulder, elbow, wrist (one joint or all joints); subluxed or dislocated hips are common. Children with distal arthrogryposis may be able to ambulate in the community. Children with involvement in all joints may use wheelchair and ambulate only at home. Physical therapy interventions: parent instruction for stretching (daily) and positioning to maintain and increase ROM; strengthening exercises (of neck, trunk, and extremity muscles) using developmental activities (prone on elbows; reaching for toys; sitting; rolling; kneeling and standing); orthotics (upper and lower extremity use of splints and orthoses; promotion of function with orthoses; maintaining ROM); maintenance of posture and prevention of scoliosis (using braces); functional mobility training (rolling; crawling; scooting; wheelchair training—power wheelchair); mobility training with assistive devices (crutches, walkers, parapodium, standers, adapted strollers); may need quads and hamstrings stretching to prevent contractures (later when the child is developmentally walking); may need surgery for club foot (when the child is developmentally ready to stand) or for contractures of the knee.

Other Pediatric Disorders/Diseases and Intervention Patterns

Table 8-29 Other Disorders/Diseases and Intervention Patterns

1. Duchenne's muscular dystrophy: X-linked recessive degenerative disease of muscle tissue; inherited by boys; carried by recessive gene from the mother. It results in destruction of muscle cells and deposits of collagen adipose tissue (laid down in calf muscles, deltoids, quadriceps, and tongue muscles), leading to

pseudohypertrophy. It begins around 2 to 3 years of age with progressive weakness from proximal to distal and can end up with death in late adolescence or early adulthood. By age 4 (and up to age 5), the child exhibits the Gower's sign: when the child pushes up from the floor on his hands, the child walks hands up his legs to be able to stand (because of weakness of knee and hip extensors). Physical therapy interventions: maintain ROM (stretching of contractures such as heel cords, hamstrings, hip flexors, and TFL; splinting; positioning in standing); maintain ambulation and standing as long as possible (using braces; crutches; standing frames; parapodium; dynamic standers; involve the child in motivating activities); maintain cardiorespiratory function and strength as long as possible (encourage recreational activities such as swimming; encourage functional activities); maintain functional skills including mobility (use assistive devices as possible; wheelchair mobility in power wheelchair; teach energy conservation techniques).

2. Down syndrome (Trisomy 21): chromosomal abnormality caused by breakage and translocation of the 21 chromosome. Types of Down syndrome: nondisjunction (over 90% of children have this type); translocation; mosaic (degree of disability is dependent on percentage of cells with abnormal characteristics). Patient can have hypotonia and decreased strength, heart defects, visual and hearing losses, feeding difficulties, speech and articulation deficits, developmental delays, cognitive deficits, and vertebral instability at C1–C2 joints (can cause C1–C2 dislocation or subluxation). Atlantoaxial dislocation is a medical emergency. If there is instability of C1–C2, teach child and family to avoid diving, tumbling, headstands, contact sports such as tackle football, and other activities that could cause hyperflexion injury to the neck. Physical therapy interventions: facilitation of gross motor skills (using positioning, feeding, and motivation—teach parents); provide activities to support oral motor skills (facilitating lip closure; inhibiting tongue protrusion); and teach energy conservation of small children (providing frequent small feedings).

3. Cerebral palsy: nonprogressive perinatal encephalopathy due to hemorrhage of ventricles in the brain, hypoxic encephalopathy, malformations, and trauma of CNS. CP can be spastic (high tone, lesion of motor cortex), athetotic (fluctuating muscle tone with lesion of basal ganglia), and ataxic (decreased balance with lesion of cerebellum). Physical therapy interventions are individualized. For hypotonia, support all limbs to prevent injury, prevent hyperextension at elbows and knees, use AROM and PROM to stimulate increased muscle output, and promote active weightbearing. For hypertonia, positioning of hips and knees greater than 90° of flexion (to inhibit reflexive extension), use midline symmetrical positioning (to inhibit abnormal reflexes), and promote active weightbearing. For

continues

Table 8-29   (continued)

athetosis, encourage midline symmetrical posture, use gentle rhythmic movements (to encourage controlled motor output), and allow abnormal movements if they contribute to functional skills. For ataxia, encourage midline symmetrical positioning, provide sensory input (to help with orientation in space), increase proprioceptive feedback (use weighted belts or vests), and use assistive devices with weights for balance.

4. Myelodysplasia/spina bifida: defective closure of vertebral column. Physical therapy interventions: (1) family education (for positioning to prevent and minimize joint deformities especially hip flexion contracture; for support of the flaccid lower extremities and reduce risk of fracture; to use assistive devices to promote optimal development; to be aware of potential shunt malfunctions causing irritability, headache, lethargy, vomiting, fever, change in behavior or seizure activity—medical emergency); (2) maximizing functional skills (strengthening through play activities; stretching tight joints and muscles; use assistive devices to promote mobility and upright positioning—dynamic or static stander, scooter or cart, wheelchair, power mobility); (3) use orthotics (HKAFO, rollator walker, standing frame, crutches, and Reciprocal Gait Orthosis—for L1–L2 lesions; KAFO, AFO, walker, forearm crutches, and wheelchair for long distances—for L3—L4; AFO, and crutches—for L4–L5; AFO—for sacral myelodysplasia).

5. Cystic fibrosis: disorder of exocrine mucous producing glands including respiratory tract, pancreas, and intestinal tract. Medical interventions: antibiotics, nutrition, and enzyme replacement. Physical therapy interventions: chest physical therapy (percussion and postural drainage), light-graded exercise program, adapted devices as needed, and aerobic activity (can help to mobilize secretions).

6. Brachial plexus injury: traction or compression injury to the unilateral brachial plexus during the birth process or due to a cervical rib abnormality. It is classified as Erb's Palsy involving C5-6 upper arm paralysis and Klumpke's Palsy involving C8-T1 lower arm paralysis (or Erb-Klumpke Palsy involving whole arm). In Erb's Palsy, the child has upper extremity in adduction, extension, internal rotation of shoulder with extension of the elbow. In Klumpke's palsy, the child has weakness or flaccidity of wrist and finger flexors and extensors and the intrinsic muscles of the hand. There is a variable recovery of traction injuries. Medical interventions: surgery to repair avulsion injuries. Physical therapy interventions: partial immobilization of limb across upper abdomen for 1 to 2 weeks (swaddle infant with arm across upper abdomen), gentle ROM to prevent contractures (after initial recovery), facilitate awareness of involved extremity (use joint

approximation, stroking, and weightbearing), and strengthening of muscles (use hand over hand activities and reaching for toys).

7. Pervasive developmental disorder (PDD) or autism—neurobiological disorders related to abnormalities in brain function; has some genetic factor; communication impairments especially expressive and receptive language skills, nonverbal communication, echolalic speech (involuntary repetition of words spoken by others), flat and monotonous or high pitched and loud voice, appears not to hear at times; socialization problems; imagination; and abnormal relationships with objects and events. Physical therapy interventions: use familiar objects and routines; use daily activities to strengthen and for functional skills (such as climbing stairs or running on the playground); and prepare the child for changes in routine.

8. Sickle cell anemia—autosomal recessive genetic trait in people of African and Mediterranean backgrounds; abnormal shape of red blood cells (sickle shaped) cannot pass through capillaries and cause blockages resulting in poor oxygen to some tissues; sickle cells break faster than normal cells causing jaundice; lack of adequate red cells causes anemia; children have fatigue caused by anemia, organ enlargement, necrosis, scarring, and pain caused by occluded blood vessels in spleen, liver, bones and kidneys; can have strokes, skin ulcers. Physical therapy interventions are dependent on the needs of the child; is a team effort; orthopedic interventions for children with fractures due to osteoporosis; wound care, including debridement for children with skin ulcers; and need general conditioning exercises (to increase strength).

9. Respiratory distress syndrome (RDS) or hyaline membrane disease: due to atelectasis (collapsed lungs) because of insufficient surfactant in premature lungs (in premature babies). Interventions: oxygen supplement and physical therapy positioning. Bronchopulmonary dysplasia of newborn: chronic lung disease from using mechanical ventilation or O_2 because RDS. Interventions: respiratory support and positioning.

10. Postnatal complications/disorders: periventricular leukomalacia (PVL) or periventricular hemorrhage: necrosis of white matter of brain and respectively bleeding, resulting in cerebral palsy. Retinopathy: due to low birth weight and high oxygen levels can have detached retina and blindness. Necrotizing enterocolitis: infected bowel (feeding problems). Physical therapy interventions in neonatal care: positioning.

References

1. Ratliffe, KT. *Clinical Pediatric Physical Therapy*. St. Louis: Mosby; 1998.
2. Rothstein, JM, Scalzitti, DA, Mayhew, TP. *The Rehabilitation Specialist's Handbook: Third Edition*. Philadelphia: F.A. Davis Company; 2005.
3. Ciccone, CD. *Pharmacology in Rehabilitation*, 3rd ed. Philadelphia: F.A. Davis Company; 2002.
4. Martin, ST, Kessler, M. *Neurologic Interventions for Physical Therapy*, 2nd ed. Philadelphia: W.B. Saunders Elsevier Company; 2007.
5. National Institute of Health. *Genetic and Rare Diseases Information Center*. National Institute of Health Web site. Available at http://www.rarediseases.info.nih.gov. Accessed November 2006.

APPENDIX A

Berg Balance Scale

Berg Balance Scale

1. Sitting to Standing
   Patient instruction: Please stand up. Try not to use your hands for support.
   ( ) 4, able to stand without using hands and stabilizes independently
   ( ) 3, able to stand independently using hands
   ( ) 2, able to stand using hands after several tries
   ( ) 1, needs minimal aid to stand or stabilize
   ( ) 0, needs moderate to maximal assist to stand

2. Standing Unsupported
   Patient instruction: Please stand for 2 minutes without holding.
   ( ) 4, able to stand safely 2 minutes
   ( ) 3, able to stand 2 minutes without supervision
   ( ) 2, able to stand 30 seconds unsupported
   ( ) 1, needs several tries to stand unsupported 30 seconds
   ( ) 0, unable to stand 30 seconds without support

3. Sitting with Back Unsupported but Feet Supported on Floor or on a Stool
   Patient instruction: Please sit with arms folded for 2 minutes.
   ( ) 4, able to sit safely and securely 2 minutes
   ( ) 3, able to sit 2 minutes with supervision
   ( ) 2, able to sit 30 seconds
   ( ) 1, able to sit 10 seconds
   ( ) 0, unable to sit without support 10 seconds

4. Standing to Sit
   Patient instruction: Please sit down.
   ( ) 4, sits safely with minimal use of hands
   ( ) 3, controls descent by using hands
   ( ) 2, uses back of legs against chair to control descent
   ( ) 1, sits independently, but has uncontrolled descent
   ( ) 0, needs assistance to sit

5. Transfers
   The PTA arranges chairs for a pivot transfer. The PTA can use either two chairs
   (one with arms and one without armrests) or a bed/mat and a chair (with armrests). The patient is asked to transfer one way toward a seat without armrests and one way toward a seat with arms.
   ( ) 4, able to transfer safely with minor use of hands
   ( ) 3, able to transfer safely with definite need of hands
   ( ) 2, able to transfer with verbal cuing and/or supervision
   ( ) 1, needs one person to assist
   ( ) 0, needs two people to assist or supervise to be safe

6. Standing Unsupported with Eyes Closed

   Patient instruction: Please close your eyes and stand still for 10 seconds.

   ( ) 4, able to stand 10 seconds safely

   ( ) 3, able to stand 10 seconds with supervision

   ( ) 2, able to stand 3 seconds

   ( ) 1, unable to keep eyes closed for 3 seconds but stands safely

   ( ) 0, needs help to keep from falling

7. Standing Unsupported with Feet Together

   Patient instruction: Place your feet together and stand without holding.

   ( ) 4, able to place feet together independently and stand safely 1 minute

   ( ) 3, able to place feet together independently and stand with supervision for 1 minute

   ( ) 2, able to place feet together independently but unable to hold for 30 seconds

   ( ) 1, needs help to assume the position but can stand for 15 seconds, feet together

   ( ) 0, needs help to assume the position and unable to stand for 15 seconds

8. Reaching Forward with Outstretched Arm while Standing

   Patient instruction: Please lift arm to 90°. Stretch out your fingers and reach forward as far as you can.

   PTA places a ruler at the tips of the outstretched fingers—patient should not touch the ruler when reaching. The distance recorded by the PTA is from the patient's fingertips (with the patient in the most forward position). The patient should use both hands when possible to avoid trunk rotation.

   ( ) 4, can reach forward confidently 20 to 30 cm (10 inches)

   ( ) 3, can reach forward safely 12 cm (5 inches)

   ( ) 2, can reach forward safely 5 cm (2 inches)

   ( ) 1, reaches forward but needs supervision

   ( ) 0, loses balance when trying, requires external support

9. Pick Up Object from the Floor from a Standing Position

   Patient instruction: Please pick up the shoe (or slipper) that is in front of your feet.

   ( ) 4, able to pick up the shoe safely and easily

   ( ) 3, able to pick up the shoe but needs supervision

   ( ) 2, unable to pick up the shoe, but reaches 2 to 5 cm (1 to 2 inches) from the shoe and keeps balance independently

   ( ) 1, unable to pick up and needs supervision while trying

   ( ) 0, unable to try and needs assistance to keep from losing balance (or falling)

10. Turning to Look behind over Your Left and Right Shoulders while Standing

    Patient instruction: Please turn and look directly behind you over toward the left shoulder. Repeat to the right.

continues

Berg Balance Scale   (continued)

The PTA, standing in the back of the patient, may pick up an object to look at directly, encouraging the patient to turn around.

( ) 4, looks behind from both sides and weight shifts well

( ) 3, looks behind one side only; other side shows less weight shift

( ) 2, turns sideways only but maintains balance

( ) 1, needs close supervision or verbal cuing

( ) 0, needs assistance while turning

11. Turn 360°

Patient instruction: Please turn completely around in a full circle, pause, and then turn a full circle in the other direction.

( ) 4, able to turn 360° safely in 4 seconds or less

( ) 3, able to turn 360° safely, one side only, 4 seconds or less

( ) 2, able to turn 360° safely, but slowly

( ) 1, needs close supervision or verbal cuing

( ) 0, needs assistance while turning

12. Place Alternate Foot on Step or Stool while Standing Unsupported

Patient instruction: Please place each foot alternately on the step stool. Continue until each foot has touched the step stool four times.

( ) 4, able to stand independently and safely and complete 8 steps in 20 seconds

( ) 3, able to stand independently and complete 8 steps in more than 20 seconds

( ) 2, able to complete 4 steps without aid with supervision

( ) 1, able to complete more than 2 steps but needs minimal assistance

( ) 0, needs assistance to keep from falling (or is unable to try)

13. Standing Unsupported, One Foot in Front

PTA needs to demonstrate the action to the patient.

Patient instruction: Please place one foot directly in front of the other. If you feel that you cannot place your foot directly in front, try and step far enough ahead that the heel of your forward foot is ahead of the toes of your other foot.

To score 3 points (at number 3), the length of the step should exceed the length of the other foot, and the width of the stance should approximate the patient's normal stance width.

( ) 4, able to place foot tandem independently and hold 30 seconds

( ) 3, able to place foot ahead of the other independently and hold 30 seconds

( ) 2, able to take a small step independently and hold 30 seconds

( ) 1, needs help to step but can hold 15 seconds

( ) 0, loses balance while stepping or standing

14. Standing on One Leg
    Patient instruction: Please stand on one leg as long as you can without holding.
    ( ) 4, able to lift leg independently and hold longer than 10 seconds
    ( ) 3, able to lift leg independently and hold 5–10 seconds
    ( ) 2, able to lift leg independently and hold 2 seconds (or longer)
    ( ) 1, tries to lift leg but unable to hold 3 seconds—patient remains standing inde-
        pendently
    ( ) 0, unable to try or needs assistance to prevent fall
    Maximum Total Score = 56

APPENDIX B

Patient Education: Borg Scale of Rating of Perceived Exertion

Patient Education: Borg Scale of Rating of Perceived Exertion

While doing exercises or physical activity, we want you to rate your perception of exertion. This feeling should reflect how heavy and strenuous the exercise feels to you, combining all sensations and feelings of physical stress, effort, and fatigue.

Try to appraise your feeling of exertion as honestly as possible without thinking about what the actual physical load is. Your own feeling of effort and exertion is important, not how it compares with other people's feelings.

Nine (9) corresponds to "very light" exercises. For a healthy person, it is like walking slowly at his or her own pace for a few minutes.

Thirteen (13) on the scale is "somewhat hard" exercise, but it still feels okay to continue. Seventeen (17) which is "very hard," is a very strenuous exercise. A healthy person can still go on, but the person needs to push himself or herself. It feels very heavy, and the person is very tired.

Nineteen (19) on the scale is an extremely strenuous exercise level. For most people, this is the most strenuous exercise that they have ever experienced.

APPENDIX C

Skin Care for Lymphedema

Lymphedema Skin Care

Avoid trauma and injury to the skin of your limb(s).

Wear loose fitting clothing and no jewelry. Wear proper, well-fitting footwear.

Avoid prolonged sitting, standing, or crossing your legs.

When traveling by air, ask for a seat with adequate leg room (for lower limb lymphedema). Get up every 30 to 60 minutes, and walk up and down the aisle of the plane. Obtain a note from your doctor for security (related to your bandages or compression garment). Increase your water intake during the air travel because the cabin is dry and your body can get dehydrated. Obtain assistance for carrying, lifting, and transporting your luggage. Wear a lymphedema alert bracelet especially when traveling out of the country. Obtain a prescription for antibiotics from your doctor, and fill it before leaving out of the country (in case an infection occurs while you are away). Consultation with your doctor is recommended before travel.

If you are wearing compression garments, make sure that they are well fitting. For strenuous activity (such as prolonged standing or sitting), support your affected limb with a compression garment (that fits well).

Avoid exposure to extreme temperatures (such as cold or heat). Do not expose your limb to hot tubs or saunas or water temperature above 102°F.

Apply moisturizer daily to prevent chapping and chaffing of skin (especially during cold weather).

Keep your limb clean and dry.

Do not cut your cuticles.

Use care with razors to avoid nicks and skin irritation and to prevent infection.

Protect exposed skin with sunscreen and insect repellant.

Avoid punctures of your skin (if possible) such as injections and blood draws.

Wear gloves while doing activities that might cause skin injury such as gardening, working with tools, or using chemicals (such as detergents).

If scratches or punctures of your skin occur, wash them with soap and water, apply antibiotic (ointment), and observe for signs of infection such as redness.

If a rash, itching, redness, pain, increased skin temperature, fever, or flu-like symptoms occur, contact your doctor immediately.

APPENDIX D

Patient Education for Skin Care (for Diabetes)

Skin Care Education

After you wash with a mild soap, make sure that you rinse and dry yourself well. Check places where water can hide, such as under the arms, under the breasts, between the legs, and between the toes.

Drink lots of fluids (such as water) to keep your skin moist and healthy.

Keep your skin moist by using a lotion or cream after you wash. Ask your doctor to suggest one.

Wear all cotton underwear. Cotton allows air to move around your body better.

Check your skin after you wash. Make sure that you have no dry, red, or sore spots that might lead to an infection.

Tell your doctor about any skin problems.

APPENDIX E

Patient Education for Foot Care (for Diabetes)

Foot Care Education

Wash your feet in warm water every day. Make sure that the water is not too hot by testing the temperature with your elbow. Do not soak your feet. Dry your feet well, especially between your toes.

Look at your feet every day to check for cuts, sores, blisters, redness, calluses, or other problems. Checking every day is more important if you have nerve damage or poor blood flow. If you cannot bend over or pull your feet up to check them, use a mirror. If you cannot see well ask someone else to check your feet.

If your skin is dry, rub lotion on your feet after you wash and dry them. Do not put lotion between your toes.

File corn and calluses gently with an emery board or pumice stone. Do this after your bath or shower.

Cut your toenails once a week or when needed. Cut toenails when they are soft from washing. Cut them to the shape of the toe and not too short. File the edges with an emery board.

Always wear socks or slippers to protect your feet from injuries.

Always wear socks or stockings to avoid blisters. Do not wear socks or knee-high stockings that are too tight below your knee.

Wear shoes that fit well. Shop for shoes at the end of the day when your feet are bigger. Break in shoes slowly. Wear them 1 to 2 hours each day for the first 1 to 2 weeks.

Before putting your shoes on, feel the insides to make sure that they have no sharp edges or objects that might injure your feet.

Tell your doctor right away about any foot problems.

Ask your doctor to look at your feet at each checkup. To make sure your doctor checks your feet, take off your shoes and socks before your doctor comes into the room.

Ask your doctor to check how well the nerves in your feet sense feeling.

Ask your doctor to check how well blood is flowing to your legs and feet.

Ask your doctor to show you the best way to trim your toenails. Ask what lotion or cream to use on your legs and feet.

If you cannot cut your toenails or you have a foot problem, ask your doctor to send you to a foot doctor (called a podiatrist).

Index

Italicized page locators indicate a figure or photo; tables are noted with a *t*.

CR. *See* Contract relax

Crackles, 354t

Cranial nerves: functions and impairments, 268–270t

abducent (CN VI), 269t

facial (CN VII), 269t

glossopharyngeal (CN IX), 269t

hypoglossal (CN XII), 270t

oculomotor (CN III), 268t

olfactory (CN I), 268t

optic (CN II), 268t

spinal accessory (CN XI), 270t

trigeminal (CN V), 269t

trochlear (CN IV), 269t

vagus (CN X), 269t

vestibulocochlear (CN VIII), 269t

Cranium, *340*

Creatinine levels, normal, 351t

Cri du chat syndrome, 545t

CRLDs. *See* Chronic restrictive lung diseases

Crohn's disease, 559t

Crutches

for children, 552t

gait training points for, 195–196t

Cryotherapy, 206t

CSF. *See* Cerebrospinal fluid

CTLSO. *See* Cervical thoracic lumbosacral orthosis

"Cuaranderos," 25t

Cultural competence, 18–26

guidelines to, 19

increasing, methods for, 19t

selected religious beliefs and health concepts, 20–23t

Cultural differences, eye contact and, 8

Cultural diversity

intervention strategies related to, 23–26

non-English speaking clients and respect for, 14t

Cultured Epidermal Autograft, 452t

Cupping, 174t

postural drainage and, 387t

Curb ascent practice, with wheelchair, 201t

Curb descent practice, with wheelchair, 202t

Curl-ups, 164t

CVA synergy patterns, 278t

Cyanosis, 355t

in brown- or black-skinned patients, 24t

Cystic fibrosis, 546t, 566t

impairments with, 367t

Cysts, 436t

Cytotoxic agents, juveniles and possible side effects with, 536t

D

DAFO. *See* Dynamic ankle-foot orthosis

DAPRE PREs, indications and contraindications with, 151–152t

DBP. *See* Diastolic blood pressure

Debridement, 448–449t

Deceleration, muscle activation pattern with, 194t

Decerebrate rigidity, 266t

Decorticate rigidity, 267t

Decubitus ulcers, 506t

Deep friction massage, 174t

Deep partial-thickness burn, 422t

Deep tendon reflexes, respiratory acidosis and decrease in, 48t

Deep tendon reflexes and grades, DTR most tested and DTR grading, 134t

Deep vein thrombosis

cerebral vascular accidents and, 291t

Homan's sign for, 140t

therapeutic heat precautions and, 54t

limitations, age-related, inter-
ventions for, 481–482t
Skier's thumb, 212t
Skin
  age-related changes in, 493t
  anatomy of, 466
  function of, 467t
Skin appendages, 467t
Skin cancers, types of, 506–507t
Skin care, patient education for, 446t
Skin characteristics: color, temperature,
      perspiration, soreness, growths,
      436–437t
Skin color, changes in, 436–437t
Skin integrity, intervention patterns for
      spinal cord injury and, 325t
SLE. See Systemic lupus erythematosus
Sleep patterns, in older persons, 476t
Slipped capital femoral epiphysis,
      563–564t
  classifications of, 549t
Slow-acting antirheumatic drugs, juve-
      niles and possible side effects
      with, 536t
Slow pulse, 355t
Slow reversals, 303t
Slow stroking, 305t
Slow vestibular stimulation, 305t
SLR. See Straight-leg raising
Smell impairments and functional limi-
      tations, age-related, interven-
      tions for, 489t
Smith's fractures, 147t
Sneezing, CDC transmission guidelines
      on, 30t
SNS. See Sympathetic nervous system
SNS deficit, with spinal cord injury,
      295t
SOAP note elements (daily/weekly),
      70–77

assessment data, 74
HIPAA documentation requirements
      and, 76–77t
objective data, 71–74
plan data, 74–75
subjective data, 71
Social Security Act, 513t
Social skills, of childhood, 530–534t
Sociological theories of aging, 476t
Sodium level, normal, 352t
Sof-Splint, 554t
Soleus and gastrocnemius test, 129
Soleus muscle, function, nerve, origin,
      insertion, and palpation,
      233t
Solid ankle AFO, 183t
Solid-back DAFO, 555t
Solid hook on back support, in wheel-
      chair, 199t
Solid insert back support, in wheel-
      chair, 198t
Solid insert (seat support), in wheel-
      chair, 197t
Somatognosia, 263t
Somatosensory balance impairments
      and functional limitations, age-
      related, interventions for,
      488–489t
S_1 heart sound ("lub"), 353t
Spasticity, 267t
  intervention patterns for cerebral
      vascular accident and decrease
      in, 314t
  intervention patterns for MS patients
      and, 321t
Spasticity stage of CVA, intervention
      strategies for, 317t
Spatial-relation deficit, 263t
Speech
  functions and impairments of, 264t